Y0-BDH-820

Fluid and Electrolytes in Pediatrics

NUTRITION AND HEALTH

Adrianne Bendich, PhD, FACN, Series Editor

For other titles published in this series, go to
http://www.springer.com/series/7659

FLUID AND ELECTROLYTES IN PEDIATRICS

A Comprehensive Handbook

Edited by

LEONARD G. FELD, MD, PhD, MMM

Levine Children's Hospital,
Charlotte, NC, USA

FREDERICK J. KASKEL, MD, PhD

Children's Hospital at Montefiore,
Bronx, NY, USA

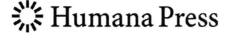 Humana Press

Editors
Leonard G. Feld
Department of Pediatrics
Levine Children's Hospital @
   Carolinas Medical Center
1000 Blythe Blvd.
Charlotte NC 28203
USA
lgfeld@yahoo.com

Frederick J. Kaskel
Department of Pediatrics
Albert Einstein College of Medicine
Children's Hospital at Montefiore
3415 Brainbridge Ave.
Bronx NY 10467
USA
fkaskel@aecom.yu.edu

Series Editor
Adrianne Bendich, PhD, FACN
GlaxoSmithKline Consumer Healthcare
Parsippany, NJ
USA

ISBN 978-1-60327-224-7   e-ISBN 978-1-60327-225-4
DOI 10.1007/978-1-60327-225-4

Library of Congress Control Number: 2009938486

© Humana Press, a part of Springer Science+Business Media, LLC 2010
All rights reserved. This work may not be translated or copied in whole or in part without the written permission of
the publisher (Humana Press, c/o Springer Science+Business Media, LLC, 233 Spring Street, New York, NY 10013,
USA), except for brief excerpts in connection with reviews or scholarly analysis. Use in connection with any form of
information storage and retrieval, electronic adaptation, computer software, or by similar or dissimilar methodology now
known or hereafter developed is forbidden.
The use in this publication of trade names, trademarks, service marks, and similar terms, even if they are not identified
as such, is not to be taken as an expression of opinion as to whether or not they are subject to proprietary rights.
While the advice and information in this book are believed to be true and accurate at the date of going to press, neither
the authors nor the editors nor the publisher can accept any legal responsibility for any errors or omissions that may be
made. The publisher makes no warranty, express or implied, with respect to the material contained herein.

Printed on acid-free paper

springer.com

Dedication

We are most appreciative for the "long-term" support and understanding from our families who have born a great deal as we have tolled through this and many other projects.

To our loved ones – *Barbara, Kimberly, Mitchell, Greg (LF), and Phyllis, Kimberly, Elizabeth, Jessica, and Erica (FK)*

Series Editor Introduction

The Nutrition and Health series of books have, as an overriding mission, to provide health professionals with texts that are considered essential because each includes (1) a synthesis of the state of the science, (2) timely, in-depth reviews by the leading researchers in their respective fields, (3) extensive, up-to-date fully annotated reference lists, (4) a detailed index, (5) relevant tables and figures, (6) identification of paradigm shifts and the consequences, (7) virtually no overlap of information between chapters, but targeted, inter-chapter referrals, (8) suggestions of areas for future research, and (9) balanced, data-driven answers to patient /health professionals questions, which are based upon the totality of evidence rather than the findings of any single study.

The series volumes are not the outcome of a symposium. Rather, each editor has the potential to examine a chosen area with a broad perspective, both in subject matter as well as in the choice of chapter authors. The international perspective, especially with regard to public health initiatives, is emphasized where appropriate. The editors, whose trainings are both research and practice oriented, have the opportunity to develop a primary objective for their book, define the scope and focus, and then invite the leading authorities from around the world to be part of their initiative. The authors are encouraged to provide an overview of the field, discuss their own research, and relate the research findings to potential human health consequences. Because each book is developed de novo, the chapters are coordinated so that the resulting volume imparts greater knowledge than the sum of the information contained in the individual chapters.

Of the 31 books currently published in the Series, only four have been given the title of Handbook. These four volumes, (1) *Handbook of Clinical Nutrition and Aging*, (2) *Handbook of Drug-Nutrient Interactions*, (3) *Handbook of Nutrition and Ophthalmology*, and (4) *Handbook of Nutrition and Pregnancy*, are comprehensive, detailed and include extensive tables and figures, appendices and detailed indices that add greatly to their value for readers. Moreover, Handbook contents cut across a wide array of health professionals' needs as well as medical specialties. The Nutrition and Health Series now will include its fifth Handbook volume, "Fluid and Electrolytes in Pediatrics: A Comprehensive Handbook."

Fluid and Electrolytes in Pediatrics: A Comprehensive Handbook edited by Leonard G. Feld, M.D., Ph.D., M.M.M. and Frederick J. Kaskel, M.D., Ph.D. is a very welcome addition to the Nutrition and Health Series and fully exemplifies the Series' goals for Handbooks. This volume is especially relevant as there is currently no comprehensive up-to-date text on the management of fluid and electrolyte disorders in pediatrics. This Handbook provides essential practice guidance that can help to improve the care of infants and young children in a wide variety of pediatric settings. This text, with over 200 relevant tables, equations, algorithms and figures, and close to 1000 up-to-date references, serves as a most valuable resource for the general practitioner, family practitioner, emergency medicine physicians, residents, medical students, nurses, physician assistants as well as many medical and surgical specialties that care for the disorders seen daily in the children admitted to neonatal intensive care units, pediatric intensive care units, inpatient units, day hospitals, surgical units, emergency care facilities, and outpatient care units. The Handbook provides detailed instructions about the signs and symptoms as well as the treatments that can help to restore the fluid balance and protect the vital organs from severe damage that can occur over a matter of hours. Health providers to the pediatric population who can benefit from the wealth of tables, figures and formulas as well as the analyses of numerous relevant case studies in the volume include specialties mentioned above as well as endocrinologists, neurologists, clinical nutritionists, gastroenterologists, neonatologists, emergency room physicians and support staff as well as researchers who are interested in the complexities of maintaining fluid and acid–base balance in the preterm, term infant, child and adolescent under acute conditions as well as for those children who have chronic conditions that predispose them to fluid and electrolyte imbalances. Moreover, graduate and medical students as well as academicians and medical staff will benefit from the detailed descriptions that are provided concerning environmental factors, such as drugs, infections, and other potential agents that can cause changes in body fluid balance. Tables of normal values for electrolytes, protein, glucose, and other components of the blood are given as detailed explanations of the compositions of the many fluids that can be provided to the patient intravenously, or by parenteral, enteral or oral routes in order to return the patient to normal levels of these essential electrolytes and fluid balance. Relevant equations are discussed and examples of how these can be helpful in treatment choices are illustrated.

This text has many unique features, such as highly detailed case studies, that help to illustrate the complexity of treating the pediatric patient with reduced capability to balance the body's fluids. There are in-depth discussions of the basic functioning of the kidneys, skin, and the lungs. Each chapter describes the etiology and demographics, biological mechanisms, patient presentation characteristics, therapy options and consequences of optimal treatment as well as delayed treatment. There are also clear, concise recommendations about fluid intakes, adverse effects of dehydration, and use of drugs and therapies that can quickly improve patient outcomes. Thus, this volume provides the broad knowledge base concerning normal fluid and electrolyte balance, kidney function, cellular physiology and the pathologies associated with changes in fluid balance, and the therapies that can help to restore normal function.

Comprehensive descriptions are provided that concentrate on the importance of various homeostatic mechanisms that interact with organ systems. Diabetes insipidus is reviewed and the differences between central and nephrogenic causes are included as well as guidance for patient management. Individual chapters containing highly relevant clinical examples and background information review the topics of water and sodium balance, potassium balance, disorders of calcium, magnesium and phosphorus balance; metabolic acidosis, metabolic alkalosis, respiratory acidosis, and respiratory alkalosis. These chapters include valuable discussions of fetal accretion of electrolytes and the consequences of preterm birth on fluid balance. The final section includes in-depth chapters on the consequences of liver disease and ascites, renal failure and transplantation, and endocrine diseases, all of which impact fluid and electrolyte balance. There are also chapters that examine genetic diseases, effects of enteral and parenteral nutrition, consequences of excess uric acid and the last chapter contains a comprehensive review of the special situations that can arise in the neonatal intensive care unit.

The editors of this volume, Dr. Leonard G. Feld and Dr. Frederick J. Kaskel are internationally recognized leaders in the fields of fluid and electrolyte balance and renal disease research, treatment, and management. Dr. Feld is the Sara H. Bissell and Howard C. Bissell Endowed Chair in Pediatrics, Chief Medical Officer at the Levine Children's Hospital and Clinical Professor of Pediatrics at the University of North Carolina School of Medicine and Dr. Kaskel is the Director of Pediatric Nephrology, Professor and Vice Chairman of Pediatrics at Albert Einstein College of Medicine in New York. Each has extensive experience in academic medicine and collectively, they have over 300 peer-reviewed articles, chapters, and reviews and Dr. Feld is the editor of the classic volume, "Hypertension in Children." Both have been recognized by their peers for their efforts to improve pediatric medicine especially under conditions where the proper acute care can have major effects on mortality and/or morbidity for preterm and term neonates, infants, and children. The editors are excellent communicators and they have worked tirelessly to develop a book that is destined to be the benchmark in the field of pediatric fluid and electrolyte balance because of its extensive, in-depth chapters covering the most important aspects of this complex field.

Fluid and Electrolytes in Pediatrics: A Comprehensive Handbook contains 18 chapters and each title provides key information to the reader about the contents of the chapter. In addition, relevant chapters begin with a list of Key Points, containing concise learning objectives as well as key words. The introductory chapters provide readers with the basics so that the more clinically related chapters can be easily understood. The editors have chosen 26 well-recognized and respected chapter authors who have included complete definitions of terms with the abbreviations fully defined for the reader and consistent use of terms between chapters. Key features of this comprehensive volume are the detailed discussions found in the more than 50 case studies. In conclusion, *Fluid and Electrolytes in Pediatrics: A Comprehensive Handbook,* edited by Leonard G. Feld and Frederick J. Kaskel provides health professionals in many areas of research and practice with the most up-to-date, well-referenced volume on the importance of the maintenance of fluid and electrolyte concentrations in the pediatric population, especially under acute care. This volume will serve the reader as the benchmark in this complex area of inter-relationships between kidney function, and the functioning of all organ systems that are intimately affected by imbalances in total body water. Moreover, the physiological and pathological examples are clearly delineated so that practitioners and students can better understand the complexities of these interactions. The editors are applauded for their efforts to develop the most authoritative resource in the field to date and this excellent Handbook is a very welcome addition to the Nutrition and Health Series.

Adrianne Bendich, PhD, FACN

Foreword

Fluid and Electrolytes in Pediatrics (a comprehensive handbook) is the latest in a series of multi-authored monographs on the Nutrition and Health Series of books from Springer/Humana.

Drs. Leonard G. Feld and Frederick J. Kaskel, pediatric nephrologists, and previous collaborators were selected as the handbook's editors. It was a wise choice, for they have each distinguished themselves as exemplary clinicians, investigators, and, most importantly, as teachers in this field for over 25 years.

A team of 28 experts in all of the topics presented was assembled with thoughtful consideration of differing writing styles and perspectives on the subject matter that is often a function of the author's depth, breadth, and duration of experience in this field. The editors are to be commended for this approach, which is rarely seen in the many publications on this general subject over the past 60 years.

Chapters 1 and 2 in Part I really "sets the stage" for all that follows, both in terms of structure/outline and content. For this reason, several important features are worth highlighting:

1. The authors are careful to highlight the critically important differences in the evaluation of disorders of water and sodium balance.
2. To the extent possible, they separate the clinical approaches to both groups of disorders while acknowledging the fact that they are inescapably linked. This is facilitated by the skillful use of clinical scenarios that the authors work through in a stepwise fashion.
3. As a natural consequence of their prior discussion of first principles of sodium and water physiology, it is particularly noteworthy in Chapter 1 that the dissociation of *total body water* from *total body sodium* is illustrated by examples of hyponatremia, isonatremia, and hypernatremia, each of which may be seen in the context of decreased, normal, or increased total body water, respectively (e.g., see Figs. 6 and 9).
4. The importance of including case scenarios in every one of the chapters underscores the time-honored importance of taking a thorough history and performing a complete physical examination; armed with this preliminary information, the astute clinician is usually able to initiate the most appropriate additional diagnostic studies and therapy.

The handbook is well organized into the four classical components of any book on this general subject, starting from the most common to the least common disorders encountered in pediatrics. Narratives are clearly expressed, tables and figures were chosen to enhance the reader's understanding of the text, and references seemed manageable in number and scope.

Fluid and Electrolytes in Pediatrics is a handbook worth having now for anyone who either plans to or is already looking after the health-care needs of all pediatric patients.

Charlotte, NC   Michael E. Norman, M.D., FAAP
December 1, 2009

Preface

One of the time-honored foundations of the practice of pediatric medicine is the understanding and application of the principles of fluid, electrolyte, and acid–base disorders. In *Fluid and Electrolytes in Pediatrics: A Comprehensive Handbook* we have selected authors with a passion, appreciation of the contributions of pioneers in pediatric medicine, and an expertise for their respective areas. Although medicine has changed enormously from the days of Gamble, Cooke, Holliday, Segar, Winters, and many other great pediatric clinical investigators, the evaluation and management of fluid, electrolyte, and acid–base disorders still form the basis of acute care and inpatient pediatrics. Today pediatric admissions are more complex and the survival of premature infants as young as 24 weeks gestation provides challenges for the generalist and specialist alike. Regardless of the location of care – from the neonatal unit, pediatric critical care, inpatient service to the emergency rooms – the clinician almost always obtains a set of electrolytes and a urinalysis on their patients and must interpret the results with regard to the specific clinical presentation.

In each chapter the authors have provided in-depth discussions, with the assistances of many scenarios in order to exemplify the major clinical pearls that will guide our continuing understanding and appreciation of the unique characteristics of pediatric fluid and electrolytes homeostasis. We have provided the authors some leeway in placing scenarios in the text or at the end of the section/chapter. In prescribing fluid and electrolyte therapies to our infants, children, and adolescents, we must apply critical analyzing skills to provide the most precise recommendations in order to assure a safe and effective environment for our precious future – our children. An example is that 5% Dextrose in Water with $\frac{1}{2}$ isotonic saline does not work for everyone. The jargon of giving 1.5 or 2 times maintenance fluid therapy is not appropriate because it is the crudest of *"estimates."*

In the first section, the chapters on Disorders of Water Homestasis by Feld, Massengill, and Friedman provide an in-depth examination of hypo- and hypernatremic disorders with detailed scenarios supported by many illustrations and tables. In the subsequent chapter on Disorders of Sodium Homeostasis, Woroniecki et al. present a discussion of sodium balance, renal regulation from the neonatal period, and the approach to assessing renal sodium excretion and the different volume states.

Disorders of Potassium Homeostasis is a key chapter because of the dire consequences of abnormal potassium balance and serum concentrations. The discussion emphasizes the practical and methodical approach to potassium abnormalities to avoid catastrophic consequences to the children.

In the second section, Charles McKay presents an elaborate review of both Disorders of Calcium and Magnesium Homeostasis. Although calcium disorders with both its low and high values are quite common, the analysis of the evaluation and treatment with detailed scenarios helps the reader to achieve a clear understanding of this important mineral. When faced with an abnormal serum magnesium concentration, this chapter will be an invaluable resource.

Valerie Johnson presents the chapter on Disorders of Phosphorus Homeostasis with an exceptional expertise and understanding. Similar to magnesium, this chapter is a ready resource to assist the clinician in the evaluation, diagnosis, and treatment of phosphorus disorders.

Part III covers Disorders of Acid–Base Homeostasis. The section editor Uri Alon has done a magnificent job in helping to guide the authors in these five chapters. Mahesh and Shuster start with an overview of normal acid–base balance, followed by Howard Corey and Uri Alon covering the ever difficult area of metabolic acidosis. Their insights in this field bring a challenging area into simpler terms. Wayne Waz reviews metabolic alkalosis and illustrates the value of the "lonely" urine electrolyte – chloride. Young and Timmons emphasize the importance of understanding respiratory disorders of acid–base physiology.

Part IV highlights Special Situations of Fluid and Electrolyte Disorders. Although it is nearly impossible to cover all areas, we have tried to include a chapter on the neonatal ICU, liver as well as renal failure, unique situations of the endocrine system, the importance of nutrition and understanding Uric Acid by Bruder Stapleton. The book would not be complete without a chapter on the genetic syndromes that affect the body's balance of water and electrolytes. In some instances there is intentional overlap of some information in this section to the first three sections of the book.

We truly hope that you will find this book an indispensable handbook and guide to the management of your patients as well as a critical resource for medical and graduate students.

SPECIAL ACKNOWLEDGEMENT AND THANK YOU

We are truly appreciative for all of the hard work and excellent efforts that were made by all of the contributing authors. The expertise in the preparation of the book is credited to Richard Hruska, Amanda Quinn and the staff at Humana/Springer. Richard was with us from the inception of this book to the final stages of production. A special thanks to Dr. Adrianne Bendich, PhD, for her helpful comments, guidance, and insightfulness in being Series Editor of the outstanding Nutrition and Health series.

Leonard G. Feld, MD, PhD, MMM
Frederick J. Kaskel, MD, PhD

Contents

Contributors

URI ALON, MD • *Professor of Pediatrics, Pediatric Nephrology, The Children's Mercy Hospital Kansas City, MO, USA*

OLUWATOYIN FATAI BAMGBOLA, MD, FMC (PAED) • *Nig, Division of Pediatric Nephrology, Percy Rosenbaum Endowed Professorial Chair in Pediatric Nephrology, Children's Hospital of New Oleans, Louisiana State University Health Science Center, New Orleans, LA, USA*

DINA BELACHEW, MD • *Resident in Pediatrics, Penn State Children's Hospital, The Milton S. Hershey Medical Center, Hershey PA, USA*

DEBORAH E. CAMPBELL, MD • *Professor of Clinical Pediatrics, Albert Einstein College of Medicine, Children's Hospital at Montefiore, Bronx, NY, USA*

HOWARD COREY, MD • *Director, Pediatric Nephrology, Goryeb Children's Hospital, Morristown NJ, USA*

LEONARD G. FELD, MD, PHD. MMM • *Chairman of Pediatrics, Carolinas Medical Center, Chief Medical Officer, Levine Children's Hospital, Charlotte, NC, USA*

AARON FRIEDMAN, MD • *Ruben/Bentson Professor and Chair, Department of Pediatrics, University of Minnesota Minneapolis, MN, USA*

BEATRICE GOILAV, MD • *Assistant Professor of Pediatrics, Albert Einstein College of Medicine of Yeshiva University Schneider Children's Hospital, New Hyde Park, New York, USA*

PAUL GOODYER, MD • *Professor of Pediatrics, McGill University Montreal, Quebec, Canada*

VANI GOPALAREDDY, MD • *Director, Pediatric Liver Transplantation, Levine Children's Hospital @ Carolinas Medical Center, Charlotte NC, USA*

ROBERTO GORDILLO, MD • *Division of Pediatric Nephrology, Children's Hospital at Montefiore, Albert Einstein College of Medicine, Bronx, NY, USA*

VALERIE L. JOHNSON, MD, PHD • *Chief, Division of Pediatric Nephrology, Associate Professor of Clinical Pediatrics Weill Medical College of Cornell University, Director, Rogosin Pediatric Kidney Center, The Rogosin Institute, New York, NY, USA*

JUHI KUMAR, MD, MPH • *Division of Pediatric Nephrology, Children's Hospital at Montefiore, Albert Einstein College of Medicine, Bronx, NY, USA*

SHEFALI MAHESH, MD • *Pediatric Nephrology, Children's Hospital at Montefiore/Albert Einstein College of Medicine, Bronx, NY, USA*

SUSAn MASSENGILL, MD • *Director, Pediatric Nephrology, Levine Children's Hospital @ Carolinas Medical Center, Charlotte NC, USA*

CHARLES MCKAY, MD • *Pediatric Nephrology, Levine Children's Hospital @ Carolinas Medical Center, Charlotte NC, USA*

MARVA MOXEY-MIMS, MD • *Director, Pediatric Nephrology Program, NIH/NIDDK/DKUH, Bethesda, MD, USA*

SHERI L. NEMEROFSKY, MD • *Assistant Professor of Pediatrics, Albert Einstein College of Medicine, Children's Hospital at Montefiore, Bronx, NY, USA*

JOEL ROSH, MD • *Director, Pediatric Gastroenterology, Goryeb Children's Hospital, Morristown, NJ, USA*

VICTOR L. SCHUSTER, MD • *Department of Medicine, Albert Einstein College of Medicine, Bronx, NY, USA*

LAWRENCE SILVERMAN, MD • *Pediatric Endocrinology, Goryeb Children's Hospital, Morristown, NJ, USA*

BRUDER STAPLETON, MD • *Professor and Chair, Pediatrics, University of Washington, Chief Academic Officer/Sr Vice President, Seattle Children's Hospital, Seattle, WA, USA*

OTWELL TIMMONS, MD • *Pediatric Critical Care, Levine Children's Hospital @ Carolinas Medical Center, Charlotte, NC, USA*

HOWARD TRACHTMAN, MD • *Professor of Pediatrics, Albert Einstein College of Medicine of Yeshiva University Schneider Children's Hospital, New Hyde Park, NY, USA*

WAYNE WAZ, MD • *Chief, Pediatric Nephrology, Children's Hospital of Buffalo, Buffalo, NY, USA*

STEVEN J. WASSNER, MD • *Vice Chair for Education, Physician Lead, Children's Hospital Safety and Quality, Chief, Division of Pediatric Nephrology and Hypertension, Penn State Children's Hospital, The Milton S. Hershey Medical Center, Hershey, PA, USA*

ROBERT WORONIECKI, MD • *Division of Pediatric Nephrology, Children's Hospital at Montefiore, Albert Einstein College of Medicine, Bronx, NY, USA*

EDWIN YOUNG, MD • *Director, Pediatric Critical Care, Levine Children's Hospital @ Carolinas Medical Center, Charlotte, NC, USA*

I DISORDERS OF WATER, SODIUM AND POTASSIUM HOMEOSTASIS

1 Disorders of Water Homeostasis

Leonard G. Feld, Aaron Friedman, and Susan F. Massengill

Key Points

1. To understand that disorders of sodium balance are related to conditions that alter extracellular fluid volume.
2. To appreciate the physiologic influences of antidiuretic hormone (ADH) and the stimuli resulting in its release.
3. To gain an understanding of the differences between *sodium status* (which determines the volume of extracellular volume) and *water status* (which determines the serum sodium concentration).
4. To recognize clinical signs and symptoms of the different forms of dehydration.
5. To appreciate that the management of hypernatremic dehydration differs from that of isonatremic/hyponatremic dehydration.

Key Words: Hyponatremia; hypernatremia; antidiuretic (ADH); vasopressin; diabetes insipidus; extracellular volume; intracellular dehydration; SIADH; osmolality

1. INTRODUCTION

The disorders of water balance of the body relate to volume control in body fluid compartments *(1)*. Osmotic shifts of water are directly dependent on the number of osmotic or solute particles (such as sodium and accompanying anions) that reside within the membranes of our body fluid compartments *(2)*. The osmolality of the body fluid compartments (extracellular and intracellular) contributes to the movement of water that occurs in a variety of disease states such as gastroenteritis/dehydration. An acute increase in the extracellular fluid osmolality due to a sodium chloride load results in a shift of water from the intracellular fluid compartment to reduce the osmolality and achieve a new, higher osmolar balance between the two compartments. The reverse would occur if there is an acute loss of osmolality from the extracellular fluid compartment. It is simple to appreciate the delicate interaction between osmolality and water balance. As discussed in Chapter 2, disorders of sodium balance are related to conditions that alter extracellular fluid volume (ECF). The simplest example is the requirement to maintain adequate extracellular volume to sustain perfusion of vital organs and tissues.

From: *Nutrition and Health: Fluid and Electrolytes in Pediatrics*
Edited by: L. G. Feld, F. J. Kaskel, DOI 10.1007/978-1-60327-225-4_1,
© Humana Press, a part of Springer Science+Business Media, LLC 2010

Impairment of tissue perfusion will lead to decreased oxygen delivery and anoxic damage resulting in organ failure (i.e., acute renal failure, hepatic failure, brain anoxia). It is therefore necessary to consider the clinical management of disorders of water (osmolality) and sodium balance (ECF volume) collectively. The identification and management of fluid and electrolyte disorders are essential in order to maintain body fluid balance.

1.1. Physiology of Water Homeostasis

Maintaining water homeostasis is an essential feature of adaptation for all mammals. Environments rarely provide water in the precise amount and at the precise time needed. A complex set of homeostatic mechanisms are at play, which regulate water intake and water excretion. These include the hypothalamus and surrounding brain, which control the sense of thirst and the production and release of arginine vasopressin (AVP), the antidiuretic hormone (ADH). AVP in turn acts on the second important organ in water homeostasis – the kidney – leading to increased reabsorption of water by the collecting duct of the kidney.

Because of the central role AVP plays in water homeostasis understanding the physiologic influences on AVP production and release is important. AVP is produced in the paraventricular and supraoptic nuclei, which project into the posterior hypothalamus. It is from the posterior hypothalamus that AVP is released. The stimuli that lead to AVP release also influence AVP production.

The elegant studies performed by Verney established the role of osmolality in the release of AVP (3). Under normal conditions, it is the osmolality of plasma and extracellular fluid as defined by the extracellular sodium concentration and associated anions along with a small contribution from glucose, which is "sensed" by osmoreceptors in the anteromedial hypothalamus. Small increases in osmolality of 1–2% (increase in 2–5 mOsm/kg H_2O) will result in the release of AVP. Conversely, a similar decrease in osmolality from approximately 290 to 280 mOsm/kg H_2O will result in cessation of AVP release and decreased production (4).

Non-osmotic stimuli will also cause AVP to be released. Gauer and Henry (5) demonstrated that a reduction in "effective circulating volume" [blood loss, hemorrhage, ECF volume depletion (dehydration, diuretics, etc.), nephrotic syndrome, cirrhosis, congestive heart failure/low cardiac output] will be "sensed" by the pressure or stretch sensitive receptors in the left atrium or large arteries of the chest then through the vagus and glossopharyngeal nerve will signal production and release of AVP. Other nonosmotic stimuli for AVP secretion include anesthetics and medications, nausea and vomiting, and weightlessness (6) (Table 1).

AVP circulates unbound, is rapidly metabolized by the liver or excreted by the kidney. The half-life is probably no more than approximately 20 minutes.

AVP plays a central role in thirst control. Thirst is the drive to consume water to replace urinary and obligate water losses such as sweating and breathing. Thirst is stimulated by an increase in serum osmolality and by extracellular volume depletion. AVP release appears to occur prior to the sensation of thirst, which is about 290 mOsm/L with maximal urinary concentration (~1200 mOsm/L) at about 292–295 mOsm/L.

The kidney plays a crucial role in the conservation of water when osmolality is increased or effective plasma volume is decreased. Similarly the kidney can excrete

Table 1
Non-osmotic Stimuli of Physiologic AVP Secretion

Hemodynamic (see text)	Non-hemodynamic	Medications
Increased Secretion	Increased Secretion	Increased Secretion
Acetylcholine	Hypoglycemia	Acetaminophen
Angiotensin II	Increased pCO_2	Beta-2 agonists
Bradykinin	hypercapnia	Chlorpropamide
Gastroenteritis	Low pO_2 _ hypoxia	Clofibrate
Histamine	Motion sickness	Cyclophosphamide
Isoproterenol	Nausea/vomiting	Epinephrine
Nitroprusside	Pregnancy	Lithium
	Stress/pain	Morphine (high dose)
		Nicotine
		NSAIDs
		Prostaglandins
		Tricyclic antidepressants
		Vincristine
Decreased Secretion	Decreased Secretion	Decreased Secretion
Atrial tachycardia	Swallowing	Alpha-adrenergic
Left atrial distention		agonists
Norepinephrine		Carbamazepine
		Clonidine
		Ethanol
		Glucocorticoids
		Morphine (low dose)
		Phenytoin
		Promethazine

NSAID – non-steroidal anti-inflammatory drugs
From Cogan (42); Robertson (43).

water rapidly in response to excess water intake. This effect is accomplished by AVP stimulating (1) interstitium through the active transport of urea from the tubule lumen to the renal epithelial cells of the thick ascending limb of the loop of Henle and the collecting duct resulting in the development of the osmotic gradient needed to reabsorb water, and (2) the transepithelial transport of water through opened water channels in the collecting duct resulting in water reabsorption (Fig. 1).

The transepithelial transport of water across the collecting duct (primary site of action is principle cell) is accomplished by the binding of AVP to its receptor (V2R) on the basolateral (non-luminal) surface of the epithelial cell. The intracellular action is mediated through cyclic AMP and protein kinase A leading to phosphorylation of aquaporin-2 water channels (7).

Aquaporins are channels that transport solute-free water through cells by permitting water to traverse cell membranes. In the kidney, aquaporin-2 is the channel through which water leaves the lumen of the tubule and enters epithelial cells of the collecting

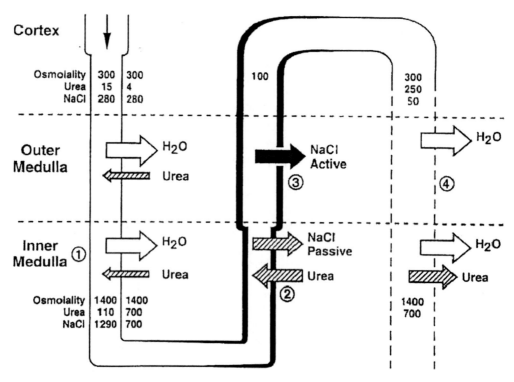

Fig. 1. Countercurrent mechanism for water reabsorption by the nephron. Reproduced with permission from *(38, Fig. 11.10)*.

duct. Water leaves these same cells through aquaporins-3 and 4. When AVP binds to the V2R receptor, aquaporin-2, which resides in intracytoplasmic vesicles, is inserted into the luminal membrane allowing water to move into the cell *(8)*. Aquaporins-3 and 4 appear to reside in the basolateral membranes and facilitate water movement from the intracellular space into the interstitium *(9)*. This movement of water into the interstitium is down a concentration gradient. The higher solute concentration in the interstitium of the kidney is facilitated by the action of AVP on epithelial sodium channels (eNaC) and the urea transporter (UT-A1) *(10, 11)*.

By 2–3 months of age, the normal infant born at term can maximally concentrate urine to 1100–1200 mOsm/kg H_2O similar to an older child or adult. AVP has been measured in amniotic fluid and is present in fetal circulation by mid-gestation. AVP levels rise (in fetal sheep) with stimuli such as increased serum osmolality *(12)*. At birth, vasopressin levels are high but decrease into "normal" ranges within 1–2 days *(13, 14)*. In neonates, AVP responds to the same stimuli as older children and adults. However, the ability to concentrate urine to the maximum achieved by older children or adults does not occur. Term infants concentrate up to 500–600 mOsm/kg H_2O and preterm infants up to 500 mOsm/kg H_2O. These low concentrating levels are probably due to a number of reasons including decreased glomerular filtration rate, decreased renal blood flow, reduced epithelial cell function in the loop of the Henle and collecting duct, reduced AVP receptor number and affinity and reduced water channel number or presence on the cell surface. Along with decreased renal capacity to reabsorb water, neonates have a reduced capacity to dilute urine so that the range of urine osmolality in the neonate is between 150 and 500 mOsm/kg H_2O as compared to the older child of 50 and 1200 mOsm/kg H_2O. Neonates have increased non-urinary water losses (skin and respiratory) as a function of weight, which are greater compared to older children and adults. The net effect is that neonates are at greater risk of dehydration either due to inadequate water provision or to high osmolar loads provided in enteral or parenteral feeds. Also, neonates are at greater risk of hyponatremia (hypo-osmolality) if water is administrated in large quantities or at too rapid rates.

2. CLINICAL ASSESSMENT OF RENAL WATER EXCRETION

Under normal conditions the "gold" standard for testing whether water homeostasis is being maintained is to measure serum and urine osmolality. Normal serum osmolality is approximately 280–290 mOsm/kg H_2O. As noted above, urine osmolality, except in neonates, can range from 50 to 1200 mOsm/kg H_2O and will depend on the physiologic circumstances. A slight increase in serum osmolytes over a short interval (i.e., NaCl) will result in AVP release (two- to fourfold increase in circulating concentration of AVP) and a marked increase in water reabsorption and urine osmolality. The concomitant measurement of an elevated serum osmolality should be matched by an appropriately elevated urine osmolality (>500 mOsm/kg H_2O >> the serum osmolality). Likewise, a decrease in serum osmolality, usually the result of water consumption or other hypotonic solutions, will reduce AVP production and secretion leading to the excretion of large volumes of water and a lowered urine osmolality. A serum osmolality below 280 mOsm/kg H_2O should be associated with urine osmolality <250 (often below 200 mOsm/kg H_2O). This physiological response depends on an intact hypothalamus–pituitary axis and normal renal function. Any stimulus (medications, anesthetics, nausea/vomiting) which directly stimulates AVP release, could interfere with normal physiologic mechanisms. Renal disease, which impairs water delivery to the kidney or affects loop of Henle or collecting duct function, could impair the response to AVP and lead to pathology.

Often in clinical situations a quick measure of serum osmolality is the equation

$$\text{serum osmolality} = 2[\text{Na}] + \frac{[\text{glucose}]}{18} + \frac{[\text{BUN}]}{2.8}$$

where [Na] is the sodium concentration in mEq/L or mmol/L (doubling the sodium value takes into account the accompanying anions – Cl^-, HCO_3^-); the glucose is measured in mg/dL and the BUN (blood urea nitrogen) in mg/dL. The BUN is often omitted if it is not rapidly changing since its impact on osmolality is muted by its ability to move freely across cell membranes. By eliminating the BUN term from the equation, the formula is a measure of effective serum osmolality or tonicity. Similarly, the specific gravity on a urine dipstick is used as a quick measure of urine osmolality. A specific gravity of 1.010 is routinely considered to correlate with a urine osmolality of

300–400 mOsm/kg H_2O (multiplying the number to the right of the decimal point by $40,000 = 0.010 \times 40,000 = 400$). The higher the specific gravity, the higher the osmolality. Unfortunately, specific gravity is a crude test that can be affected by solutes such as albumin (patients with proteinuria have high urinary specific gravity) or glucose. In order to aid in the diagnosis of diabetes insipidus, direct measurement of osmolality is required.

2.1. Measurement of the Diluting and Concentrating Ability of the Kidney

The defense of tonicity (effective osmolality) involves the thirst mechanism and the ability of the kidneys to excrete or conserve solute-free water depending upon the presence of ADH. Urine can be divided into two components. One component is the urine volume containing a solute concentration equal to that of plasma. This isotonic component has been termed the osmolar clearance (C_{osm}) and is an index of the kidney's ability to excrete solute particles. The second component is the volume of solute-free water (C_{H_2O}). It is this latter volume that effectively changes the osmotic concentration of the extracellular fluid compartment and is an index of the kidney's ability to maintain the serum in an iso-osmolar state *(15, 16)*.

Free-water clearance, abbreviated C_{H_2O}, is calculated as shown:

$$C_{H_2O} = \dot{V} - C_{osm},$$

where

$$C_{osm} = \frac{(U_{osm}) \times (\dot{V})}{(P_{osm})}$$

and where $\dot{V}$ is the urine flow rate (mL/min), P_{osm} is the plasma osmolality, and U_{osm} is the urine osmolality.

When the kidney reabsorbs equal proportions of water and solute as they exist in the plasma, the urine has a osmolality equal to plasma, therefore, $C_{osm} = \dot{V}$. In this situation, the osmolality of the ECF remains unchanged. When ADH is present or elevated, then solute-free water is reabsorbed in a greater proportion than filtered solute thereby resulting in a concentrated (hypertonic) urine ($C_{osm} > \dot{V}$) or a negative C_{H_2O} value. For example, consider a situation where the urine flow rate is 1 L/day, serum osmolality of 300 mOsm, and urine osmolality of 600 mOsm:

$$
\begin{aligned}
C_{H_2O} &= 1\text{L/day} - (600\,\text{mOsm} \times 1\text{L/day})/300\,\text{mOsm} \\
&= 1\text{L/day} - 2\text{L/day} \\
&= -1\text{L/day (or 1L of free water was reabsorbed)}
\end{aligned}
$$

On the other hand, when ADH levels are low, then solute-free water is excreted in a greater proportion than the filtered solute thereby resulting in a dilute (hypotonic) urine

($C_{osm} < \dot{V}$) or a positive C_{H_2O} value. For example, consider a situation where the urine flow rate is 1 L/day, serum osmolality of 300 mOsm, and urine osmolality of 150 mOsm:

$$C_{H_2O} = 1\text{L/day} - (150\,\text{mOsm} \times 1\text{L/d})/300\,\text{mOsm}$$
$$= 1\text{L/day} - 0.5\text{L/day}$$
$$= 0.5\text{L/day free water excreted}$$

Changes in the free-water excretion and reabsorption occur independent of changes in the solute excretion (C_{osm}).

2.2. Composition of Body Fluids

As individuals age, the proportion of total body water (TBW) to body weight decreases. Water accounts for 60% of TBW in men and 50% in women while infants have a higher proportion of water, 70–80%, due to the lower proportion of muscle in comparison to adipose *(17)*. The higher proportion of TBW to whole body weight in younger children is mainly due to the larger ECF volume when compared to adults. The disproportionate weight of brain, skin, and the interstitium in younger children contributes to the variability in the ECF volume. Water is distributed between two main compartments, the intracellular fluid compartment (ICF) and extracellular fluid compartment (ECF) (Fig. 2). The intracellular compartment makes up approximately 2/3

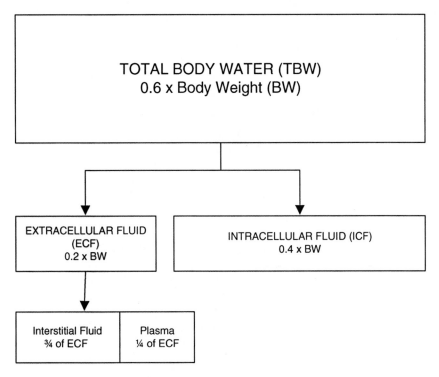

Fig. 2. Body fluid compartments.

of the TBW. The ECF constitutes 1/3 of the TBW composed of plasma and interstitial fluid. Abnormal accumulation of plasma ultrafiltrate, also referred to as "third spaced fluids," can result in edema, ascites, or pleural effusions.

Sodium along with Cl⁻ and HCO₃⁻ are the primary determinants of the ECF and provide the osmotic drive to maintain the ECF volume (Fig. 3, Table 2). Water moves freely across cell membranes between the ICF and ECF compartments to maintain osmotic

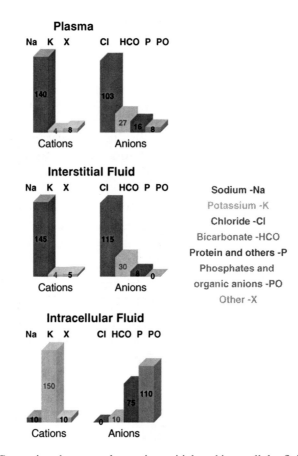

Fig. 3. Comparison between plasma, interstitial, and intracellular fluid (ICF).

Table 2
Approximate Mineral Composition of the ECF and ICF

	ECF (mEq/L)	ICF (mEq/L)
Na⁺	135–145	10–20
K⁺	3.5–5	120–150
Cl⁻	95–105	0–3
HCO₃⁻	22–30	10
Phosphate	2	110–120

equilibrium. For example, an increase in the water content of the ECF causes movement of water into the ICF from the ECF resulting in an expansion of both the ICF and ECF and a new osmolar balance (Fig. 4). If extensive, volume overload is clinically recognized as edema, ascites, or pleural effusions. In contrast, loss of sodium from the ECF results in ECF depletion with some relative ICF expansion and presents as signs of dehydration (Fig. 5). The kidneys are responsible for regulating the water balance and eliminate the majority of water from the body.

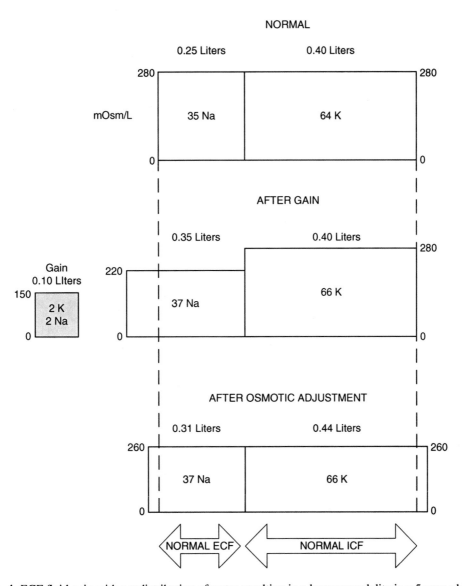

Fig. 4. ECF fluid gain with a redistribution of water resulting in a lower osmolality in a 5-year-old.

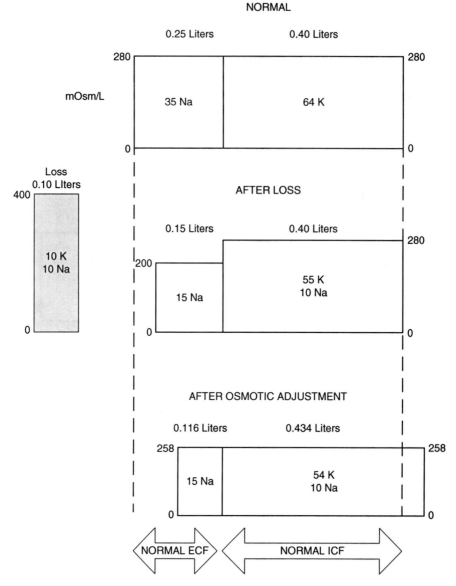

Fig. 5. Loss of hypertonic fluid and sodium from the ECF secondary to dehydration in a teenager. Reproduced with permission from Winters *(39)*.

2.3. Maintenance Requirements

For nearly 50 years, we have estimated the caloric and fluid requirements each day based on the Holliday and Segar method *(18)*. It is based on caloric requirement each day and the amount of fluid needed based on caloric expenditure (Table 3).

Table 3
Caloric, Water, and Basic Electrolyte Requirements Based on Weight

Body weight (kg)	Calories	Water	Sodium mEq/100 mL H₂O	Chloride mEq/100 mL H₂O	Potassium mEq/100 mL H₂O
3–10 kg	100/kg	100/kg Or 4 mL/kg/h	3	2	2
11–20 kg	50/kg	1000 mL + 50 mL/kg for each kg above 10/ Or 40 mL/h + 2 mL/kg/h	3	2	2
>20 kg	20/kg	1500 mL + 20 mL/kg for each kg above 20 Or 60 mL/h + 1 mL/kg/h	3	2	2

EXAMPLE of a calculation for maintenance fluid requirements for a 15 kg child

BW = 15Kg

Calories: 100 calories/kg for 1st 10 kg + 50 calories/kg for 5 kg (15–10 kg) = 1250 calories/day

Water: 100 mL/kg for 1st 10 kg + 50 mL/kg for 5 kg (15–10 kg) = 1250 mL/day

Sodium: 3 mEq/100 mL water = 3 mEq × 12.5 = 36.5 mEq/day or 30 mEq/L of solution

Potassium: 2 mEq/ 100 mL water = 2 mEq × 12.5 = 25 mEq/day or 20 mEq/L of solution

The child requires intravenous fluids ~ 1250 mL/day

5% Dextrose with 30 mEq/L of NaCl and 20 mEq/L of KCl at 50 mL/h

5% dextrose is provided to deliver 5 g of carbohydrate per 100 mL of solution or 50 g/L or 200 calories/L (50 g × ~4 calories/g of carbohydrate).

NOTE: This solution will only deliver 20% of the daily caloric requirement of 250 calories at the maintenance rate. For a limited period of time (generally under 5–7 days) this amount of carbohydrate will be sufficient to prevent protein breakdown. If it is anticipated that there will be a need for prolonged parenteral therapy, a higher dextrose solution will be required and provided through a central venous access if the dextrose concentration in the final solution will exceed 10–12.5%.

Recently, a modification to maintenance therapy was proposed substituting isotonic saline for the hypotonic solution recommended by Holliday and Segar *(19)*. The case for this modification is based on the observation that some children have been seriously injured [cerebral edema, brain injury and death] by the inappropriate use of maintenance solutions [hypotonic] especially in situations of unappreciated volume contraction or nonosmotic release of antidiuretic hormone. To date, studies regarding the use of isotonic saline as maintenance fluid therapy across the full range of hospitalized pediatric patients are lacking *(20)*.

Intravenous fluids that are safe to administer parenterally based on their osmolality are shown in Table 4. Each solution is selected based on the clinical status of the patient. Solutions without dextrose (0.45% isotonic saline) or without electrolytes 5% dextrose in water are only administered under special clinical situations.

Table 4
Solutions Used for Intravenous Administration

Solution	Osmolality mOsm/L	Sodium mEq/L	Potassium Eq/L	Chloride mEq/L	Dextrose mOsm/L
0.9% Isotonic saline (normal saline)	308	154		154	
0.45% Isotonic saline* (1/2 Normal)	154	77		77	
5% Dextrose in Water					278
5% Dextrose + 0.33% isotonic saline	378	50		50	278
5% Dextrose + 0.45% isotonic saline	432	77		77	278

*The lowest intravenous solution that can be used safely is 0.45% isotonic saline with an osmolality of 154 mOsm/L or approximately 50% of plasma. Any solution with an osmolality under this value will result in cell breakdown with a large potassium load to the extracellular space resulting in severe hyperkalemia leading to cardiac arrhythmias and possibly death.

3. HYPONATREMIA AND HYPO-OSMOLALITY

A low serum sodium less than 130 mmol/L (hyponatremia) is nearly always associated with water retention by the kidney. Hyponatremia can occur with extracellular volume depletion or even extracellular volume expansion such as in the syndrome of inappropriate antidiuretic hormone (AVP) release or SIADH. The presence of elevated levels of AVP in blood alone does *not* result in hyponatremia. Patients must have an intake of water or receive a hypotonic solution under the influence of high or excessive AVP to become hyponatremic or hypo-osmolar. Rarely, hyponatremia is the result of excessive salt loss. Recently an expert panel provided guidelines for hyponatremia in adults *(21)*. The evaluation and approach to hyponatremia in children is shown in Fig. 6a,b.

3.1. Hyponatremic Dehydration

Hyponatremic dehydration is a common condition usually associated with acute gastroenteritis. The pathophysiology of this condition involves loss of fluid and electrolytes in stool (sodium, bicarbonate, water usually hypo-osmolar to extracellular fluid) and emesis. This extrarenal loss results in extracellular volume depletion leading to the release of aldosterone and the non-osmotic release of AVP. Aldosterone will increase renal sodium reabsorption with a loss of urinary potassium eventually leading to hypokalemia. AVP will increase water reabsorption, and if the extracellular volume depletion is allowed to persist with the patient provided hypo-osmolar fluids either by mouth (clear liquids) or intravenously (5% dextrose + 0.225 (1/4) isotonic saline or 5% dextrose + 0.45 (1/2) isotonic saline), the patient develops a hypo-osmolar or hyponatremic state.

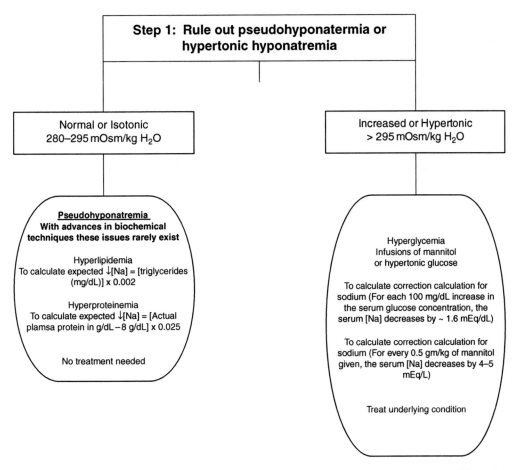

Fig. 6. Suggested evaluation of hyponatremia based on plasma osmolality or tonicity. Modified with permission from Feld *(40)*.

(Continued)

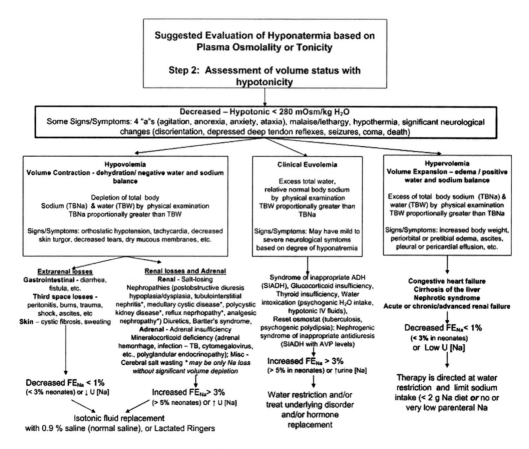

Fig. 6. (Continued)

The signs and symptoms of hyponatremic dehydration are primarily those of dehy-dration. Table 5 describes the generally accepted clinical signs and symptoms of dehydration as a percent of body weight lost. In general, with hyponatremia (hypo-osmolality) the symptoms/signs are more pronounced than the actual percent of body weight lost. This occurs because the extracellular fluid space is more signifi-cantly impacted than in iso-osmolar (normal serum sodium) or hyperosmolar (hyper-natremic) dehydration. If the serum sodium falls rapidly (>10 mEq/L per 24 h) or decreases below 125 mEq/L, the patient may experience more significant cen-tral nervous system symptoms – more profound lethargy, obtundation, and seizures. Seizures associated with hyponatremia are more refractory to treatment with antiepilep-tics and requires an increase in serum osmolality or reversal of the hypo-osmolality (hyponatremia).

The approach to hyponatremic dehydration involves treatment of the underlying con-dition, administration of oral or intravenous therapy to correct the dehydration and direct treatment of the hyponatremia, if necessary (Scenario 1). For mild to moderate dehy-dration providing oral restoration usually is sufficient unless vomiting is frequent and there is lack of evidence that fluids consumed in a therapeutic fashion (5–15 mL every

Table 5
Severity of Dehydration

Characteristics			
Infants	*Mild – 1–5%*	*Moderate – 6–9%*	*Severe – >10% (=> 15% = shock)*
Older Children	*Mild – 1–3%*	*Moderate – 3–6%*	*Severe – >6% (=> 9% = shock)*
Pulse	Full, normal	Rapid	Rapid, weak
Systolic BP	Normal	Normal, Low	Very Low
Urine output	Decreased	Decreased (<1 mL/kg/h)	Oliguria
Buccal mucosa	Slightly dry	Dry	Parched
Ant fontanel	Normal	Sunken	Markedly sunken
Eyes	Normal	Sunken	Markedly sunken
Skin turgor/capillary refill	Normal	Decreased	Markedly decreased
Skin	Normal	Cool	Cool, mottling, Acrocyanosis
Infants < 12 months of age			

Reproduced with permission from Feld *(41)*.

Table 6
Restoration Oral Solutions

	Restoration (rehydration) oral solutions			
Solution	*Carbohydrate g/L*	*Na mmol/L*	*K mmol/L*	*Osmolality mOsm/kg H_2O*
URS (WHO)	20 (dextrose)	90	25	310
Pedialyte®	25	45	20	250
Rehydralyte	25	75	20	210

5–10 min) would be retained. Tables 6 and 7 describe commonly used oral and intravenous restoration (rehydration) fluids. For moderate dehydration, the World Health Organization recommends oral rehydration solutions. However, many clinicians will initiate intravenous treatment followed by oral therapy. The restorative, intravenous treatment for extracellular volume depletion is isotonic saline (normal saline). For moderate to severe dehydration, an intravenous bolus of 20–40 mL/kg of isotonic saline should be provided over 30–60 min depending on the clinical state (more rapid administration

Table 7
Intravenous Restoration (Rehydration) Solutions

Solution	Na mmol/L	K mmol/L	Cl mmol/L	Ca mmol/L	Lactate mmol/L
NS (normal saline)	154		154		
LR (Lactated Ringers)	130	4	109	3	28

in patients with hypotension, decreased turgor or tachycardia). The vast majority of patients will improve and the institution of oral fluids can be started. With improvement in extracellular volume depletion in patients with gastroenteritis, gut perfusion improves and oral rehydration is better tolerated (22). This approach will not only restore extracellular volume but allow the serum sodium concentration to approach normal values.

Case Scenario 1. Hyponatremia with Sodium and Water Deficits = Hypovolemia

A 4-month-old infant presents to her pediatrician with a 4–5 day history of low-grade fever (38–38.5°C), numerous watery diarrhea, and decreased activity. Since the child refused to take her usual breast milk volume or solid foods, the mother and grandmother substituted non-carbonated soda (coca-cola, ginger ale, apple juice, or orange juice will have ~550–700 mOsm/kg H_2O with less than 5 mEq/L of sodium) and "sweet" (sugar-added) iced tea. Over the last 12 h there were a few episodes of emesis and there were less wet diapers.

On examination the child was lethargic, dry mucous membranes, no tears, sunken eyeballs, and reduced skin turgor. Vitals signs were the following: blood pressure 74/43 mmHg, temperature of 38°C, respiratory rate of 36/min, and pulse of 175 beats/min. The weight was 6 kg. Weight at the time of her immunization 7 days ago was 6.6 kg. There were no other significant findings.

With the magnitude of dehydration and lethargy, the decision by the clinician was to initiate parenteral fluid replacement rather than oral rehydration therapy. The child was admitted to the hospital with diagnosis of dehydration. On admission the laboratory studies were as follows:

Sodium 124 mEq/L, chloride 94 mEq/L (normal 98–118 mEq/L), potassium 4 mEq/L (normal 4.1–5.3 mEq/L), bicarbonate (or total CO_s) 12 mEq/L (normal 20–28 mEq/L or mmol/L), serum creatinine 0.8 mg/dL (normal ~0.3–0.5 mg/dL), blood urea nitrogen 40 mg/dL, blood glucose 70 mg/dL; complete blood count was normal except for a hematocrit of 38% (normal ~36%);
Urinalysis/chemistries: specific gravity of 1.030, trace protein, no blood or glucose, small ketones; urine creatinine 40 mg/dL and sodium 15 mEq/L.

Fractional excretion of sodium (FE$_{Na}$)

([urine sodium $\times$ serum creatinine]/[serum sodium $\times$ urine creatinine] $\times$ 100%) =
  ([15 mEq/L $\times$ 0.8 mg/dL]/[129 mEq/L $\times$ 40 mg/dL]) = 0.23%
Normal values for FE$_{Na}$ = $\sim$ 1 $-$ 2% ; decreased renal perfusion
  (dehydration, decreased intravascular volume) < 1%

3.2. Assessment

The clinical and laboratory information suggest *hyponatremic dehydration* secondary to extrarenal losses from diarrhea with administration by the family of hypotonic or dilute fluids. The child has lost proportionally more sodium than water or a relatively hypertonic fluid loss. The result is a lower extracellular fluid osmolality compared to the intracellular fluid osmolality. The magnitude of the dehydration is about *10% or moderate to severe*. The pre-illness weight was 6.6 kg with a current weight of 6 kg or a 0.6 kg loss over the last week. Estimated guidelines for vital signs at this age: the normal respiratory rate for children is approximately 36; normal pulse is about 130 (standard deviation is $\sim$45) beats/min; normal blood pressure is approximately 89/54 mmHg. As noted above, the decision by the clinician was to initiate parenteral fluid replacement rather than oral rehydration therapy. The relative contraindications for oral rehydration therapy would include a young infant less than 3–4 months of age, the presence of impending shock or markedly impaired perfusion (increased capillary refill time/decreased skin turgor), inability to consume oral fluids due to intractable vomiting, marked irritability or lethargy/unresponsiveness or the judgment of the clinician.

3.3. Therapeutic Plan

1. Volume deficit, electrolyte calculations: traditionally, treatment has been divided into three phases: an emergent or acute phase – isotonic saline fluid infusion over about 1 h; replacement phase – over 24 h unless there are on-going losses that are not replaced adequately in the first day of treatment; and the maintenance phase – day 2 continuing to home management.

Emergent or acute phase – Over about 1 h (this may need to be prolonged in cases of more significant volume depletion). In order to re-establish circulatory volume to prevent prolonged loss of perfusion to the key organs such as kidney, brain, gastrointestinal tract, the fluid choices would be isotonic (0.9%) saline (normal saline) or another isotonic/hypertonic solution such as 5% albumin, Ringer's lactate, or a plasma preparation. With the availability of isotonic saline, this is the usual fluid choice.

Weight (kg) $\times$ fluid bolus of 20 mL/kg over 30–60 min.
(If the patient was in shock the fluid delivery would be a more rapid infusion to prevent organ failure.)
6 kg $\times$ 20 mL = 120 mL over 30–60 min. This only replaces 20% of the losses [total losses 600 mL].

Acute – Repletion/Replacement/Restoration Phase – Over 24 h; in this period the daily fluid/electrolyte maintenance requirements and deficit calculation are derived from standard estimates.

1. *Maintenance fluid/electrolyte calculations for 24 h:*
   Calculations based on daily caloric requirements.

Body weight (BW) in kg	Caloric needs calories/kg BW	Water needs mL/100 calories used per day – each mL equals about 1 calorie*	Electrolyte needs mEq/100 calories used per day (alternate method is mEq/kg per day)	Calories derived from glucose/dextrose
3–10	100	100	Sodium =	5 g/100 calories
11–20	1000 + 50 calories/kg for each kg above 10	1000 + 50 mL/kg for each kg above 10	2.5–3 mEq (or 3 mEq/kg) Potassium = 2–2.5 mEq	used
>20	1500 + 20 calories/kg for each kg above 20	1500 + 20 mL/kg for each kg above 20	(or ~ 2 mEq/kg)	

*Kidney losses are about 45–75 mL/100 calories expended; sweat losses usually 0; stool losses are about 5–10 mL/100 calories expended, and insensible losses (skin ~30 mL + respiratory ~15 mL) are about 45 mL/100 calories expended – 100 mL of total daily water losses = 100 calories expended per day or *1 mL = 1 calorie.*

For this 6.6 kg infant
Maintenance requirements for 24 h

Water	100 mL/kg × 6.6 kg = 660 mL
Sodium	3 mEq/100 mL × 660 mL = 20 mEq
Potassium	2 mEq/100 mL × 660 mL = 13 mEq

2. *Deficit Replacement of water and electrolytes:* In most circumstances the acid–base disorder is a simple metabolic acidosis that does not require bicarbonate replacement unless there is severe tissue/impaired circulatory compromise such as shock (generally 15% dehydration). In general, there is only partial replacement of potassium deficits that are fully corrected over 2–4 days following resumption of oral intake.

There are two approaches to calculate deficits in hyponatremic dehydration.
Approach 1: Use of the table below for 10% dehydration

Type of dehydration* based on serum [Na] in mEq/L	Water (mL/kg)	Sodium (mEq/kg)	Potassium (mEq/kg)
Isonatremic [Na] 130–150	100	10	8
Hyponatremic [Na] < 130	100	10–12	8
Hypernatremic [Na] > 150	100		2–2

*Isonatremic dehydration is the most common accounting for 70–80% of infants and children; hypernatremic dehydration accounts for about 15%, and hyponatremic dehydration for about 5–10% of cases. Adapted from Winter RW: Principles of Pediatric Fluid Therapy, 2nd Ed, Little Brown and Co., Boston, 1982, p 86.

For this 6 kg infant with hyponatremic dehydration at 10%
Deficits for 24 h

Water   Pre-illness weight – Illness weight = 6.6–6 kg = 0.6 kg = 600 mL
Sodium   10 mEq × 6.6 kg = 66 mEq
Potassium   8 mEq × 6.6 kg = 53 mEq

Total First 24 h Requirements
The total amount of maintenance and deficit amounts are given 50% over the first 8 h
and the remainder over the next 16 h.

Component of therapy	Water	Sodium	Potassium	Hourly rate Round number up or down to the nearest 5 increment
Acute phase	120	18 (154 mEq/L × 0.12 L)	0	Entire amount over 20–60 min
Maintenance	660	20	13	
Deficit	600	66	53	
Ongoing losses of diarrhea or vomiting*				
TOTAL	1280	104	66	
Emergent phase therapy	(120)	(18)		
FINAL THERAPY	1160	86	66	
Hours 1–8	580	43	33	72 mL/h
Hours 9–24	580	43	33	36 mL/h

- From clinical experience the gastrointestinal losses tend to resolve or decrease significantly following the initiation of parenteral therapy. If it does continue these losses will need to be added to the ongoing loss row.
- For each liter of IV solution there would be 43 mEq/0.58 L = ~75 mEq/L for the 1st 8 h, then about 35 ml/h for the next 16 h.
- *Fluid selection – 5% dextrose + 0.45% isotonic saline + 40 mEq KCl/L*

Generally the final solution potassium concentration is about 30– 40 mEq/L (*it should not exceed 40 mEq/L* without close intensive care monitoring). Some clinicians have recommended using a lower concentration of 20–25 mEq/L since potassium stores will be replenished when the child restart oral feeds. The 5% dextrose provides 50 g of carbohydrate per liter of 50 g × ~4 calories/g = 200 calories. This would be about 20% of the daily caloric intake which is sufficient to prevent protein breakdown over a short treatment period (less than 1 week).

Approach 2: Direct Deficit Calculation

a. Sodium deficit: Fluid deficit (L) × 0.6 (sodium distribution factor) × normal serum sodium concentration = 0.6 L × 0.6 × 140 mEq/L = 50 mEq

b. Additional sodium = (Desired serum sodium − actual serum sodium) × 0.6 L/kg × kg body weight = (135 − 124 mEq/L) × 0.6 L/kg × 6.6 kg = 43.6 mEq*
c. Total sodium deficit = 50 + 43.6 = 94 mEq
d. Total potassium deficit = Fluid deficit (L) × 0.4 (potassium distribution factor) × normal intracellular potassium concentration = 0.6 L × 0.4 × 120 mEq/L = ~ 29 mEq

- In cases of isonatremic dehydration, the calculation is identical except the additional sodium deficit (b. above) is excluded from the calculation.

Total First 24 h Requirements

The maintenance is provided equally over the entire 24 h period, and deficit amounts are given 50% over the first 8 h (emergent phase is usually excluded from the 24 h calculations) and the remainder over the next 16 h.

Component of therapy	*Water*	*Sodium*	*Potassium*	*Hourly rate Round number up or down to the nearest 5 increment*
Acute phase	120	18 (154 mEq/L × 0.12 L)	0	Entire amount over 20–60 min
Maintenance	660	20	13	
Deficit	600	94	29	
Ongoing losses of diarrhea or vomiting*				
TOTAL	1280	132	42	
Emergent phase therapy	(120)	(18)		
FINAL THERAPY	1160	114	42	
Hours 1–8	520 mL	64	20	
	1/3 Maintenance = 220 mL	7	5	
	1/2 Deficit = 300 mL	57	15	
Hours 9–24	740 mL	71	22	
	2/3 Maintenance = 440 mL	14	8	
	1/2 Deficit = 300 mL	57	14	

- For the first 8 h, each liter of IV solution there would be 64 mEq/0.52 L = 123 mEq of sodium per liter = *Fluid selection – 5% dextrose + isotonic saline + 40 mEq KCl/L at a rate of 520 mL/7 h = ~75 mL/h*

- For the remaining 16 h, each liter of IV solution there would be 71 mEq/0.74 L = 95 mEq/L = *Fluid selection – 5% dextrose + 0.45% isotonic saline + 40 mEq KCl/L at a rate of 740 mL/16 h = ~45 mL/h*

The major difference in the two approaches is the provision of isotonic saline rather $\frac{1}{2}$ isotonic saline in the first 8 h. Thereafter, the approaches are nearly identical. As stated above, using a lower intravenous potassium concentration of 20–25 mEq/L is also acceptable.

Signs and symptoms (Fig. 6b) attributable to hyponatremia include anorexia, weakness, lethargy, confusion, seizures, and coma. It seems appropriate here to point out that although hyponatremia is not unusual, the central nervous system (CNS) manifestations are fortunately quite uncommon. What protects the CNS from swelling whenever the osmolality falls (in situations of hyponatremia or in situations of decreasing osmolality when the serum osmolality starts above normal such as the correction of hypernatremia) are at least 5 physiological process recently reviewed by Chesney *(23)*. These processes include diminished ADH secretion unless volume contraction exists simultaneously; reduced movement of brain cell aquaporins (aquaporin-4) thus reducing water movement into brain cells; movement of ionic and nonionic osmolytes out of cells especially in the brain; existing mechanisms that regulate cell volume; and existing mechanisms that sense intracellular osmolality. The interchanges between these processes help keep the brain from swelling when the osmolality falls but they can be overwhelmed when the rate of water ingested by the patient or infused into the patient exceeds these regulatory controls. However, in situations with significant neurological symptoms (seizures, coma) associated with hyponatremia, a more rapid increase in the serum sodium and osmolality needs to be considered. Under those conditions, the use of a hypertonicsaline solution may be necessary. Three percent NaCl (500 mEq NaCl/L – 0.5 mEq/mL) is the preferred solution. The recommended change in serum sodium *should not* exceed 10 mEq/L/24 h (approximately 20 mOsm/kg H_2O/24 h – Na and Cl each contributes 10 mOsm/kg H_2O). To calculate the amount of sodium required to change the serum sodium concentration, the following equation can be used:

$$(\text{Desired [Na]} - \text{Measured [Na]}) \times \text{BW} \times 0.6$$

EX: To raise the serum sodium concentration from 123 to 130 mEq/L for a 10 kg child – (130–123) × 10 kg × 0.6 = 42 mEq

[Na] is the sodium concentration in mEq (or mmol/L). BW is bodyweight in kilograms and 0.6 represents the 60% of BW (except newborns and young neonates) that is water. The entire body water space is used for this calculation since sodium added to the extracellular space raises extracellular (ECF) osmolality drawing water from the intracellular space into the extracellular to equalize osmolality in the body fluid compartments. In most patients, 3% saline correction is only administered until symptoms are abated which usually occurs when the serum sodium is raised by approximately 5–10 mEq (osmolality – 10–20 mOsm/kg H_2O). Ultimately, patients can be corrected near the lower limit of the normal range for serum sodium – approximately 130 mEq/L. An infusion 6 mEq/kg/h (there is 0.5 mEq/mL in the 3% NaCl solution which implies a delivery volume of 12 mL/kg/h) of a 3% NaCl solution will raise the serum sodium approximately 5 mEq/h.

3.4. Syndrome of Inappropriate Antidiuretic Hormone (SIADH) Release

In the classic description by Bartter and Schwartz, SIADH release includes hyponatremia and hypo-osmolality of the serum, a urine osmolality that is inappropriately greater than serum, normal renal, thyroid and adrenal function and increased urine sodium excretion *(24)*. Another way to view SIADH release is as a *non-physiologic* condition of AVP excess. Thus release of AVP due to hyperosmolality or volume depletion does not represent inappropriate ADH release because both represent physiologic release of AVP. So SIADH cannot occur in a state of negative water balance. SIADH release can be viewed as having three basic causes – (a) ectopic production, (b) exogenous administration of vasopressin, or (c) "abnormal" release of AVP from neurohypophysis. Table 8 lists some of the more common causes of SIADH release.

In SIADH AVP is released despite a normal or low serum osmolality. As noted above, the excess AVP results in a further reduction in serum sodium and osmolality only if the patient continues to consume water in excess to urine and insensible losses (sweating and respiration). Because patients are not volume depleted (in fact they are volume expanded), urinary sodium losses are high. SIADH release is associated with total body water expansion; high urine sodium concentration without evidence of heart, liver, or kidney diseases; and no edema. The diagnostic criteria for SIADH are listed in Table 9.

The treatment of choice for SIADH release is to treat the underlying cause such as a direct therapy for ectopic AVP production, removal of an offending drug agent; or reduction in the dose or lengthening the interval of exogenous AVP administration. Since treatment of the underlying cause may not be possible, fluid restriction is often effective. The total fluid intake should be less than that excreted in urine and from insensible loss (approximately 40% of maintenance calculation). This therapy will raise the serum sodium by 2–3 mEq/L/24 h. Other proposed therapies for a more rapid increase in sodium (osmolality) include (a) doxycycline, a tetracycline derivative that interferes with the action of AVP but cannot be used in young children, (b) fludrocortisone, which increases sodium retention but leads to hypokalemia and hypertension, and (c) AVP antagonists. AVP antagonists appear effective in short-term trials but are untested in children *(25)*. Finally, prevention of hyponatremia by limiting water intake in situations where one might expect SIADH to occur, such as neurological surgery, is warranted.

Case Scenario 2. Patient with Meningitis and SIADH

A 10-month-old infant presents to the pediatric emergency room with a generalized tonic clonic seizure. The child had a fever to 39–40°C for the past 24–36 h, lethargy, vomiting, decreased oral intake, and less wet diapers. The child did not receive Prevnar (pneumococcal vaccine).

On examination the child appeared ill and irritable resisting any movement. Vitals signs were the following: blood pressure 94/58 mmHg; temperature of 39°C, respiratory rate of 40/min, and pulse of 175 beats/min. The weight was 10 kg. There were no

Table 8
Causes of SIADH

Tumors	Chest disorders	CNS disorders	Drugs
Bronchogenic	Infection	Infection/	Adenine
AdenoCarcinoma	TB	inflammatory	Arabinoside
Duodenum	Bacterial	TB meningitis	Amitriptyline
AdenoCarcinoma	Mycoplasma	Bacterial meningitis	Barbiturates
of pancreas	Viral	Encephalitis	Carbamazepine
Ca of ureter	Fungal	Head trauma	Chlorpropamide
Hodgkin's	Positive pressure	Subarachnoid	Clofibrate
Thymoma	ventilation	hemorrhage	Colchicine
Acute leukemia	Dec left atrial	Hypoxia–ischemia	Diuretics
Lymphosarcoma	pressure	Acute psychosis	Fluphenazine
Histiocytic	Pneumothorax	Brain tumor/mass lesions	Isoproterenol
lymphoma	Atelectasis	Miscellaneous	Morphine
	Asthma	Guillain–Barré	Nicotine
	Cystic fibrosis	syndrome	Tricyclics
	Mitral valve	Spinal cord	Vinblastine
	Commissuro-	lesions	Vincristine
	tomy	VA shunt Obstruction/	
	PDA ligation	hydrocephalus	
	Malignancy	Acute intermittent	
		porphyria	
		Cavernous sinus	
		thrombosis	
		Stress/extensive	
		exercise	
		(running a	
		marathon, etc.)	
		Idiopathic	

Ca – cancer; VA – ventriculo-atrial shunt
Reproduced with permission from Feld *(41)*.

focal neurological findings. The impression was meningitis, probably pneumococcal, and hyponatremia.

On admission the laboratory studies were as follows:

Sodium 126 mEq/L, chloride 95 mEq/L (normal 98–118 mEq/L), potassium 4 mEq/L (normal 4.1–5.3 mEq/L), bicarbonate (or total CO_s) was 19 mEq/L (normal 20–28 mEq/L or mmol/L), serum creatinine 0.3 mg/dL (normal ~0.3–0.5 mg/dL), blood urea nitrogen 6 mg/dL, uric acid of 2.4 mg/dL, blood glucose 85 mg/dL; white blood count was elevated at 26,000/mm^3 with 255 immature cells (bands). Lumbar puncture showed a protein concentration of 140 mg/dL, glucose of 30 mg/dL and 2000 leukocytes/mm^3 with more than 80% polymorphonuclear leukocytes. Blood and urine

Table 9
Diagnostic Criteria for SIADH

1)	Hypotonic hyponatremia
2)	Inappropriate urine osmolality compared to plasma osmolality. In patients with an medical condition associated with the occurrence of SIADH, a urine osmolality greater than maximal dilution (75–125 mOsm/L) and a low plasma osmolality is "inappropriate" to state of water balance
3)	Absence of thyroid, adrenal, cardiac, or renal disease
4)	Absence of volume contraction
5)	High urinary sodium concentration (increased FE_{Na})

Reproduced with permission from Feld *(41)*.

culture pending. Serum osmolality 262 mOsm/kg (this was a measured value, although the effective osmolality or tonicity is [2 × serum sodium + glucose/18 = 252 + 5 = 257]).

Urinalysis/chemistries: specific gravity of 1.018 (estimated osmolality = 720 mOsm/kg), no blood, protein, or glucose, small ketones; urine sodium 100 mEq/L, urine creatinine 15 mg/dL; fractional sodium excretion (FE_{Na}) – 1.6%.

3.5. Assessment

The clinical and laboratory information suggest meningitis with SIADH. The presentation of neurological findings with hyponatremia suggests this diagnosis. There is no evidence of volume depletion or expansion/excess of the extracellular fluid compartment. The presence of hyponatremia with a decreased serum osmolality (effective osmolality/tonicity) with a urine osmolality, which is not maximally dilute ($<\sim$125 mOsm/kg) without evidence of renal, thyroid, or adrenal disease is consistent with SIADH. Additional information supports the diagnosis: a low serum uric acid and BUN in the face of clinical euvolemia, elevated FENa (>1%) – inconsistent with hypovolemia when the FE_{Na} should be <1%, lack of evidence of diuretic use, pseudohyponatremia (secondary to increased plasma proteins or lipids) or hypertonic hyponatremia (hyperglycemia or mannitol infusions).

3.6. Therapeutic Plan

SIADH will not resolve until the underlying disease process has significantly improved or resolved (treatment of meningitis will not be discussed). The approach is a three-step process.

1. Acute presentation (neurological manifestations such as coma, encephalopathy, and seizures).

    a. There are two approaches for *symptomatic presentation* that can be used to increase the serum sodium concentration/serum osmolality.
    Increase the serum sodium by 10 mEq/L or the serum osmolality by 20 mOsm/kg (10 mOsm from sodium and 10 mOsm from chloride) with the use of hypertonic or

3% saline (513 mEq/L of sodium or ~0.5 mEq/mL). Regardless of the approach, when the symptoms are improved the 3% infusion should be discontinued.

  i. For sodium correction = 10 mEq/kg Na × body weight (BW) × 0.6 (distribution factor for sodium) = 6 BW = # of mEq to be infused. Since there is 0.5 mEq Na/mL or 1 mEq/2 mL, *the amount of 3% saline to be infused over about 60–90 min would be 2 mL/mEq × 6 mEq × BW = 12 BW.*
  ii. The alternative method is to provide 2–4 mL/kg /h to increase the serum sodium by 2–4 mEq/L/h.
  iii. Furosemide has been used in a dosage of 0.5 mg/kg up to a maximum of 20 mg given intravenously which may enhance free-water excretion, increase the serum sodium concentration, and avoid ECF volume expansion/excess.

  b. If the symptoms are absent or mild – *asymptomatic presentation,* a lower infusion rate of 0.5–2 mL/kg of body weight may be used which will increase the serum sodium from 0.5 to 2 mEq/L/h. Some centers will select to use isotonic saline in asymptomatic patients for patients with a serum sodium above 123–125 mEq/L.
  c. In either case, the *serum sodium should be monitored every 2–3 h* to prevent overcorrection of the serum sodium concentration.
  d. The *maximum serum sodium correction per 24 h should not exceed 10 mEq/L* (some clinicians limit the increase to 8 mEq/L/24 h).

3.7. Hyperosmolar Hyponatremia

In general, when the serum sodium is found to be below normal, serum osmolality is also below normal. However, as noted above, serum osmolality reflects the concentration of electrolytes (with sodium the major extracellular cation) and other osmolytes such as glucose and urea. The best example of a clinical situation where a low serum sodium is associated with an elevated serum osmolality is diabetes mellitus especially diabetic ketoacidosis.

Illustrative of this point is the following case scenario. A patient with Type 1 diabetes mellitus presents with a 3 day history of fever and abdominal pain. The patient complains of anorexia and nausea. As a result, the patient used less insulin. The patient is febrile, ill appearing, and weak with a respiratory rate of 20 and deep breaths, heart rate of 130 beats/min, and a blood pressure of 84/54 mmHg. Laboratory assessment includes serum sodium 125 mEq/L, potassium 3.8 mEq/L, chloride 90 mEq/L, bicarbonate 10 mEq/L, glucose 900 mg/dL, and urea 20 mg/dL. Urinalysis reveals a specific gravity of 1.035, pH 5, glucose 4+, ketones 3+, protein 1+, and no blood. At first glance the low serum sodium would suggest a low serum osmolality. However, if we use the formula above to estimate osmolality we would find 2× [Na] equals 250 plus glucose of 900/18 equals 50 plus a urea of 20/2.8 equals approximately 7 making the serum osmolality 307 – well above the normal range.

What is the pathophysiology of hyperosmolar hyponatremia? Why is the serum sodium low in this condition? As the extracellular glucose concentration increases in the face of low available insulin, glucose cannot enter cells. The extracellular osmolality increases and provides an osmotic force for water to leave the intracellular space for the extracellular space. No additional sodium is added to the extracellular space. This results in a decrease in the concentration of sodium in the extracellular space. There may also be some loss of sodium in urine but the major cause of a low serum sodium in diabetic ketoacidosis is the "dilutional effect" of glucose drawing water from the intracellular to extracellular space.

In a recent publication, the above observation was examined in patients treated for diabetic ketoacidosis. The authors found that during initial management when the serum glucose concentration fell and the serum sodium concentration rose [resulting in little change in osmolality] central nervous system morbidity was lower (26). Recognizing that hyponatremia in this setting is associated with hyperosmolality, then managing the hyperosmolality carefully and in concert with serum glucose concentration will improve outcome in this type of clinical scenario.

3.8. Cerebral Salt Wasting

Cerebral salt wasting is far less understood cause of hyponatremia/hypo-osmolality. Cerebral salt wasting occurs within a few days of a central nervous system insult, such as a brain injury or brain surgery. Like SIADH release, hyponatremia and hypo-osmolality are noted. However unlike SIADH release, urine volumes are high (urine sodium concentration are very high), extracellular volume is contracted along with high measurable serum levels of natriuretic peptides (brain and cardiac), and low levels of renin and aldosterone despite volume contraction. Although both SIADH release and cerebral salt wasting can follow brain injury, differentiating the entities is important since one is treated with fluid restriction and in the other (cerebral salt wasting) fluid restriction could be detrimental (Table 10). Cerebral salt wasting should be considered in a child following brain injury or surgery with hyponatremia, when there is evidence of volume

Table 10
Differences Between SIADH and Cerebral Salt Wasting (CSW)

	SIADH	CSW
Weight	Increased	Decreased
Extracellular fluid volume	Increased	Decreased
Signs of dehydration	Not present	Present
Hematocrit	Normal	Increased
Serum sodium concentration	Decreased	Decreased
Plasma osmolality	Decreased	Decreased
Urine sodium concentration	Increased	Increased
Urine volume	Decreased	Increased
Plasma [arginine vasopressin]	Increased	Normal or decreased
Serum uric acid concentration	Decreased	Normal
Serum albumin concentration	Normal or decreased	Increased
BUN and serum [creatinine]	Both decreased	Both increased
Treatment	Fluid restriction	Isotonic saline

Modified with permission from Feld (41). Adapted from Chonchol and Berl (44), and Ingelfinger (45).

contraction, very *high* urine output with urinary sodium losses >80 mEq/L and negative sodium balance, suppressed antidiuretic hormone (why this is true is unclear) and low plasma aldosterone concentration (along with low plasma renin activity) *(27)*.

The treatment of cerebral salt wasting includes providing salt and water – often very large sodium infusions while awaiting resolution, which usually occurs in 2–4 weeks. Other potential therapies include providing AVP while administering sodium and the use of fludrocortisone to help enhance sodium reabsorption. Additional potassium may also be needed with fludrocortisone administration.

4. HYPERNATREMIA AND HYPERTONICITY

4.1. Definition and Pathophysiology

Hypernatremia (serum sodium > 150 mEq/L) occurs less frequently than hyponatremia and reflects a net water deficit through water losses or inadequate water replacement. Since sodium is the predominant element in the serum osmolality formula, hypernatremia is always a state of increased effective tonicity or hyperosmolality. Infrequently, it results from a pure sodium gain. Protective mechanisms against the development of hypernatremia include the ability of the kidney to excrete concentrated urine through ADH release and an intact thirst mechanism leading to increased water intake (Fig. 7). Young infants have higher maintenance water requirements related to their large surface area for size and given their dependence on others to provide necessary fluids, they are particularly vulnerable to hypernatremia.

The consequences of hypernatremia are often severe due to cellular dehydration from water shifting from the intracellular to extracellular space in an attempt to reestablish osmotic equilibrium. The brain in infants and young children is particularly susceptible to injury because of its large water content.

4.2. Symptoms

The typical features of dehydration (Table 3) are often lacking due to the preservation of the intravascular volume at the expense of intracellular dehydration (Fig. 8). The signs and symptoms of hypernatremia are typically neurologic in nature from CNS injury and consist of irritability, high-pitched cry, seizures, lethargy, intense thirst, altered mentation and coma *(28, 29)*. In fatal cases, patients may experience intracranial hemorrhages, cranial thrombosis, and infarctions as the brain shrinks away from the meninges and calvarium, placing tension on bridging veins. In those infants and children who survive hypernatremic dehydration, rates of persistent neurologic impairment range from 11 to 15%.

4.3. Diagnosis and Causes

A variety of causes leading to free water losses result in hypernatremia if fluid intake or thirst is impaired (Fig. 9). Hypernatremia may result from either extrarenal water loss or renal water loss. Examples of non-renal water loss include insensible water losses through perspiration or the respiratory tract (hyperventilation, mechanical ventilation).

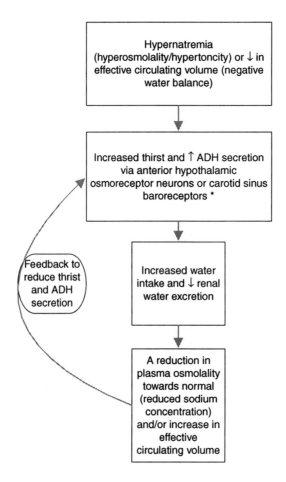

* The opposite scenario of hypoosmolality (hyponatremia) and/or increased effective circulating volume (positive water balance) would have the opposite effect. There would be decreased oral intake and water intake leading to water excretion to restore plasma osmolality and circulatory volume (water balance).

Fig. 7. Protective mechanisms against the development of hypernatremia.

Historically, acute infectious diarrhea is the most common cause of hypernatremia in children due to hypotonic fluid losses in stool in conjunction with low water intake or vomiting. In addition, osmotic diarrhea from enteral feeds in acutely or chronically ill infants/children or in those with neurologic impairment may also lead to hypernatremia. The presence of fever or elevated ambient temperatures accentuates the water losses (there is a 12% loss per degree increase in body temperature). Hypotonic fluid losses in these situations are accompanied by losses from the extracellular fluid volume compartment adding to the total body sodium as well as water deficit. Urine will have a high osmolality and urinary sodium concentration < 20 mEq/L.

Renal water loss is accompanied by polyuria due to the inability to conserve water appropriately. Polyuria can either result from the excretion of a large solute load, i.e.,

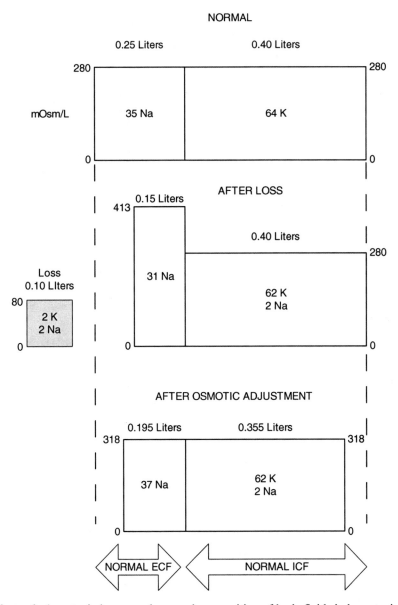

Fig. 8. Effects of a hypotonic loss on volume and composition of body fluids in hypertonic dehydration. The normal situation is altered after the loss followed by an osmolar readjustment with a resulting higher osmolality in both the ECF and ICF. Reproduced with permission from Winters *(39)*.

glucose, or from the excretion of very dilute urine. Evaluating the urine osmolality assists in distinguishing between these two clinical settings (Fig. 10). Osmotic diuresis occurs with poorly controlled diabetes and resulting glucosuria, administration of mannitol for cerebral edema, or excessive urea excretion seen in those receiving hyperalimentation with high protein content or those with a high catabolic rate. Urine osmolality will exceed >300 mOsm/L with a urine sodium concentration >20 mEq/L. In

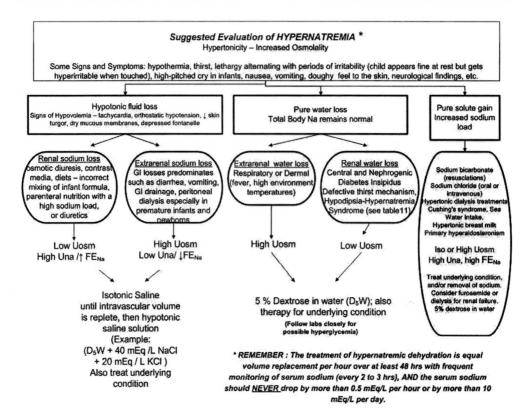

Fig. 9. Suggested evaluation of hypernatremia.

contrast, the polyuria from diabetes insipidus results from the inability of the kidney to excrete concentrated urine due to either deficient vasopressin secretion (central diabetes insipidus) or renal resistance to vasopressin (nephrogenic diabetes insipidus). In contrast to osmotic diuresis, the urine osmolality in diabetes insipidus is <150 mOsm/L and a low sodium concentration in face of an elevated serum sodium levels.

Central diabetes insipidus (DI) may be idiopathic or may result from trauma, infections, neoplasms, intracranial hemorrhages, neurosurgical procedures, or granulomatous conditions as seen with sarcoid and histiocytosis X *(30)* (Table 11). It is characterized by excessive polydipsia and polyuria and the inability to concentrate urine despite a hypovolemic stimulus. A strong preference for cold fluids is a unique feature of this form of polyuria. Diminishing urine volume and increasing urine osmolality in response to exogenous vasopressin confirms the diagnosis of central DI. Intramuscular injections of vasopressin have been replaced by desmopressin delivered either by intranasal or oral routes with the former having greater potency due to absorption *(31)*.

Nephrogenic DI is characterized by the inability to concentrate urine due to unresponsiveness of the distal renal tubule to circulating vasopressin *(32–34)*. There are two different receptors for ADH: the V1 (AVPR1) and V2 (AVPR2) receptors with the latter being located on the X-chromosome (Xq-28). Familial nephrogenic DI that accounts for 90% of all hereditary forms occurs with an X-linked mode of inheritance due to

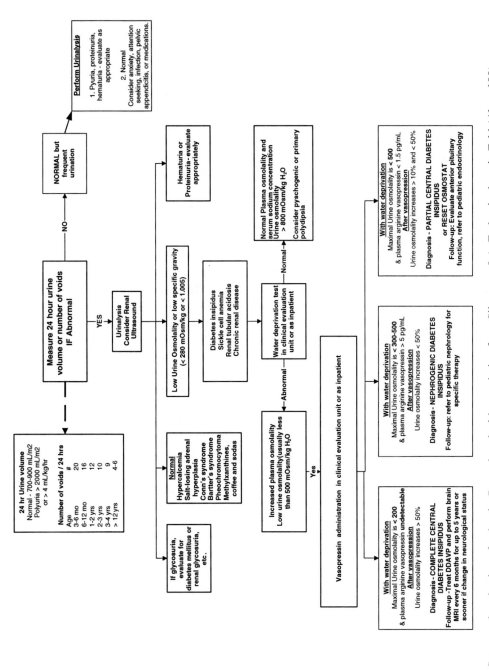

Fig. 10. Suggested evaluation of polyuria. Reproduced with permission from Silverman LA, Endocrinology in Feld (*41, p. 188*).

Table 11
Causes of Central and Nephrogenic Diabetes Insipidus

Central diabetes insipidus	Nephrogenic diabetes insipidus
Idiopathic	**Congenital**
Hereditary – autosomal recessive or dominant	ADH receptor – X-linked Aquaporin defect
Head trauma or skull fracture	**Renal Disease**
Supracellular or intracellular tumors (craniopharyngioma, glioma, pinealoma)	Obstructive uropathy Renal dysplasia
Granulomatous disease – sarcoid, TB,	Medullary cystic disease
Wegener's granulomatosis, syphilis	Pyelonephritis and reflux nephropathy
Histiocytosis	Polycystic disease
Guillain–Barré syndrome	Uric acid nephropathy
Sickle cell disease	**Systemic disease with renal involvement**
Cerebral hemorrhage, thrombosis or aneurysm	Sickle cell disease
Ischemic encephalopathy – cardiac arrest or shock	Sarcoidosis Amyloidosis
Infection – meningitis or encephalitis	Multiple myeloma Sjögren disease
Associated with cleft lip and palate	**Medications**
Leukemia or lymphomas	Aminoglycosides
Anorexia nervosa	Amphotericin
	Diuretics
	Isophosphamide
	Lithium
	Methicillin
	Methoxyflurane
	Phenytoin
	Vinblastine
	Miscellaneous
	Hypokalemia
	Hypercalcemia
	Excessive water intake or decreased protein intake

Reproduced with permission from Feld *(41)*.

mutations in the gene *AVPR2* gene, resulting in the loss of function or dysfunction of the V2 receptor. The disease presents in the neonatal period with polyuria, excessive thirst, poor weight gain, unexplained fever, and recurrent episodes of hypernatremic dehydration. A less common form of nephrogenic DI is seen with an aquaporin-2 gene mutation, which encodes the vasopressin-regulated water channel, aquaporin-2 (*AQP2*), in renal collecting ducts. Mutations in the *AQP2* gene may have either an autosomal dominant or recessive mode of inheritance. Molecular genetic testing is available to distinguish between the two forms of diabetes insipidus. Testing is particularly important where there is a known history of families with X-linked nephrogenic DI and prenatal mutation analysis can be performed. Acquired forms of nephrogenic DI are more common than the hereditary forms. Typically, causes in the pediatric population include chronic kidney disease from cystic kidney disease, renal dysplasia, obstructive uropathies, or chronic pyelonephritis; and with metabolic disturbances as seen with hypokalemia and hypercalcemia.

Unlike central DI, administration of vasopressin will not affect urinary volume or osmolality in situations of nephrogenic DI. Paramount to dealing with a child with NDI is to ensure unrestricted amounts of water. Therapeutic management is aimed at decreasing urinary volume through a low osmolar load (low protein and low sodium diet – 0.7 mEq/kg/day). Additionally, hydrochlorothiazide (1–2 mg/kg/day) acts to block sodium reabsorption in the distal tubule leading to a modest extracellular fluid volume contraction and consequently increased proximal tubular reabsorption of water (Table 12). Long-term monotherapy with hydrochlorothiazide commonly results in hypokalemia. This potentially serious complication can be avoided by the addition of amiloride. Indomethacin (0.75–1.5 mg/kg/d) can provide further reduction of urinary volume. Collectively, these maneuvers diminish free-water clearance by approximately 50%. Early recognition of this condition averts recurrent episodes of hypernatremic dehydration, hyperthermia, and mental retardation, which are well-described complications.

Least commonly observed as a cause of hypernatremia is sodium gain. Administration of hypertonic sodium bicarbonate solutions in situations of cardiopulmonary resuscitation (less common), inadvertent fluid boluses with hypertonic sodium chloride solutions, and seawater drowning can lead to hypernatremia. Boiled skim milk, once commonplace in the treatment of infants with diarrhea, resulted in hypernatremia *(35, 36)*. Large outbreaks of hypernatremia have been reported in the past due to improper preparation of powdered infant formulations. Urine studies show normal or high osmolality and urinary sodium excretion >20 mEq/L.

4.4. Treatment

The objectives of managing hypernatremia involve identifying the underlying cause, limiting further water loss, and replacing the water deficit. Evaluation of volume status is critical to the therapeutic management of patients with hypernatremia. In addition, ongoing water losses through insensible losses, diarrhea, or polyuria must be taken into account.

When hypernatremia is accompanied by depletion of extracellular volume, restoring this space with isotonic solution (normal saline, lactated Ringer's solution, 5% albumin) takes precedence regardless of the serum sodium concentration. Treatment of hypernatremia requires cautious lowering of serum sodium by no more than 0.5 mEq/L/h or 10 mEq/24 h. In states of hypernatremia, fluid shifts out of brain cells to establish osmotic equilibrium leading to cellular shrinkage. Too rapid of a correction of serum sodium results in osmotic water movement back into brain cells leading to cerebral

Table 12
Suggested Management of Diabetes Insipidus

Central diabetes insipidus
Desmopressin acetate (DDAVP, vasopressin)
- *Oral*
  - ≤12 years: Initial: 0.05 mg once a day or twice daily; titrate to desired response (range 0.1–0.6 mg daily or twice daily)
  - >12 years: 0.05 mg twice daily; titrate to desired response (range 0.1–1.2 mg divided 2–3 times daily)
- *Intranasal solution*
  - Children 3 months to ≤ 12 years: Initial 5 mcg/day divided 1–2 times/day (range 5–30 mcg/day)
  - Children > 12 years: Initial 5–40 mcg/day divided 1–2 times/day
- *Subcutaneous*
  - Children > 12 years: 2–4 mcg/day divided 1–2 times/day

Some of the adverse reactions: Desmopressin acetate: facial flushing, palpitations, headache, dizziness, hyponatremia, nausea, abdominal cramps, rhinitis, nasal congestion, etc.; vasopressin: circumoral pallor, vertigo, water intoxication, abdominal cramps, nausea, flatus, wheezing, diaphoresis, etc.

Nephrogenic Diabetes Insipidus
- Salt restriction ≤ 100 mEq/d (2.3 g sodium)
- Protein restriction ≤ 1 g/kg/day*
- Diuretics
  - Hydrochlorothiazide (HCTZ) 1–2 mg/kg/day divided 1–2 times/day
  - Amiloride 0.2–0.4 mg/kg/day
- Indomethacin 0.75–1.5 mg/kg/day
- Ample fluid via mouth or G-Tube; if necessary intravenous such as 5% dextrose with ¼ (0.225%) isotonic saline to achieve normal or high normal serum sodium concentrations.
Some of the adverse reactions: Hydrochlorothiazide: hypotension, headache, hypokalemia, hyperglycemia, hyperlipidemia, hyperuricemia, metabolic alkalosis, muscle weakness, etc. Amiloride: headache, dizziness, hyperkalemia, hyperchloremic metabolic alkalosis, nauseas, diarrhea, vomiting, abdominal pain, weakness, muscle cramps, etc. Indomethacin: fatigue, hyperkalemia, epigastric or abdominal pain, gastrointestinal bleeding, ulcers, renal failure, etc.

---

*Caution in infants and young children

edema with the potential complications of seizures, cerebral herniation, and death. Water deficit in hypernatremia can be calculated by the following equation:

$$\text{Water deficit} = \text{TBW} \times ([\text{Na}^+_{(measured)}] - [\text{Na}^+_{(desired)}]/[\text{Na}^+_{(desired)}])$$

where TBW is total body water, $[\text{Na}^+_{(measured)}]$ is the measured sodium concentration, and $[\text{Na}^+_{(desired)}]$ is the desired sodium concentration.

Total body water (TBW) is 0.6 × body weight in kilograms.

For example, to estimate the water deficit in a 10 kg infant with a serum sodium of 160, first calculate the total body water of a 10 kg infant, which is estimated at 6 L (TBW = 0.6 × 10 kg). The water deficit can then be calculated as follows:

$$H_2O \text{ deficit} = TBW \times (\text{Actual Serum [Na]} - \text{Desired Serum [Na]})/\text{Desired Serum [Na]}$$
$$H_2O \text{ deficit} = 6L \times (160 - 145)/145 = 0.6L$$

REMEMBER, in the first 24 h, fluid calculations should be adjusted to include the replacement of the free-water deficit, ongoing losses plus maintenance requirements.

A patient with hypernatremia due to pure water losses and euvolemia needs replacement with 5% dextrose solution in water (D_5W). If the hypernatremia has developed over a short course of time (<24 h), then rapid correction does not risk the development of cerebral edema. As noted above, if hypernatremia is secondary to central DI, administration of a vasopressin analogue is indicated (Table 12).

Treatment of hypernatremia due to sodium gains is targeted at removal of excess sodium through administration of diuretics such as furosemide or by dialysis if there is associated renal impairment.

Case Scenario 3. Hypernatremia with Sodium and Water Deficits = Hypovolemia

A 6-month-old infant presents to her pediatrician in December with a 4-day history of fever (up to 40°C), along with mild upper respiratory symptoms. On the evening and night prior to presentation, she began to have diarrhea and emesis with cessation of formula and solid foods. The child had a wet diaper this morning.

On examination, the child appeared quiet but became irritable during the exam, mucous membranes were mildly dry, and the skin felt doughy. Vitals signs were the following: blood pressure 85/58 mmHg, temperature of 39°C, respiratory rate of 40/min, and pulse of 175 beats/min. The weight was 7.5 kg. A previous weight about 2 weeks ago was 8.4 kg. There were no other significant findings and the child appears to have good turgor and skin elasticity.

With the magnitude of dehydration, high fever, and irritability, the decision by the clinician was to initiate parenteral fluid replacement rather than oral rehydration therapy. The child was admitted to the hospital with diagnosis of dehydration. On admission, the laboratory studies were as follows:

Sodium 162 mEq/L, chloride 126 mEq/L (normal 98 –118 mEq/L), potassium 4 mEq/L (normal 4.1–5.3 mEq/L), bicarbonate (or total CO_2) was 12 mEq/L (normal 20–28 mEq/L or mmol/L), serum creatinine 1 mg/dL (normal ~0.3–0.5 mg/dL), blood urea nitrogen 29 mg/dL, blood glucose 85 mg/dL; complete blood count was normal without immature cells.

Urinalysis/chemistries: specific gravity of 1.030, no blood, protein or glucose, small ketones; urine creatinine 30 mg/dL and sodium 30 mEq/L;

Fractional excretion of sodium (FE$_{Na}$)

([urine sodium $\times$ serum creatinine]/[serum sodium $\times$ urine creatinine] $\times$ 100%) =
   ([30 mEq/L $\times$ 1 mg/dL]/[161 mEq/L $\times$ 30 mg/dL]) = 0.62%
Normal values for FE$_{Na}$ = $\sim 1 - 2\%$;decreased renal perfusion
   (dehydration, decreased intravascular volume) < 1%

4.5. Assessment

The clinical and laboratory information suggest *hypernatremic dehydration*. In many cases there is extrarenal losses from diarrhea and vomiting with predisposing factors being young age, fever, curtailment of oral intake and possibly, high solute fluids such as concentrated or improper preparation of formula or other fluid with a high sodium content. The child has lost proportionally more water than sodium or a relatively hypotonic fluid loss. The result is a higher extracellular fluid osmolality, which results in a fluid shift from the intracellular fluid compartment to the extracellular fluid compartment. This provides for better organ perfusion compared to iso- or hyponatremic dehydration of comparable degrees. The child on examination appears better perfused and provides a history of urine output rather than oliguria. This may lead to an underestimate of the degree of dehydration. In this case, the magnitude of the dehydration is about *10% or moderate*. The pre-illness weight was ~8.3 kg with a current weight of 7.5 kg or a 0.8 kg loss over the last week. Estimated guidelines for vital signs at this age: the normal respiratory rate for children is approximately 36; normal pulse is about 130 (standard deviation is ~45) beats/min; normal blood pressure is approximately 89/54 mmHg.

As noted above, the decision by the clinician was to initiate parenteral fluid replacement rather than oral rehydration therapy. The relative contraindications for oral rehydration therapy would include a young infant less than 3–4 months of age, the presence of impending shock or markedly impaired perfusion (increased capillary refill – turgor), inability to consume oral fluids due to intractable vomiting, marked irritability or lethargy/unresponsiveness or the judgment of the clinician.

4.6. Therapeutic Plan

1. Volume deficit, electrolyte calculations: Traditionally, treatment has been divided into three phases: an emergent or acute phase – isotonic saline; replacement phase – over 24 h unless there are on-going losses, which are not replaced adequately in the first day of treatment; and the maintenance phase – day 2 continuing to home management. However, in hypernatremic dehydration, the hyperosmolality results in the formation of idiogenic osmoles (organic and inorganic) such as taurine, glutamate, glutamine, urea, and inositol within the brain cells to assist in maintaining osmotic equilibrium between the two fluid compartments. If the adjustment in osmolality (lowering) occurs to quickly in the extracellular compartment, the osmotic changes will result in the brain cells to swell with resultant neurologic manifestations such as hemorrhage.

Emergent or acute phase – This may need to be prolonged in cases of more significant volume depletion. In some cases of hypernatremic dehydration the emergent phase is not necessary. If there are significant findings of decreased perfusion or hypotension, then therapy would be reasonable. Otherwise the process is for a slow restoration of the serum sodium concentration in order to allow the idiogenic osmols to dissipate over a few days. Similar to other forms of dehydration, if it is necessary to reestablish circulatory volume to prevent prolonged loss of perfusion to the key organs such as kidney, brain, gastrointestinal tract, etc., the fluid choices would be isotonic (0.9%) saline (normal saline) or another isotonic/hypertonic solution such as 5% albumin, Ringer's lactate, or a plasma preparation. With the availability of isotonic saline, this is the usual fluid choice.

Acute – Repletion/Replacement/Restoration Phase – Over 48 h; in this period the daily fluid/electrolyte maintenance requirements and deficit calculation are derived from standard estimates. Even though there are objective clinical signs of dehydration and estimated volume deficits, subjectivity will always to be a factor. For hypernatremic dehydration there are two basic rules – *slow correction and close monitoring*. Slow correction means that the serum sodium concentration should not be reduced by more than about 10 mEq/day. Correct the patient over 48 h for a serum sodium concentration of less than 165 mEq/L; correct the patient over 72 h for values above 165 mEq/L.

1. Maintenance fluid/electrolyte calculations for 24 h: Since the patient has a serum sodium concentration of 161mEq/L, the correction is over 2 days so 2 days of maintenance fluids needs to be added to the total fluid requirements for 48 h.

Calculations based on daily caloric requirements

Body weight (BW) in kg	Caloric needs Calories/kg BW	Water needs mL/100 calories used per day – each mL equals about 1 calorie*	Electrolyte needs mEq/100 calories used per day (alternate method is mEq/kg/day)	Calories derived from glu- cose/dextrose
3–10	100	100	Sodium = 2.5–3 mEq (or 3 mEq/kg) Potassium = 2–2.5 mEq (or ~2 mEq/kg)	5 g/100 calories used
11–20	1000 + 50 calories/kg for each kg above 10	1000 + 50 mL/kg for each kg above 10		
>20	1500 + 20 calories/kg for each kg above 20	1500 + 20 mL/kg for each kg above 20		

*Kidney losses are about 45–75 mL/100 calories expended; sweat losses usually 0; stool losses are about 5–10 mL/100 calories expended, and insensible losses (skin ~30 mL + respiratory ~15 mL) is about 45 mL/100 calories expended – 100 mL of total daily water losses = 100 calories expended per day or *1 mL = 1 calorie.*

For this 8.3 kg infant

Maintenance requirements for 48 h

Water	100 mL/kg × 8.3 kg = 830 mL × 2 days = 1660 mL
Sodium	3 mEq/100 mL × 830 mL = 25 mEq × 2 days = 50 mEq
Potassium	2 mEq/100 mL × 830 mL = 17 mEq × 2 days = 34 mEq

There are two approaches to replace the deficit. Both have a similar intravenous rate and time period (at least 48 h), they only differ in the method of calculation.

Approach 1: Use Table Below

Deficit replacement of water and electrolytes: in most circumstances the acid–base disorder is a simple metabolic acidosis, which does not require bicarbonate replacement unless there is severe tissue/impaired circulatory compromise such as shock (generally 15% dehydration). In general there is only partial replacement of potassium deficits, which are fully corrected over 2–4 days following resumption of oral intake.

Type of dehydration* based on serum [Na] in mEq/L	Water (mL/kg)	Sodium (mEq/kg)	Potassium (mEq/kg)
Isonatremic [Na] 130–150	120	10	8
Hyponatremic [Na] < 130	100	10–12	8
Hypernatremic [Na] > 150	100	4	2

*Isonatremic dehydration is the most common accounting for 70–80% of infants and children; hypernatremic dehydration accounts for about 15%, and hyponatremic dehydration for about 5–10% of cases. Adapted from Winter RW: Principles of Pediatric Fluid Therapy, 2nd Ed, Little Brown and Co., Boston, 1982, p 86.

For this 8.3 kg infant with hypernatremic dehydration at 10%

Deficits

Water	Pre-illness weight – Illness weight = 8.3 – 7.5 kg = 0.8 kg = 800 mL
Sodium	4 mEq × 8.3 kg = 33 mEq
Potassium	2 mEq × 8.3 kg = 17 mEq

2. Total 48 h Requirements

The total amount of maintenance (2 days) and deficit amounts are given equally over the 48 h period with frequent monitoring of electrolytes in order to adjust the intravenous rate or sodium concentration based on the rate of decline of the serum sodium concentration.

$$\text{Fluid selection} - 5\% \text{ dextrose} + 1/4 \text{ } isotonic \text{ } saline(\sim 30 - 40 \text{ mEq/L of Na})$$
$$+ 20 \text{ mEq KCl/L at 50 mL/h given equally over 48 h.}$$

Generally the final solution potassium concentration is about 20 mEq/L, it should not exceed 40 mEq/L without close intensive care monitoring. The 5% dextrose provides 50 g of carbohydrate per liter of 50 g × ~4 calories/g = 200 calories. This would be about 20% of the daily caloric intake, which is sufficient to prevent protein breakdown over a short treatment period (less than one week).

Component of therapy	Water	Sodium	Potassium	Hourly rate Round number up or down to the nearest 5 increment
Maintenance – 2 days	1660	50	34	
Deficit	800	33	17	
Ongoing losses of diarrhea or vomiting*				
TOTAL	2460	83	51	50 mL/hr

* From clinical experience the gastrointestinal losses tend to resolve or decrease significantly following the initiation of parenteral therapy. If it does continue, these losses will need to be added to the ongoing loss row.

Approach 2: Use a Free-Water Deficit Calculation
Total 48 h Requirements

The total amount of maintenance (2 days) and deficit amounts are given equally over the 48 h period with frequent monitoring of electrolytes in order to adjust the intravenous rate or sodium concentration based on the rate of decline of the serum sodium concentration.

$$\text{Water deficit} - 4\,\text{mL/kg} \times \text{body weight}$$
$$\times (\text{Ideal Serum [Sodium]} - \text{Actual serum [sodium]})$$

Component of therapy	Water	Sodium	Potassium	Hourly rate Round number up or down to the nearest 5 increment
Maintenance – 2 days	1660	50	34	
Water deficit 4 mL × 8.3 kg × (162–145 mEq/L)	564			
Sodium deficit 0.56 L × 0.6 × 140 mEq/L		47		
Potassium deficit 0.56 L × 0.4 × 120 mEq/L			26	
Ongoing losses of diarrhea or vomiting*				
TOTAL	2224	97	60	46 mL/h

Table 13
Treatment Summary for Dehydration

Body weight (kg)	Water needs mL/100 calories used per day – each mL equals about one calorie*	Sodium need mEq/100 calories used per day (alternate method is mEq/kg/day)	Potassium needs mEq/100 calories used per day (alternate method is mEq/kg/day)
A. Maintenance			
3–10	100 mL/kg	Sodium = 2.5–3 mEq (or 3 mEq/kg)	Potassium = 2–2.5 mEq (or ~2 mEq/kg)
11–20	1000 + 50 mL/kg for each kg above 10		
>20	1500 + 20 mL/kg for each kg above 20		

B. Type of Dehydration based on serum [Na] in mEq/L Calculations do not include an emergent therapy phase

	Water (mL/kg)	Sodium (mEq/kg)	Potassium (mEq/kg)
B.1. Isonatremic [Na] 130–150 mEq/L – Provide maintenance needs plus one of the following			
Approach 1	100 mL/kg	10 mEq/kg	8 mEq/kg
Approach 2	Based on % dehydration Dry weight × %	Fluid deficit (L) × 0.6 × 135 mEq/L	Fluid deficit (L) × 0.4 × 120 mEq/L

Fluid selection: 5% dextrose +1/3 (0.33%) isotonic saline + 40 mEq KCl/L OR
5% dextrose + 1/2 (0.45%) isotonic saline + 40 mEq KCl/L
Rate: 1/2 of the maintenance and 1/2 fluid deficit delivered over 8 h and the remainder over the next 16 h

B.2. Hyponatremic [Na] < 130 mEq/L – Maintenance plus one of the following			
Approach 1	100–120 mL/kg	10–12 mEq/kg	8 mEq/kg
Fluid selection – 5% dextrose + 0.45% isotonic saline + 40 mEq KCl/L			
Approach 2	Based on % dehydration Dry Weight × %	Fluid deficit (L) × 0.6 × 140 mEq/L	Fluid deficit (L) × 0.4 × 120 mEq/L

PLUS sodium deficit – (desired sodium (135) – actual sodium) × 0.6 L/kg × BW kg

First 8 h, Fluid selection: 5% dextrose + isotonic saline + 40 mEq KCl/L; In both approaches the Fluid Selection for the next 16 hrs (9–24 h) is 5% dextrose + ½ isotonic saline + 40 mEq KCl/L

B.3. Hypernatremic [Na] > 150 mEq/L

| Approach 1 | 100 mL/kg | 4 mEq/L | 2 mEq/L |

Fluid selection: 5% dextrose + ¼ isotonic saline (~30–40 mEq/L of Na) + 20 mEq KCl/L
1st 24 h: 24 h of Maintenance + ½ deficit
2nd 24 h: 24 h of Maintenance + ½ deficit with close monitoring of serum sodium every 2–3 h.

| Approach 2 | 4 mL × (actual – desired mEq Na/L) × BW kg | Fluid deficit (L) × 0.6 × 140 mEq/L | Fluid deficit (L) × 0.4 × 120 mEq/L |

1st 24 h: 24 h of Maintenance + ½ deficit
2nd 24 h: 24 h of Maintenance + ½ deficit
Fluid selection – 5% dextrose + 1/4 isotonic saline (~40 mEq/L of Na) + 30 mEq KCl/L
(some recommend using 5 dextrose with ½ isotonic saline + potassium)

4 mL/kg is derived from the relationship as follows: How much water is required to reduce 1 mEq of sodium?

$$145\,\text{mEq}/1000\,\text{mL} = 145 + \text{X}/1000\text{mL} = 6.9\,\text{mEq}; 6.9\,\text{mEq}$$
$$\times\,0.6\,(\text{distribution factor}) = 4\,\text{mL} \qquad (37)$$

$$\text{Water Deficit} - 4\,\text{mL} \times (162 - 145\,\text{mEq Na/L}) \times 8.3\,\text{kg} = 560\,\text{mL}$$

SodiumDeficit: $0.56\text{L} \times 0.6 \times 140\,\text{mEq/L}$

PotassiumDeficit: $0.56\text{L} \times 0.4(\text{distributionfactorforpotassium}) \times 120\,\text{mEq/L}$
(intracellular[K])

- From clinical experience the gastrointestinal losses tend to resolve or decrease significantly following the initiation of parenteral therapy. If it does continue these losses will need to be added to the ongoing loss row.
- 1st 24 h: 24 h of Maintenance + ½ deficit = 880 mL + 282 mL = 1162 mL; Na = 25 mEq (maintenance) + 24 (deficit) = 49 mEq; K = 17 (maintenance) + 13 (deficit) = 30 mEq.
- 2nd 24 h: 24 h of Maintenance + ½ deficit = 880 mL + 282 mL = 1162 mL; Na = 25 mEq (maintenance) + 23 (deficit) = 48 mEq; K = 17 (maintenance) + 13 (deficit) = 30 mEq.
- Fluid selection – 5% dextrose + ¼ isotonic saline (~40 mEq/L of Na) + 30 mEq KCl /L at 46 mL.

In both approaches, it is strongly suggested to monitor serum sodium concentration every 2–3 h and adjust the fluid rate and sodium concentration as appropriate. In cases of severe hypernatremic dehydration with marked circulatory compromise or shock, it is reasonable to provide 5% dextrose with ½ isotonic saline without potassium for the first 24 h. If circulatory status is restored, then a lower intravenous concentration of sodium can be used and potassium can be added, if appropriate, to the solution (37).

Two other viewpoints that are in the literature: Laurence Finberg has suggested the use of 2.5% dextrose with 25 mEq/L of sodium plus 40 mEq/L of KCl and one ampule of 10% calcium gluconate per 500 mL of intravenous fluid to prevent hypocalcemia. The rate would be about 6–7 mL/kg/h.

Some have suggested using a higher sodium concentration – 0.45% isotonic saline or even isotonic saline to restore extracellular fluid volume then moving to a lower sodium containing solution to restore the water deficit. This approach may also reduce the possibility of dropping the serum sodium too quickly and preventing neurological problems.

Table 13 provides a summary of the treatment for Isonatremic, hyponatremic, and hypernatremic dehydration.

REFERENCES

1. Gamble JL. Chemical Anatomy Physiology and Pathology of Extracellular Fluid. Harvard University Press, 1950.
2. Winters RW. The Body Fluids in Pediatrics. Little, Brown & Co, Boston, 1973, p. 102.
3. Verney EB. The antidiuretic hormone and the factors which determine its release. Proc R Soc London 135 (Series B) (1947) 25.

4. Robertson GL. Antidiuretic hormone: Normal and disordered function. Endocrinol Metab Clin N Am (2001) 30:671.

5. Gauer OH, Henry JP. Circulatory basis of fluid volume control. Physiol Rev (1963) 43:423.

6. Baylis PH, Robertson GL. Arginine vasopressin response to insulin-induced hypoglycemia in man. J Clin Endocrinol Metab (1981) 53:935.

7. Robben JH, Knoers NVAM, Deen PMT. Cell biological aspects of vasopressin type-2 receptor and aquaporin-2 water channel in nephrogenic diabetes insipidus. Am J Physiol Renal Physiol (2006) 291:F257–F270.

8. Borgnia M, Nielsen S, Engel A, Agre P. Cellular and molecular biology of aquaporin water channels. Annu Rev Biochem (1999) 68:425.

9. Kim SW, Gresz V, Rojek A, et al. Decreased expression of AQP2 and AQP4 water channels and Na, K, ATPase in kidney collecting duct in AQP3 null mice. Biol Cell (2005) 97:765–778.

10. Ecelbarger CA, Kim GH, Wang W, et al. Vasopressin mediated regulation of epithelial sodium channel abundance in the rat kidney. Am J Physiol Renal Physiol (2000) 279:F46–F53.

11. Sands JM. Molecular mechanisms of urate transport. J Membr Biol (2003) 191:149–163.

12. Robillard JE, Matson JR, Sessions C, et al. The dynamics of vasopressin release and blood volume regulation during fetal hemorrhage in the lamb fetus. Pediatr Res (1979) 13:606.

13. Popjavuori M, Raivio KO. The effects of acute and chronic perinatal stress on plasma vasopressin concentrations and renin activity at birth. Biol Neonate (1985) 47:259.

14. Wiriyathian S, Rosenfeld CR, Arant BS, et al. Urinary arginine vasopressin: Pattern of excretion in the neonatal period. Pediatr Res (1986) 20:103.

15. Vander A. Control of sodium and water excretion: Regulation of extracellular volume and osmolality. In: Renal Physiology, 3rd edition. McGraw-Hill Inc., New York: 1985, pp. 136–4016.

16. Keoppen BM, Stanton BA. Regulation of body fluid osmolality: Regulation of water balance. In: Renal Physiology, 2nd edition. Mosby-Year Book Inc., St. Louis: 1997, pp. 90–91.

17. Finberg L, Kravath RE, Hellerstein S. Composition – Chemical Anatomy. In: Water and Electrolytes in Pediatrics: Physiology, Pathology, and Treatment, 2nd edition. 2WB Saunders Company, Philadelphia: 1993, pp. 11–16.

18. Holliday MA, Segar WE. The maintenance need for water in parenteral fluid therapy. Pediatrics (1957) 19:823–832.

19. Moritz ML, Ayus JC. Prevention of hospital acquired hyponatremia, a case for using isotonic saline. Pediatrics (2003) 111:227–230.

20. Friedman AL, Ray PE. Maintenance fluid therapy. What it is and what it is not. Pediatric Nephrol (2008) 23:677–680.

21. Verbalis JG, Goldsmith SR, Greenberg A, et al. Hyponatremia treatment guideline 2007: Expert Panel Recommendations. Am J Med (2007) 120:S1–S21.

22. Hirschorn N. The treatment of acute diarrhea in children: an historical and physiological perspective. Am J Clin Nutr (1980) 33:637.

23. Chesney RW. The role of the kidney in protecting the brain against cerebral edema and neuronal cell swelling. J Pediatr (2008) 152:4–6.

24. Bartter FC, Schwartz WB. The syndrome of inappropriate secretion if antidiuretic hormone. Am J Med (1967) 42:790.

25. Chen S, Jalandhara N, Batlle D. Evaluation and management of hyponatremia: an emerging role for vasopressin receptor antagonists. Nature Clin Pract (2007) 3:82.

26. Hoorn EJ, Carlotti APC, Costa LAA, McMahon B, et al. Preventing a drop in effective plasma osmolality to minimize the likelihood of cerebral edema during treatment of children with diabetic ketoacidosis. J Pediatr (2007) 150:467–473.

27. Kappy MS, Ganong CA. Cerebral salt wasting in children: The role of atrial natriuretic hormone. Adv Pediatr (1996) 43:271–307.

28. Finberg L. Hypernatremic (hypertonic) dehydration in infants. N Eng J Med (1973) 289:196–198.

29. Finberg L. Pathogenesis of the lesion in the central nervous system in hypernatremic states: I. Clinical observations of infants. Pediatrics (1959) 23:40–45.

30. Greger NG, Kirkland RT, Clayton GW, et al. Central Diabetes Insipidus: 22 years' experience. AJDC (1986) 140:551–554.

31. Richardson DW, Robinson AG. Desmopressin. Ann Intern Med (1985) 103:228.

32. Knoers N, Monnens LAH. Nephrogenic diabetes insipidus: clinical symptoms, pathogenesis, genetics and treatment. Pediatr Nephrol (1992) 6:476–482.

33. Deen PMT, Knoers N. Vasopressin type-2 receptor and aquaporin-2 water channel mutants in nephrogenic diabetes insipidus. Am J Med Sci (1998) 316:300–309.

34. Kirchlechner V, Koller DY, Seidl R, et al. Treatment of nephrogenic diabetes insipidus with hydrochlorothiazide and amiloride. Arch Dis Child (1999) 80:548–552.

35. Anand SK, Sandborg C, Robinson RG, et al. Neonatal hypernatremia associated with elevated sodium concentration of breast milk. J Peds (1980) 96:66–68.

36. Colle E, Ayoub E, Raile R. Hypertonic dehydration (hypernatremia): The role of feedings high in solutes. Pediatrics (1958) 22:5.

37. Hochman HI, Grodin MA, Crone RK. Dehydration, diabetic ketoacidosis and shock in the pediatric patient. Pediatric Clin NA (1979) 26:803–826.

38. Czernichow P, Friedman AL, Kappy M. Posterior Pituitary and Water Metabolism. In: Principles and Practice of Pediatric Endocrinology, Kappy M, Allen D, Geffner M (eds.), 1st edition, Charles C. Thomas Co., Springfield, IL: 2005, pp. 815–856.

39. Winters RW. Principles of Fluid Therapy. Abbott Laboratories, North Chicago: 1970.

40. Feld LG. Hyponatremia in infants and children: A practical approach. J Nephrology (1996) 9:5.

41. Feld LG. Nephrology. In: Fast Facts in Pediatrics, 1st edition, Feld LG, Meltzer AJ (eds.), Elsevier, Amsterdam, 2006, p. 451.

42. Cogan MG. Fluid & Electrolytes: Physiology & Pathophysiology. Appleton & Lange, Norwalk: 1991, p. 85.

43. Robertson GL. Thirst and Vasopressin. In: The Kidney Physiology and Pathophysiology, 4th edition, Alpern RJ, Hebert SC (eds.), 1985, pp. 1131–1135.

44. Chonchol M, Berl M. Hyponatremia. In: Acid–Base and Electrolyte Disorders, DuBose TD, Hamm LL (eds.), WB Saunders, Philadelphia: 2002, p. 233.

45. Ingelfinger JR. Diabetes Insipidus, SIADH and Cerebral Salt Wasting. In: Current Pediatric Therapy, Burg F, Ingelfinger JR, Polin R, Gershon AA (eds.), WB Saunders, Philadelphia: 2006, p. 1002.

2 Disorders of Sodium Homeostasis

*Roberto Gordillo, Juhi Kumar,
and Robert P. Woroniecki*

Key Points

1. Renal sodium excretion is the primary determinant of sodium homeostasis.
2. Changes in sodium concentration in extracellular fluid (ECF) are associated with disorders of water balance.
3. Hypovolemia refers to losses of salt and water from the ECF, whereas dehydration is defined as primarily water loss from ECF.
4. Hypervolemia results when fluid accumulates in the ECF at a higher rate than the output due to either sodium and water retention or abnormal sodium and water intake.
5. Activation of sympathetic nervous system, renin–angiotensin–aldosterone, and epithelial sodium channel contributes to renal sodium and water retention.

Key Words: Isovolemia; atrial natriuretic hormone; hypovolemia; hypervolemia; Starling's forces; cirrhosis; congestive heart failure; renin–angiotensin system; nephrotic syndrome; dehydration

1. SODIUM REGULATION IN ISOVOLEMIA

Regulation of sodium and water homeostasis is one of the major functions of the kidney *(1, 2)*. Sodium balance is the result of sodium intake, extra-renal sodium loss, and renal sodium excretion. Renal sodium excretion is the primary determinant of sodium homeostasis *(2)*. Since sodium is a main cation of extracellular fluid (ECF), changes in sodium concentration are linked to changes in ECF volume *(3)* and are associated with disorders of water balance. The extracellular fluid compartment is subdivided into the intravascular and interstitial compartment, commonly referred to as a "third space." The chemical composition and the interdependence of fluid compartments were discussed in Chapter 1: Water Homeostasis. Estimates of intravascular volume distribution indicate that 85% of blood circulates on the low pressure (venous side of the circulation) and an approximately 15% of blood is on the high pressure (arterial circulation) *(4)*.

Although the term "effective circulatory volume" has been used in medical literature for decades, its definition remains unclear *(4)*. Peters *(5)* referred to "effective blood

From: *Nutrition and Health: Fluid and Electrolytes in Pediatrics*
Edited by: L. G. Feld, F. J. Kaskel, DOI 10.1007/978-1-60327-225-4_2,
© Humana Press, a part of Springer Science+Business Media, LLC 2010

volume" as that portion of the total circulating volume that is "somehow sensed," and thus responds to too little or too much volume. In an underfilled body fluid compartment, there must be signals, coming from extra-renal locations promoting retention of sodium and water by the kidney, in response to a decreased effective blood volume *(6)*. Since the kidney can normally regulate sodium and water *(5, 7)*, if heart failure or cirrhosis is reversed (transplantation), the afferent signal for sodium and water retention in patients with heart failure and cirrhosis must come from extra-renal sites *(6)*. Although low cardiac output was proposed to explain low effective circulatory volume *(8)*, sodium and water retention still occur in high-output heart failure and in pregnant women, who also have an increased cardiac output *(3)*.

The "underfilling hypothesis" was subsequently proposed *(9)*. If 85% of the total blood volume is on the venous circulation (low pressure) and 15% of the total blood volume resides on the arterial circulation (high pressure), then an increase in total blood volume and an "underfilling" of the arterial circulation can occur, by an expansion of the venous compartment *(10)*. Underfilling may also occur with low cardiac output (heart failure) or arterial vasodilatation (pregnancy, cirrhosis, sepsis). When arterial underfilling is the result of arterial dilatation or low cardiac output, the neurohumoral axis is stimulated and renal sodium and water retention occurs to maintain perfusion to vital organs *(3)*. These mechanisms include activation of the renin–angiotensin–aldosterone system, activation of the sympathetic system, and nonosmotic vasopressin release *(3)*, which initially maintain perfusion, although in patients with advanced edematous states, sodium and water retention leads to pulmonary edema and ascites *(6)*. The high-pressure (arterial) circulation response to increase pressure and stretch is mediated by baroreceptors located in the aortic arch, left ventricle, carotid sinus, and juxtaglomerular apparatus (glomerular afferent arteriole) *(6)*. Baroreceptors signal the appropriate areas in the brain leading to the release of arginine vasopressin (AVP) *(6)*. In patients with congestive heart failure, who have hyponatremia and low osmolality along with detectable serum concentrations of AVP, there is a nonosmotic AVP release similar to the phenomenon in cirrhotic patients *(11)*. When arterial "underfilling" is detected, secondary to low-output heart failure (arterial baroreceptor stretch) or arterial vasodilatation (high-output heart failure, cirrhosis), an increase in sympathetic tone and nonosmotic AVP release occurs *(6)*. The increase in sympathetic tone stimulates the renin–angiotensin–aldosterone system (RAAS) through renal β-adrenergic stimulation and by an increase in sympathetic tone and RAAS to increase systemic vascular resistance compensating for arterial "underfilling" *(6)*. The nonosmotic release of AVP stimulates the V1a receptors (V1aR) on vascular smooth muscle, which contributes to the compensatory response to arterial "underfilling" *(6)*. The AVP receptors V2 on the collecting tubules, when stimulated, activate the adenylate cyclase and cyclic AMP, increasing the number of aquaporin-2 water channels in the apical membrane of the collective tubules, leading to an increased water reabsorption responsible for hyponatremia in patients with edematous states *(6)*.

Low-pressure receptors located in the atria, in response to an increase in transmural atrial pressure, inhibit the release of AVP, decrease vascular resistance in the kidney, and increase water and sodium excretion *(3)*. Atrial stretch associated with heart failure results in secretion of atrial natriuretic peptides such as C-terminal-ANP,

N-terminal-ANP, B-type natriuretic peptide (BNP). This increase in the synthesis of atrial natriuretic hormones in heart failure patients results in less retention of water, thereby decreasing edema by inhibition of RAAS and sodium absorption (3). Although in heart failure atrial pressure is increased, sodium and water retention occurs (3). This may be explained by "underfilling" that activates arterial stretch receptors, which in turn activate the sympathetic system and the renin–angiotensin–aldosterone system (RAAS) as well as nonosmotic vasopressin release, dominating the response, over the atrial pressure receptor reflex in patients with heart failure (3).

In the first trimester of pregnancy, the systemic arterial vasodilatation and decrease in blood pressure are associated with increased cardiac output (3). When arterial "underfilling" is detected, RAAS is activated, resulting in water and sodium retention and nonosmotic release of AVP (3). In this scenario, there is an increase in renal blood flow and glomerular filtration rate, which does not occur in patients with heart failure or cirrhosis (3). Estrogen upregulates endothelial nitric oxide synthase (eNOS), increasing nitric oxide, which may be also responsible for the systemic and renal vasodilatation observed in pregnancy (3).

ECF volume and total body sodium are assessed by a thorough history, physical examination and measurement of serum sodium concentration and fractional urinary sodium excretion (12). If not corrected, sodium loss causes volume depletion (hypovolemia) and increased sodium intake leads to volume expansion (hypervolemia).

2. HYPOVOLEMIA

2.1. Definition and Pathophysiology

Hypovolemia occurs when the loss of fluid from the ECF exceeds the ability to replenish the deficit by enteral or parenteral sources. Decrease in effective circulating volume occurs due to losses from the gastrointestinal tract, kidneys, skin, respiratory system, or third-space sequestration (Table 1).

Table 1
Sources of ECF Volume Loss

Gastrointestinal losses	Vomiting, diarrhea, prolonged nasogastric suction, fistulas, ostomies, bleeding
Renal losses	Diuretics, salt wasting nephropathies, osmotic diuresis, adrenal insufficiency, central or nephrogenic diabetes insipidus
Skin losses	Burns, extensive skin lesions, sweat losses in endurance exercise
Respiratory losses	Large pleural effusions, bronchorrhea
Third space sequestration	Crush injuries, intestinal obstruction, acute pancreatitis, bleeding, sepsis, anaphylaxis

Volume depletion due to gastrointestinal losses generally leads to a hypotonic state. In addition, when replacement is hypotonic, this leads to hyponatremia and hypotonicity. The volume depletion stimulates the baroreceptors releasing AVP leading to fluid retention with an exacerbation of the hyponatremia. Prolonged loss of stomach contents results in loss of hydrogen and chloride ions resulting in a state of metabolic alkalosis (see Chapter 9). Since bicarbonaturia obligates excretion of sodium, patients with prolonged vomiting have a urine sodium concentration that may be paradoxically elevated. This is true at the start of the metabolic alkalosis but if losses and volume depletion persist patients have a paradoxical aciduria and they do not have ongoing bicarbonate losses, hence increasing serum bicarbonates. In this situation urine chloride concentration or fractional excretion of chloride is a more reliable marker of volume depletion. Hypokalemia is also commonly observed with vomiting and diarrhea *(2)*.

Diuretics are known to cause hyponatremia. Thiazide diuretics act at the distal nephron by inhibiting sodium chloride reabsorption and are more likely to cause hyponatremia than the loop diuretics (73% vs. 8%; thiazides compared to furosemide) *(3)*.

Salt wasting nephropathy is frequently found in children with tubular and interstitial diseases, such as medullary cystic kidney disease, obstructive uropathy, hypoplastic kidneys, and in patients with renal insufficiency. Salt wasting results from tubular epithelium injury causing aldosterone resistance, osmotic diuresis due to increased urea load on the remaining functioning nephrons, and an inability to "shut off" natriuretic forces (i.e., atrial natriuretic peptides) when sodium intake is reduced *(13, 14)*.

Primary adrenal insufficiency leads to renal sodium wasting, hypovolemia, and hyperkalemia associated with an increased urine sodium concentration (Chapter 14). When patients ingest hypotonic fluids or are treated with hypotonic fluids intravenously, severe hyponatremia may develop *(6)*.

Vigorous endurance exercises like running a marathon may result in hyponatremia either due to excessive loss of sodium and chloride in the sweat or due to overhydration secondary to excessive hypotonic fluid ingestion, along with AVP secretion (due to osmotic and nonosmotic stimulation – decreasing water excretion) *(15)*. The consensus statement of the Second Exercise Induced Hyponatremia conference recommends to drink liquids only when thirsty and to avoid weight gain during exercise to prevent hyponatremia *(15)*.

Hypovolemia should not be considered synonymous with dehydration. Hypovolemic losses usually refer to losses of salt and water from the ECF, whereas dehydration is defined as primarily water loss from ECF, often resulting in hypernatremia, although these patients are also hypovolemic *(3)*.

2.1.1. CARDIAC AND RENAL RESPONSES TO HYPOVOLEMIA

Decrease in effective circulating volume elicits cardiac and renal responses to restore volume back toward normal. Initially hypovolemia results in decreased venous return to the heart sensed by the receptors in the atria and the pulmonary vessels, triggering activation of the sympathetic nervous system leading to selective vasoconstriction of the skin and skeletal muscle's vasculature. Further volume loss causes a decrease in cardiac output and fall in blood pressure activating the baroreceptors in the carotid sinus and aortic arch. Stimulation of the baroreceptors leads to activation of three major neurohormonal vasoconstrictor mechanisms: increase in sympathetic activity, activation of renin–angiotensin system, and release of arginine vasopressin. These act in concert to increase venous return, cardiac contractility, vascular resistance, and renal retention of sodium and water, leading to normalization of effective circulating volume (Fig. 1) *(2)*.

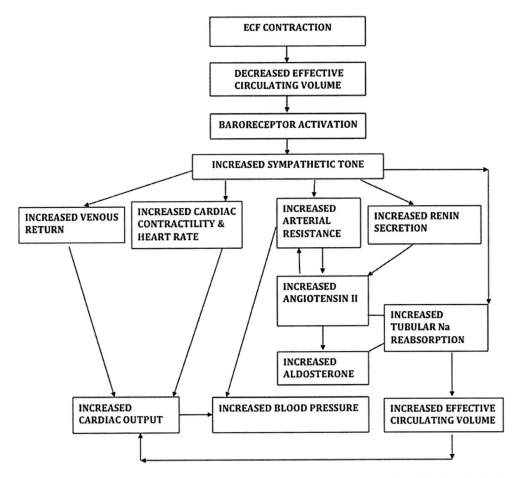

Fig. 1. Hemodynamic responses induced by the sympathetic nervous system after effective circulating volume depletion. (Adapted from Rose BD and Post TW *(40)* with permission.)

2.1.2. RENAL RESPONSE TO HYPOVOLEMIA

Renal sodium excretion is altered with changes in effective circulating volume. In states of severe volume depletion the urine is almost devoid of any sodium. Glomerular filtration rate (GFR) and more importantly tubular reabsorption play a key role in sodium conservation. With decrease in effective circulating volume, there is increased circulating norepinephrine and angiotensin II concentrations leading to efferent arteriolar constriction and increase in the filtration fraction, which is defined as the ratio of the glomerular filtration rate (GFR) to the renal plasma flow (RPF). An increase in filtration fraction results in increased protein concentration and increase in oncotic pressure in the efferent arterioles and peritubular capillaries surrounding the proximal tubules contributing to an increase in sodium and water reabsorption. The proximal tubule and distal tubule/collecting ducts are the primary sites of sodium reabsorption. Sodium reabsorption is regulated by increased norepinephrine and angiotensin II activity in the proximal tubule and increased aldosterone in the collecting ducts. If there is a defect in any of ECF regulation mechanisms, then the phenomenon of pressure natriuresis becomes important in maintaining sodium balance. The increase in sodium and water excretion occurs even with slight elevations of blood pressure. Decreased reabsorption in the proximal tubule and loop of Henle and increased release of vasodilating renal prostaglandins and nitric oxide (from the macula densa) are thought to lead to pressure natriuresis *(1, 9)*.

2.1.3. Serum Sodium Concentration in Hypovolemia

Serum sodium concentrations under hypovolemic conditions depend upon a multitude of factors: from underlying etiology of hypovolemia, sodium and water content of the fluid lost, sodium content of the restoration fluid provided, and co-existing conditions. Restoration fluid provided in severe hypovolemia should be generally isotonic (0.9% saline) at first, until measurement of serum electrolytes is available, and then adjusted accordingly. Iatrogenic hyponatremia may develop during administration of hypotonic fluids. In secretory diarrheas the sodium content is similar to plasma, so serum sodium concentrations generally do not change. In osmotic diarrheas more water is lost than sodium, hypernatremia may develop if the thirst mechanisms are not intact. Low urine sodium concentration or fractional excretion of sodium (FENa) is always an indicator of decreased effective circulating volume, unless there is a defect in the kidney that precludes sodium reabsorption *(10)*. In certain conditions like nephritic syndrome, heart failure, and cirrhosis, patients may develop edema, decreased effective circulating volume without total body water volume depletion. In these situations, the kidneys respond by increasing sodium and water reabsorption with a low FENa. Urine sodium concentrations can vary in hypovolemia based on the underlying etiology of the hypovolemic state (Table 2).

2.2. Symptoms and Signs of Hypovolemia

Most of the symptoms are due to the underlying etiology of the hypovolemia. Loss of fluid from the ECF compartment results in decreased tissue perfusion, which produces similar symptomatology regardless of the underlying cause (Table 3).

2.3. Diagnosis

Diagnosis of hypovolemia requires a detailed history and physical examination to elicit the etiology and extent of hypovolemia (Chapter 1). Laboratory tests help to con-

Table 2
Classification of Hypovolemic Disorders Based on Urine Sodium Excretion (Chapter 1)

Low urine sodium concentration (UNa < 10 mol/L)	*Normal or increased urine sodium concentration (UNa > 20 mmol/L)*
Vomiting	Diuretics
Diarrhea	Osmotic diuresis (glucose, mannitol, urea)
Nasogastric aspiration	Mineralocorticoid deficiency
Fistulae	Postobstructive diuresis
Ostomies	Non-oliguric acute renal failure
Gastrointestinal bleeding	Salt wasting nephropathy
Burns	Bicarbonaturia
Extensive skin lesions	Ketonuria
Heat exposure	
Cystic fibrosis	
Large pleural effusion	
Third space	
Crush injuries	

Table 3
Symptoms and Signs of Hypovolemia

Symptoms	*Signs*
Abdominal pain	Weight loss
Chest pain	Decreased skin turgor/prolonged capillary refill
Confusion	Dry mucus membranes
Decreased p.o. oral intake	Orthostatic hypotension
Decreased urine output	Sunken eyes
Diarrhea	Sunken fontanelle (in infants)
Disorientation	Tachycardia
Fatigue	Weak pulse
Increased thirst	
Irritability	
Muscle weakness	
Postural dizziness	
Salt craving (primary adrenal insufficiency)	
Seizures	
Vomiting	

firm the diagnosis and the co-existing electrolyte abnormalities. The most direct sign of volume depletion is weight loss. The severity of volume depletion can be assessed if the pre-illness and illness weight are known, using the formula

$$\% \text{ Dehydration} = (\text{pre} - \text{illness weight} - \text{illness weight})/\text{pre} - \text{illness weight} \times 100$$

If the weights are not known, then other clinical signs can be used to approximate the severity of dehydration.

Laboratory tests help to confirm the diagnosis and the co-existing electrolyte abnormalities (Table 4).

Table 4
Laboratory Signs of Hypovolemia

Complete blood count	Elevated hematocrit, but possibly low if bleeding
Serum chemistry	Serum sodium, potassium, bicarbonate may be increased or decreased
	Elevated plasma albumin (unless nephrotic syndrome)
Urine analysis	High specific gravity and osmolality
Urine electrolytes	Usually less than sodium <20 mEq/L (unless renal sodium losses) Fractional excretion of sodium <1%

The *goals* of treatment are twofold:

• restore normovolemia
• correct electrolyte abnormalities.

2.4. Hypovolemia Clinical Case Scenarios (See Case Scenarios in Chapter 1)

Case Scenario One:
A 9-month-old baby boy has been sick for the past 2 days. He has had fever for 2 days, temperature maximum of 103°F, four to five loose, non-bloody stools/day, decreased oral intake, and decreased activity. In the emergency room he refused to take any oral fluids for the past 12 h. He vomited 2 days ago, but not in the past 24 h. Parents deny any decrease in urine output.

On physical examination he is afebrile, BP 100/70 mmHg, HR 90/min, RR 26/min. His weight is 10 kg. Mucus membranes are moist, skin turgor is normal, capillary refill is <2 s, and he cries on physical examination with tears but is consolable. There is some urine in his diaper. No prior weight is available. Laboratory studies reveal a normal CBC, normal chemistries, and a normal urinalysis.

Clinical assessment of this baby suggests mild dehydration. He is given a trial of Pedialyte p.o. (250 ml over 2 h), which he is able to tolerate without further emesis in the next 2 h. He has one more episode of diarrhea in the ER, but no emesis. He has urine output as evidenced by a wet diaper.

2.4.1. MANAGEMENT

This is a 9-month-old baby boy with gastroenteritis and mild dehydration. He does not have any vomiting now, so he should be given a trial of p.o. oral rehydration fluids in the ED. As he tolerated the oral challenge he can be sent home with the following instructions to the family:

- Give Pedialyte 250 ml over the next 2 h (deficit correction for mild dehydration – 50 ml/kg over 4 h, he has already received half the correction in the ER).
- For every episode of diarrhea give 100 ml of Pedialyte (10 ml/kg/episode).
- Continue to encourage breast feeding and other foods the baby eats.
- If baby is not taking anything else by mouth, he will need 40ml/hr of Pedialate (maintenance requirement).
- If patient starts vomiting and unable to take p.o., then return to the ER.
- Monitor urine output and other signs of dehydration as explained, similar to Scenario in Chapter 1.

Case Scenario Two:

A 17-month-old boy with prune belly syndrome and chronic kidney disease presents to the ER with a 2 day history of fever, vomiting, and diarrhea. His mother reports a decreased urine output since the morning. He was seen in clinic a week ago and weighed 10 kg and had an estimated GFR of 50 ml/min/1.73 m^2. In the ER he was irritable but consolable, had a blood pressure of 90/70 mmHg, HR 120/min, T 102°F, RR 28/min, and the weight was 9 kg. Physical examination showed a toddler with dry mucus membranes, decreased tears, sunken eyes, tenting of the skin, and a capillary refill of 2 s. Patient was given a 10ml/kg intravenous bolus of normal saline after his blood was sent for analysis. Initial reports showed a serum sodium of 125 mEq/L, K –3.7 mEq/L, HCO_3^- 18 mmol/L, BUN/Cr 71/2.6, CBC showed anemia with hemoglobin of 9.8 g/dL, white count was normal. UA: SG 1010, pH 7.0, protein 100 mg/dL, large blood, no ketones or glucose, nitrite positive, leukocytes were positive, many WBCs and RBCs under high power field. Urine and blood cultures were sent.

2.4.2. MANAGEMENT

A 17-month-old boy with gastroenteritis, 10% dehydration, asymptomatic hyponatremia, worsening renal function (estimated GFR 20 ml/min), anemia, and a possible urinary tract infection.

FLUID AND SODIUM requirements for 24 h (deficit + maintenance + ongoing losses):

FLUID REQUIREMENTS for 24 h:

Deficit: 10 kg × 100 ml/kg = 1000 ml
Maintenance: 1000 ml
TOTAL fluid requirement = 2000 ml

SODIUM REQUIREMENTS: Na deficit in hyponatremia patient has two components:

- Na deficit independent of any volume deficit: Na required to normalize serum Na without replacing a volume loss

Deficit: (expected–observed serum sodium) × 0.6 (fraction of total body water) × wt (kg)

- 10 kg non-dehydrated patient with Na 125 mEq/L: Na deficit = (135 mEq – 125 mEq) × 0.6 × 10 = 60 mEq
- Na deficit associated with volume loss: Na concentration of deficit volume in isonatremic dehydration is 140 mEq/L: Na deficit = 140 mEq/L × 1 L (1000 ml) = 150 mEq
- Maintenance sodium: 3 mEq/100 ml = 30 mEq

Hence TOTAL sodium requirement = 60 + 140 + 30 mEq = 230 mEq.

The patient requires 2000 ml of fluid and 230 mEq of sodium in the next 24 h to correct his hypovolemia and hyponatremia. Half of the correction can be given in the first 8 h and the rest in the next 16 h. Initial fluid should have a higher sodium content. There is no need for rapid correction of sodium as patient is asymptomatic. Patient received a 100 ml bolus of normal saline (has 15.4 mEq sodium), which will be deducted from the total sodium requirements.

First 8 h: 900 ml of fluid and 120 mEq sodium = 0.78 NS ≈ Normal saline

Next 16 h: 1000 ml of fluid and 100 mEq of sodium = 0.68 NS ≈ ½ Normal saline

So give D5 with NS for the first 16 h, and then change to D5 with 1/2 NS for the next 8 h.

- Monitor serum electrolytes every 3–4 h.
- Replace ongoing losses in addition to the above fluids. Diarrheal fluid usually is close to half normal saline and that can be used for ongoing losses.
- Once urine output is confirmed add potassium to the fluids as patient is losing potassium in the diarrheal fluid.
- If the serum bicarbonate is very low, some of the sodium can be added as sodium bicarbonate.

With the above regimen the patient's dehydration and hyponatremia were corrected in 36 h. He required IV antibiotics for an *Escherichia coli* UTI. His serum creatinine returned to baseline after 2 weeks.

3. HYPERVOLEMIA

3.1. Definition and Pathophysiology

Hypervolemia results when fluid accumulates in the ECF at a higher rate than the output due to either sodium and water retention or abnormal sodium and water intake. Since the ECF volume compartment is largely determined by its quantity of $[Na^+]$, the most reliable way to assess the sodium content in the ECF compartment is to measure the plasma sodium concentration and to multiply this value by the estimated ECF volume (quantitative and clinical assessments of the ECF volume were provided in Chapter 1).

Sodium concentration in the ECF compartment (mEq/L) = Plasma sodium (mEq/L) × ECF volume (liters) For example, if the serum sodium concentration is 140 mEq/L in 10 kg child, whose estimated ECF (ECF ≈ 0.2 × body weight) is 2 L, then the sodium content of ECF is 2 L × 140 mEq/L = 280 mEq. Another clinically useful method to assess changes in ECF volume is using hematocrit values. Hematocrit is defined as the ratio of red blood cells (RBCs) volume to the blood volume. Hematocrit = RBC volume/total blood volume. For example, assuming that patient has no bleeding, anemia or erythrocytosis, and that normal total blood volume is ~ 80 ml/kg, if the normal hematocrit is 0.40, then normal blood volume in child with weight of 20 kg is 1600 ml, with RBC volume = 0.4 × 1600 ml = 640 ml, and plasma volume = 0.6 × 1600 ml = 960 ml. In contrast if the measured hematocrit is 0.50, and RBC volume remains the same (640 ml), his/her plasma volume would be reduced to from 960 ml to 800 ml (0.5 × 1600 ml), or 16.6% *(16)*.

Clinical hypervolemia may result in edema or hypertension. Edema is defined as the palpable swelling produced by expansion of the interstitial fluid volume. Edema is usually accompanied by weight gain if it results from increase in total body sodium content. Increased capillary permeability may be the main mechanism of edema in inflammatory states (i.e., insect bites), but the edema in these circumstances is usually localized. For generalized edema (anasarca) there are two main mechanisms that are required:

1. *Disruption of the Starling's forces*: It is an alteration in capillary hemodynamics favoring movement of fluid from the vascular space into the interstitium.

$$\text{Net filtration} = LpS(\Delta \text{ hydraulic pressure} - \Delta \text{ oncotic pressure}), \text{ or}$$
$$\text{Net filtration} = LpS[(P_{cap} - P_{int}) - (\pi_{cap} - \pi_{int})]$$

where L_p is the measure of unit porosity and S is the surface area, P_{cap} is the hydraulic pressure in the capillary, P_{int} is the hydraulic pressure of the interstitium, π_{cap} is the oncotic pressure in the capillary, and π_{int} is the oncotic pressure in the interstitium *(17)*. In a physiologic state edema does not form since the forces along the capillary are balanced so that any net fluid filtration into the interstitial space does not exceed the ability of the lymphatic system to remove it. Situations favoring edema formation are increased capillary permeability, decreased capillary oncotic pressure, increased capillary hydraulic pressure, increased interstitial oncotic pressure, and impairment of lymphatic drainage.

2. *Sodium and water retention by the kidney*: Retention of water most commonly occurs due to conditions that impair renal sodium excretion *(6)*. These conditions result in increase in ECF volume and are characterized by high concentrations of plasma arginine vasopressin, despite hypotonicity (the exception is renal insufficiency where high urea concentration contributes to increased tonicity) *(18, 10)*. Table 5 lists these conditions.

In sodium retaining disorders secondary to systemic arterial vasodilatation (cirrhosis), the compensatory mechanism includes increase in shortening fraction due to the reduced cardiac afterload *(19)*. However, with uncompensated arterial underfilling, there

Table 5
Hypervolemic Disorders Asso-
ciated with Impaired Sodium
Excretion by the Kidneys

Increased ECF volume

Renal insufficiency
Cirrhosis
Congestive heart failure
Nephrotic syndrome

---

is a stimulation of sympathetic nervous system and humoral system (vasopressin release and renin–angiotensin–aldosterone system) resulting in sodium and water retention by the kidney *(20)*.

Accidental or iatrogenic sodium load may be the result in hypervolemia. This condition may self-correct if the renal function is normal. In edema associated with primary hyperaldosteronism, aldosterone initially induces sodium and water retention, followed by a spontaneous diuresis (aldosterone escape), which partially lowers the extracellular fluid volume toward normal *(19, 21)*. This response is induced by the volume expansion *(21)*.

3.1.1. HEART FAILURE

Heart failure (HF) is a complex syndrome that results from structural or functional cardiac disorder that impairs heart ventricle to fill or eject blood *(22)*. In healthy individuals, increase in total blood volume is associated with increase in sodium and water excretion by the kidney *(23)*. However, in patients with heart failure, the water and sodium excretion depends on the integrity of the arterial system, not the total body volume *(23)*. As mentioned previously, 85% of the total blood volume circulates in the venous system; therefore in the states of low cardiac output that causes arterial underfilling, the increase in total body volume occurs mainly in the venous circulation *(23)*. When there is an increase in sodium reabsorption in the proximal tubule secondary to the arterial underfilling and neurohumoral activation, there is decreased delivery of sodium to the distal collecting tubule (site of action of aldosterone and natriuretic peptides). Therefore in patients with heart failure there is an escape from the sodium–water retaining effect of aldosterone and natriuretic peptides *(23)*. When the neurohumoral axis is stimulated, secondary to decreased distention of the arterial baroreceptors, renal sodium and water retention occurs as a compensatory mechanism to maintain adequate tissue perfusion *(3)*. There is an adrenergic discharge, leading to the activation of the renin–angiotensin–aldosterone system (RAAS) *(23)*. The adrenergic response and the elevation of angiotensin II activate the receptors in the proximal tubule, resulting in the increased absorption of sodium in the proximal tubule and decreasing the delivery of sodium to the distal collective tubule *(23)*. The adrenergic discharge is also responsible for the release of the nonosmotic release of AVP, which is responsible for heart failure-induced hyponatremia *(16, 23–25)*. As mentioned earlier AVP causes activation of the V2 receptors in the collecting tubule, increasing the number of aquaporin-2 water channels, but the V1a receptors in the smooth muscle are also activated, leading to constriction of the coronary vessels, proliferation of cardiac myocytes, therefore, increasing ventrical wall stress, dilatation, and hypertrophy *(22)*.

The activation of RAAS and the sympathetic nervous system is the normal response to low cardiac output, which occurs in patients with heart failure *(22)*. This neurohormonal activation of RAAS and the adrenergic discharge increases the afterload by increasing peripheral vascular resistance and the retention of sodium, potassium, and water, enhancing the preload *(22)*.

Angiotensin II contributes to the retention of sodium and water by

1. Stimulating the release of aldosterone, causing the reabsorption of sodium in the distal tubule/collecting duct
2. Renal efferent arteriolar constriction, causing a decreased renal blood flow by increasing the renal filtration fraction *(1)*
3. Stimulation of thirst through central nervous system mechanism

An increase in filtration fraction results in an increase in oncotic pressure (increased protein concentration) in the efferent arterioles and peritubular capillaries around the proximal tubules *(1)*. This increase in the oncotic pressure has been proposed to increase the absorption of sodium and water in the proximal tubules *(1)*. Angiotensin II also stimulates myocyte hypertrophy and fibrosis, contributing to the deterioration of the heart function. Therefore, treatment with angiotensin convertase inhibitors (ACEi) that inhibit the conversion of angiotensin I to angiotensin II improves cardiac remodeling *(23)*.

The natriuretic peptides, atrial natriuretic peptide (ANP) and brain natriuretic peptide, or B-type natriuretic peptide (BNP), are elevated in patients with heart failure *(1)*. These hormones have natriuretic properties, vasorelaxant properties, and renin–aldosterone inhibiting properties *(1)*. BNP is produced by the ventricular myocardium as a response to stretching of the myocardium; its effects, vasodilatory and natriuretic, oppose the actions of aldosterone and angiotensin II *(26)*. Atrial natriuretic peptide (ANP) is primarily released from the atria in response to volume expansion. ANP triggers an increase in intracardiac pressure *(27)*, which is thought to play a counterbalancing role in congestive heart failure, limiting the accumulation of edema. ANP increases the glomerular filtration rate (GFR) without raising renal blood flow *(28)* and directly reduces sodium reabsorption in the inner medullary collecting duct, activating cyclic GMP closing sodium channels in the luminal membrane that normally allow luminal sodium to enter the tubular cell *(29, 30)*.

Renal prostaglandins do not regulate sodium excretion by the kidney in healthy individuals *(1)*. Prostaglandin activity is elevated in heart failure patients and is correlated with the severity of the disease and degree of hyponatremia *(1)*. The exact role of prostaglandins in the sodium handling by the kidney in edematous states, similar to heart failure, is not clear *(1)*.

3.1.2. CIRRHOSIS (SEE CHAPTER 12)

Cirrhosis is commonly caused by hepatitis C or alcoholism in adults and in children it is due to cholestasis, inborn errors of metabolism, and chronic hepatitis. Ascites is the most common complication of cirrhosis *(31)*. Splanchnic vasodilatation is the main factor contributing to ascites *(9)*. In cirrhosis portal hypertension is produced, most importantly, by nitric oxide, and to a lesser extent, prostaglandins leading to splanchnic arterial vasodilatation *(32)*. In these situations there is an up-regulation of endothelial nitric oxide synthase (eNOS) *(6)*. In experimental cirrhosis in rats, inhibition of eNOS until normal vascular resistance is achieved results in a reversal in the elevation of plasma AVP, renin, and aldosterone concentrations *(33)*. Splanchnic vasodilatation has only a small effect on the effective circulatory volume (ECV), which is maintained within normal limits secondary to increased cardiac output and plasma volume. These effects happen early in the onset of cirrhosis. In the late stages of cirrhosis, splanchnic arterial vasodilatation causes the ECF volume to decrease markedly and, subsequently, the arterial blood pressure to fall *(31)*. The dilated circulation acts as an "underfilled" compartment, stimulating the activation of the renin–angiotensin–aldosterone system (RAAS) and the sympathetic nervous system, maintaining the arterial blood pressure resulting in sodium and water retention. Portal hypertension and splanchnic arterial vasodilatation alter the intestinal capillary pressure and permeability, facilitating the leaking and accumulation of retained fluid within the abdominal space *(31)*. As the disease progresses, there is an impairment in renal excretion of free water, causing dilutional hyponatremia, and renal vasoconstriction, leading to the hepatorenal syndrome *(31)*.

The hepatorenal syndrome results often in irreversible renal failure with a very poor prognosis. However, the hepatorenal syndrome is a functional, rather than a structural type of renal failure, as liver transplantation can reverse the syndrome. There is evidence to support the hypothesis that primary arterial vasodilatation explains the retention of sodium and water, and the ascites in cirrhotic patients *(6)*. In the splanchnic circulation, there is an elevated concentration of V1a receptors. Therefore, when terlipressin (V1a agonist) and albumin are provided for about 1 week, the hepatorenal syndrome is reversed in more than half of cirrhotic patients *(6)*.

Increased sodium reabsorption in the proximal and distal tubule in cirrhotic patients and in heart failure patients is secondary to activation of the neurohormonal system promoting sodium and water retention, endogenous increased reabsorption by the nephron segments, and loss of tubuloglomerular feedback (the mechanism increasing glomerular filtration rate when the distal tubule is reached by a reduced sodium load) *(1)*. An increase in renal vascular resistance and filtration fraction is frequently observed in decompensated cirrhotic patients *(1)*. For this reason, decreased hydrostatic pressure and increased oncotic pressure in the peritubular spaces may be responsible for the increased sodium and water reabsorption seen in cirrhosis *(1)*.

Evidence suggests that inhibition of aldosterone with spironolactone, or the removal of aldosterone source (the adrenal gland), results in natriuresis consistent with the increased levels of aldosterone contributing to water and sodium retention in the distal tubule of cirrhotic patients *(1)*.

Nonosmotic release of vasopressin plays an important role in water and sodium retention in cirrhotic patients. The increased secretion of vasopressin is the major factor responsible for the inability to excrete water and sodium in the cirrhotic rats *(34)*. When cirrhotic patients present with ascites and/or edema, they may have an abnormal response to fluid administration, contrary to cirrhotic patients without ascites or edema, who can excrete water and sodium adequately *(1)*. Two possible explanations are as follows:

a) Nonosmotic release of vasopressin.
b) Decrease in water and sodium delivery to the distal tubule since interventions that improve the delivery of sodium and water to the distal tubule of cirrhotic patients, like infusion of albumin with saline, mannitol, or water immersion, improve water and sodium excretion *(1)*.

Similar to patients with heart failure, the escape of the aldosterone effect and the resistance to natriuretic peptides in cirrhotic patients are mediated by the decreased delivery of water and sodium to the distal tubule *(1)*.

3.1.3. NEPHROTIC SYNDROME

The principal clinical presentation of nephrotic syndrome is edema, and its pathogenesis remains controversial *(35)*. The classical theory is that edema formation is secondary to a decrease in plasma oncotic pressure due to loss of albumin in the urine, causing water to shift into the interstitial space secondary to decreased oncotic pressure. That reduces the intravascular volume leading to renal hypoperfusion and stimulation of the renin–angiotensin–aldosterone (RAA) system, leading to increased reabsorption of sodium, especially at the distal segments of the nephron. This hypothesis is not fully supported by clinical findings. Plasma volume has been shown to be decreased only in some children with minimal change disease, particularly during the initial phase of a relapse, but absent in others and almost always absent in adults with nephrotic syndrome *(36)*. Studies have failed to demonstrate elevation of RAAS hormones, and increased sodium reabsorption is still present when albumin or ACEi were given to suppress the renin production. It has been postulated that there is an intrinsic nephron abnormality with increased activity of Na/K-ATPase leading to retention of sodium. Patients with nephrotic syndrome can have several types of intrinsic renal lesions *(1)*. The nephron site responsible for the increased sodium reabsorption in nephrotic patients is not clear. From clinical and animal studies, the distal nephron seems to be the site of the increased sodium retention, although increased sodium retention in the proximal tubule occurs in selected cases *(1)*. If oncotic and hydrostatic pressures are the primary physical forces in the peritubular capillaries responsible for the renal water and sodium retention, it is likely they act at the level of the convoluted proximal tubule *(1)*. The low filtration fraction, elevated renal plasma flow, and normal vascular resistance observed in patients with nephrotic syndrome suggest that other factors, besides the oncotic and hydrostatic pressures, must be involved in the enhanced sodium retention *(1)*. The role of natriuretic peptides in patients with nephrotic syndrome is not clear yet, as well as other humoral factors such as kinins and prostaglandins *(1)*.

In rats with nephrosis induced by aminonucleosides, the decreased plasma volume, normal GFR, and edema could be prevented with the removal of the adrenal glands *(1)*. In contrast patients with nephrotic syndrome induced by nephrotoxic serum have increased plasma volume, low GFR, and edema independently of the adrenal glands *(1)*. Meltzer et al. *(37)* identified two groups of patients with nephrotic syndrome. One group with hypovolemia and with stimulation of RAAS was characterized by minimal change disease and normal GFR *(37)*. The other group included patients with hypervolemia who had low or normal plasma renin activity and aldosterone level; this group was characterized by chronic glomerulopathy and low GFR *(37)*. Patients with nephrotic syndrome and low GFR usually show enhanced sodium retention *(37)*.

Contrary to heart failure and cirrhosis patients, hyponatremia is not commonly associated with nephrotic syndrome *(1)*. Elevated serum lipid concentration may cause *pseudohyponatremia*. Abnormal water excretion has been shown in children with nephrotic syndrome *(38)* and increased levels of vasopressin also contribute to the retention of water *(39)*. Water immersion and albumin infusion can reduce the plasma concentration of vasopressin and induce diuresis in these patients *(1)*.

Summarizing, a fall in GFR, changes in oncotic and hydrostatic pressures, stimulation of sympathetic nervous system and RAAS, and nonosmotic release of vasopressin are involved in the retention of sodium and water in the nephrotic syndrome *(1)*.

3.1.4. TREATMENT

Diuretics are usually effective in reducing edema of congestive heart failure, although effective fluid removal should be carefully monitored *(26)*. Patients with heart failure should be treated with diuretics as part of their initial therapy *(27)*. Loop diuretics are most often used (furosemide, bumetanide, torsemide). Patients who are chronically treated with loop diuretics usually require a higher dose in the acute setting *(27)*. The addition of a thiazide diuretic potentiates the effects of the loop diuretics.

In patients with cirrhosis and ascites, fluid accumulation in the peritoneal cavity is sufficient to cause discomfort *(11)*. Free water excretion by the kidney and GFR are normal in most patients and the serum sodium and creatinine concentrations are within normal limits *(11)*. Usually, a negative sodium balance and, subsequently, loss of peritoneal fluid are easily achieved with diuretics, in patients with mild to moderate volume ascites *(28)*. The diuretic of choice is spironolactone or amiloride *(11)*. Furosemide is used with caution, because the risk of renal failure secondary to excessive diuresis and hypovolemia *(11)*, and the response to treatment should be monitored by evaluation of urine output and changes in body weight *(11)*. The measurement of urine sodium may be helpful to assess the response to diuretics *(11)*. An important part of the therapy of cirrhotic ascites is the avoidance of non-steroidal anti-inflammatory drugs (NSAID). These medications inhibit the synthesis of renal prostaglandins, and this leads to renal vasoconstriction, a lesser response to diuretics, and increased risk of acute renal insufficiency *(29)*. In children with nephrotic syndrome, diuretics should only be given for severe edema and in the absence of intravascular volume depletion. Dietary sodium restriction (less that 2 g/day in adults) is also recommended *(31)*, since diuretic effects may be overcome by high sodium intake. Non-adherence to a low-sodium diet is often linked to diuretic failure. Another reason for diminished diuretic effectiveness in edematous states may be reduced absorption of oral diuretics due to gastrointestinal mucosal edema. Reduced blood flow to the kidneys in states with decreased ECF decreases the amount of sodium delivered to the loop of Henle, and thus loop diuretic effectiveness. In addition in hypoalbuminemic states loop diuretics that are albumin bound are less effectively delivered to the site of action. Patients with anasarca or diuretic resistance may be treated with furosemide (1–2 mg/kg per dose) together with 25% albumin (0.5–1 g/kg) IV infusion, given over 4 h once to twice a day with careful monitoring of urine output and respiratory status, as IV albumin has been associated with pulmonary edema *(30)*. Albumin binds furosemide improving its delivery to site of action in the ascending loop of Henle increasing sodium excretion. Albumin also prevents intravascular volume depletion. Spironolactone (1.0–3.5 mg/kg/day, adult maximal dose 400 mg), thiazide diuretics, and amiloride (0.2–0.625 mg/kg/day, adult maximal dose 20 mg) may be used in combination with a loop diuretic *(31)*.

Case Scenarios (See Scenarios in Chapter 1)

1. A 7-year-old girl presents to the emergency department with vomiting and cough for 3 days. The mother also reports weight loss, approximately 4 kg over the last 4 months and the development of bilateral lower extremity edema over the past week. The girl is urinating, but less than usual. She was a full-term neonate, born by uneventful normal spontaneous vaginal delivery. The child was diagnosed with acute lymphoblastic leukemia at 4 years of age. The medical records indicate the use of doxorubicin and methotrexate as part of the consolidation chemotherapy, and she has responded very well to the treatment and is in remission. Past family history is significant for maternal grandmother with insulin-dependent diabetes mellitus, on dialysis. Initial exam shows a thin 8-year-old girl, 10th percentile for weight and 25th percentile for height, jugular venous distention is noted to the angle of the jaw when seated at 90°, an S3 gallop and ventricular heave, tachypnea, diffuse rales, and 3+ pitting edema to the mid-calf bilaterally are present. Electrocardiogram reveals sinus tachycardia, left atrial enlargement, and T-wave abnormalities. All these findings are clinically diagnostic of left heart failure. The girl's symptoms improve after the initial treatment with intravenous furosemide 1 mg/kg twice a day for 24 h and she is transferred to the cardiology service. Her echocardiogram demonstrates severe global hypokinesis and a 20% ejection fraction.

   Doxorubicin is a drug well known for its cardiac toxicity. The girl's treatment is likely the etiology of her heart failure. The compensatory mechanisms associated with low cardiac output, secondary to left heart failure, include up-regulation of sympathetic tone and the renin–angiotensin axis, causing increased release of vasopressin, aldosterone, and atrial natriuretic peptide, leading to sodium and water retention, resulting in volume expansion.

2. A 12-year-old boy with history of steroid-sensitive nephrotic syndrome, diagnosed when he was 6 years old, presents to the emergency department with the chief complain of

abdominal distention and edema of lower extremities. Mother reports that 5 days ago, the boy had cold symptoms that included runny nose, non-productive cough, and low-grade fever that resolved. Two siblings had the same symptoms and recovered. The boy noticed the swelling of both legs 3 days ago. On physical examination, the boy has no fever and is normotensive. Weight is 55 kg; the last weight according to mom in the pediatrician office 3 weeks ago was 48 kgs. There is pitting edema of both legs to the level of the knees, and generalized abdominal distension, flank fullness, and shifting dullness, consistent with ascites. Urine analysis shows a specific gravity of 1.025, no blood detected, and 3+ protein. Urine protein to creatinine ratio is 7. Basic metabolic panel shows normal renal function and electrolytes.

Albumin 25% – 1 g/kg – is infused over 4 h and furosemide 1 mg/kg is also given 2 h into infusion and at the end of the infusion. The boy voids approximately 500 ml and abdominal distention improves; he is also started on prednisone 60 mg/m^2 for probable steroid responsive nephrotic syndrome.

REFERENCES

1. Berl T, Schrier RW: *Renal Sodium Excretion, Edematous Disorders and Diuretic Use*. Philadelphia, PA, Lippincott Williams & Wilkins, 2002
2. Simpson FO: Sodium intake, body sodium, and sodium excretion. *Lancet* 2:25–29, 1988
3. Schrier RW: Decreased effective blood volume in edematous disorders: what does this mean? *J Am Soc Nephrol* 18:2028–2031, 2007
4. Schrier RW: Body fluid volume regulation in health and disease: a unifying hypothesis. *Ann Intern Med* 113:155–159, 1990
5. Peters JP: The role of sodium in the production of edema. *N Engl J Med* 239:353–362, 1948
6. Schrier RW: Water and sodium retention in edematous disorders: role of vasopressin and aldosterone. *Am J Med* 119:S47–53, 2006
7. Singer DR, Markandu ND, Buckley MG, et al.: Blood pressure and endocrine responses to changes in dietary sodium intake in cardiac transplant recipients. Implications for the control of sodium balance. *Circulation* 89:1153–1159, 1994
8. Borst JG, De Vries LA: The three types of "natural" diuresis. *Lancet* 2:1–6, 1950
9. Schrier RW, Arroyo V, Bernardi M, et al.: Peripheral arterial vasodilation hypothesis: a proposal for the initiation of renal sodium and water retention in cirrhosis. *Hepatology* 8:1151–1157, 1988
10. Rose BD PT: *Edematous States*, 5th edition New York, McGraw-Hill, 2001
11. Bichet D, Szatalowicz V, Chaimovitz C, et al.: Role of vasopressin in abnormal water excretion in cirrhotic patients. *Ann Intern Med* 96:413–417, 1982
12. Schrier R: Body fluid volume regulation in health and disease: a unifying hypothesis. *Ann Intern Med* 113, 1990
13. Wright F: Flow-dependent transport processes: Filtration, absorption, secretion. *Am J Phys* 243:F1, 1982
14. Greger R, Velazquez H: The cortical thick ascending limb and early distal convoluted tubule in the urine concentrating mechanism. *Kidney Int* 31, 1987
15. Hew-Butler T, Ayus JC, Kipps C, et al.: Statement of the Second International Exercise-Associated Hyponatremia Consensus Development Conference, New Zealand, 2007. *Clin J Sport Med* 18: 111–121, 2008
16. Szatalowicz VL, Arnold PE, Chaimovitz C, et al.: Radioimmunoassay of plasma arginine vasopressin in hyponatremic patients with congestive heart failure. *N Engl J Med* 305:263–266, 1981
17. Verney EB: The antidiuretic hormone and the factors which determine its release. *Proc R Soc Lond B Biol Sci* 135:25–106, 1947

18. Friis-Hansen B: Body water compartments in children: changes during growth and related changes in body composition. *Pediatrics* 28:169–181, 1961

19. Adrogue HJ, Madias NE: Hyponatremia. *N Engl J Med* 342:1581–1589, 2000

20. Anderson RJ, Chung HM, Kluge R, et al.: Hyponatremia: a prospective analysis of its epidemiology and the pathogenetic role of vasopressin. *Ann Intern Med* 102:164–168, 1985

21. Taylor AE: Capillary fluid filtration. Starling forces and lymph flow. *Circ Res* 49:557–575, 1981

22. Ho KK, Pinsky JL, Kannel WB, et al.: The epidemiology of heart failure: the Framingham Study. *J Am Coll Cardiol* 22:6A–13A, 1993

23. Chen HH, Schrier RW: Pathophysiology of volume overload in acute heart failure syndromes. *Am J Med* 119:S11–16, 2006

24. Schrier RW, Berl T: Nonosmolar factors affecting renal water excretion (first of two parts). *N Engl J Med* 292:81–88, 1975

25. Schrier RW, Berl T: Nonosmolar factors affecting renal water excretion (second of two parts). *N Engl J Med* 292:141–145, 1975

26. Jessup M, Brozena S: Heart failure. *N Engl J Med* 348:2007–2018, 2003

27. de Zeeuw D, Janssen WM, de Jong PE: Atrial natriuretic factor: its (patho)physiological significance in humans. *Kidney Int* 41:1115–1133, 1992

28. Weidmann P, Hasler L, Gnadinger MP, et al.: Blood levels and renal effects of atrial natriuretic peptide in normal man. *J Clin Invest* 77:734–742, 1986

29. Cogan MG: Atrial natriuretic peptide. *Kidney Int* 37:1148–1160, 1990

30. Ujiie K, Nonoguchi H, Tomita K, et al.: Effects of ANF on cGMP synthesis in inner medullary collecting duct subsegments of rats. *Am J Physiol* 259:F535–538, 1990

31. Gines P, Cardenas A, Arroyo V, et al.: Management of cirrhosis and ascites. *N Engl J Med* 350:1646–1654, 2004

32. Martin PY, Gines P, Schrier RW: Nitric oxide as a mediator of hemodynamic abnormalities and sodium and water retention in cirrhosis. *N Engl J Med* 339:533–541, 1998

33. Martin PY, Ohara M, Gines P, et al.: Nitric oxide synthase (NOS) inhibition for one week improves renal sodium and water excretion in cirrhotic rats with ascites. *J Clin Invest* 101:235–242, 1998

34. Claria J, Jimenez W, Arroyo V, et al.: Blockade of the hydroosmotic effect of vasopressin normalizes water excretion in cirrhotic rats. *Gastroenterology* 97:1294–1299, 1989

35. Eddy AA, Symons JM: Nephrotic syndrome in childhood. *Lancet* 362:629–639, 2003

36. Constantinescu AR, Shah HB, Foote EF, et al.: Predicting first-year relapses in children with nephrotic syndrome. *Pediatrics* 105:492–495, 2000

37. Meltzer JI, Keim HJ, Laragh JH, et al.: Nephrotic syndrome: vasoconstriction and hypervolemic types indicated by renin-sodium profiling. *Ann Intern Med* 91:688–696, 1979

38. Gur A, Adefuin PY, Siegel NJ, et al.: A study of the renal handling of water in lipoid nephrosis. *Pediatr Res* 10:197–201, 1976

39. Sala C, Bedogna V, Gammaro L, et al.: Central role of vasopressin in sodium/water retention in hypo- and hypervolemic nephrotic patients: a unifying hypothesis. *J Nephrol* 17:653–657, 2004

40 Rose BD and Post TW. Regulation of the effective circulating volume. In: Clinical Physiology of Acid-Base and Electrolyte disorders. McGraw Hill, 2001: 8.5

3 Disorders of Potassium Balance

Beatrice Goilav and Howard Trachtman

Key Points

Potassium homeostasis:

- K^+ is the most essential intracellular cation, generating the resting potential in neuronal and muscle cells.
- Extracellular K^+ levels are tightly regulated.
- Any disturbances of serum K^+ levels can affect the resting potential and lead to arrhythmias or muscular abnormalities.

Renal K^+ handling and changes during maturation:

- The kidneys are primarily responsible for excreting excess K^+.
- The goal of adult kidneys is to maintain a zero K^+ balance, while newborn kidneys retain K^+ to allow somatic growth.
- Premature infants are prone to develop hyperkalemia, because they cannot rapidly eliminate exogenous excess K^+.

Disturbances in K^+ balance:

- Serum K^+ levels can be abnormal due to abnormal intake or abnormal excretion of K^+, but can also be caused by abnormal distribution of K^+ between the extra- and intracellular space.
- Clinical symptoms vary and do not allow distinguishing between hypo- and hyperkalemia.

Hypokalemia:

- Mild hypokalemia is a common finding in clinical practice.
- Administration of diuretics is the most common acquired cause of hypokalemia.
- Decreased intake of K^+ can lead to total body K^+ depletion and hypokalemia.

Hyperkalemia:

- Hyperkalemia is rare in individuals with normal renal function.
- ECG findings with hyperkalemia occur individually and cannot be correlated with the serum K^+ level per se.
- Medications are a common cause of hyperkalemia in susceptible individuals

---

This chapter is dedicated to my beloved parents, Florenza and Yoan Goilav-Glück.

From: *Nutrition and Health: Fluid and Electrolytes in Pediatrics*
Edited by: L. G. Feld, F. J. Kaskel, DOI 10.1007/978-1-60327-225-4_3,
© Humana Press, a part of Springer Science+Business Media, LLC 2010

Key Words: Hypokalemia; hyperkalemia; Gitelman's syndrome; Bartter's syndrome; congenital adrenal hyperplasia

1. GENERAL OVERVIEW OF POTASSIUM BALANCE

Potassium (K^+) is the most abundant intracellular cation. About 98% of the total body K^+ content in the adult is located within cells, where its concentration ranges from 100 to 150 mEq/L. The remaining 2% resides in the extracellular fluid *(1)*. Extracellular K^+ concentration, ranging from 3.5 to 5.0 mEq/L, is tightly regulated by mechanisms that control the distribution between the intra- and extracellular compartments and whole body K^+ balance. The serum K^+ level is dependent on the net sum of K^+ intake, distribution of K^+ between the intracellular (ICF) and extracellular (ECF) space, and K^+ excretion.

K^+ has two major physiologic functions: (1) the difference in the K^+ concentration between intracellular and extracellular fluid is the major determinant of the resting membrane potential of a cell. This transcellular K^+ gradient is maintained by the action of the enzyme sodium–potassium–adenosine triphosphatase (Na^+–K^+-ATPase) located in the cell membrane *(2)*. The resting potential allows for an action potential to be generated, which is essential for normal neuronal and muscular function, and exocrine secretion of hormones. (2) Maintenance of an intracellular K^+ concentration within the normal range is essential for a variety of cellular functions, including cell growth and division, DNA and protein synthesis, enzymatic activity, and cellular volume regulation *(2)*.

Total body K^+ content depends on the balance between intake and output, the latter being regulated primarily by renal and, to a lesser extent, fecal excretion. The homeostatic goal of the adult is to remain in zero K^+ balance. Thus, K^+ excretion matches dietary intake, with about 90% of the daily K^+ intake ($\sim$1.5 mEq/kg body weight) eliminated by the kidneys and the remaining 10% lost through the stool *(1)*. Children maintain a positive net K^+ balance, because the cation is required for somatic growth.

2. DISTRIBUTION OF POTASSIUM BETWEEN ICF AND ECF

Regulation of the internal distribution of K^+ between the intracellular and extracellular spaces is extremely efficient. An ingested K^+ load initially leads to uptake of most of the K^+ by muscle, liver, bone, and red cells. This rapid process is followed by renal excretion of excess K^+ that was not mobilized into cells. The net effect is that all excess K^+ is excreted within 6–8 h *(3)*.

2.1. Sodium–Potassium-ATPase

The difference between intracellular and extracellular K^+ concentration is maintained by the activity of the Na^+–K^+-ATPase. The pump transports 3 Na^+ ions out of the cell in exchange for 2 K^+ ions into the cell, generating a negative intracellular voltage and consuming energy (ATP) during this process (Fig. 1) *(2)*. The Na^+–K^+-ATPase activity is regulated by hormones as well as the extracellular K^+ concentration per se *(2)*.

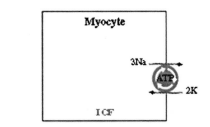

Fig. 1. Schematic illustration of a cell model for a muscle cell. The Na^+–K^+-ATPase is located in the cellular membrane. It continuously moves 2 K^+ into the cell in exchange for 3Na^+ out of the cell, which generates an electrical gradient with the intracellular space being negatively charged relative to the extracellular space. This difference in electrical gradient allows a cell to depolarize when stimulated. The enzyme is regulated by several different hormones including insulin, epinephrine, and thyroid hormone. ECF: extracellular fluid; ICF: intracellular fluid; ATP: adenosine triphosphate.

2.2. Hormones

Catecholamines. Catecholamines influence K^+ distribution with α-receptors inhibiting and $β_2$-receptors promoting the cellular entry of K^+. The $β_2$-receptor-induced stimulation of K^+ uptake is mediated partly by activation of the Na^+–K^+-ATPase pump. Administration of a $β_2$-adrenergic agonist, such as albuterol or dobutamine, can induce a hypokalemic response. Basal catecholamine levels permissively promote K^+ entry into cells and increases in catecholamine levels during exercise enhance cellular K^+ uptake *(4)*.

Insulin. Insulin promotes the entry of K^+ into cells by increasing Na^+–K^+-ATPase activity directly *(2)*. Basal insulin levels permissively facilitate K^+ entry into cells and enhanced insulin secretion in response to a dietary carbohydrate load further increases cellular K^+ uptake *(4)*.

Aldosterone. Aldosterone promotes K^+ uptake into cells, and increases excretion of K^+ in the urine and the gut *(5)*. Hyperkalemia raises aldosterone levels.

Other Hormones. Thyroid hormone, glucocorticoids, and growth hormone also promote cellular uptake of K^+ by chronically stimulating Na^+–K^+-ATPase *(6)*.

2.3. Plasma K^+ Concentration

After a K^+ load, intracellular movement of K^+ occurs independent of hormonal and other factors *(5)*. On the other hand, loss of K^+ from the ECF due to increased gastrointestinal or renal losses as seen for example in diarrhea or during an osmotic diuresis, respectively, results first in a fall in the plasma K^+ concentration followed by the movement of K^+ from the cells into the ECF. This indicates that the plasma K^+ concentration varies directly with total body K^+ stores and vice versa *(7)*.

2.4. Exercise

Exercise causes release of K^+ from muscle cells due to depolarization and is followed by reuptake of K^+ by the Na^+–K^+-ATPase pump *(2)*. With strenuous exercise, the reduction in ATP within muscle cells leads to opening of K^+ channels, promoting K^+ release from cells (8). However, this effect is counterbalanced by the exercise-induced release of catecholamines, which in turn decreases extracellular K^+ levels.

2.5. Extracellular pH

Any changes in acid–base balance can have an effect on the plasma K^+ concentration. In metabolic acidosis, excess H^+ ions are buffered in the cells (9). To preserve electroneutrality, K^+ moves out of the cells. This results in an increase in the plasma K^+ concentration. A common rule of thumb is that, for every 0.1-unit decrease in blood pH, the plasma K^+ concentration increases by $\sim$0.6 mEq/L (9).

In diarrheal states or renal tubular acidosis, the presence of other factors (increased gastrointestinal or urinary K^+ losses, respectively) can modulate the increase in plasma K^+ and result in hypokalemia. This is due to net negative K^+ balance leading to depletion of K^+ stores, masking the relative hyperkalemia. Correcting the acidosis may lead to clinically relevant hypokalemia, unless K^+ supplements are administered (9).

Conversely, metabolic alkalosis causes a shift of K^+ ions into the cells in exchange for H^+ ions. However, the change in plasma K^+ concentration is much less pronounced (0.2–0.4 mEq/L). This is due to the smaller degree of intracellular buffering and transcellular movement of H^+ in this condition. More prolonged metabolic alkalosis can result in hypokalemia due to a shift of K^+ into the renal collecting duct cells, and subsequent urinary K^+ secretion (10).

2.6. Other Conditions

Hyperosmolality causes a rise of plasma K^+ by 0.3–0.8 mEq/L for every 10 mosmol/kg increase in effective plasma osmolality (11). This is attributed to movement of K^+ out of cells in response to osmotically induced water movement.

3. RENAL POTASSIUM HANDLING

Renal K^+ excretion plays the dominant role in responding to changes in K^+ intake and maintaining serum K^+ levels within the homeostatic range. In individuals with normal renal function, dietary K^+ is largely excreted in the urine. K^+ handling by the adult kidney involves three processes: filtration, reabsorption, and secretion (10). In the healthy adult kidney, K^+ secretion predominates over K^+ absorption. In children, the opposite is true with the kidneys avidly retaining K^+ needed for growth.

The following section will detail the processes involved in K^+ handling by specific segments of the nephron.

3.1. Proximal Tubule

K^+ is freely filtered at the glomerulus. Thus, the concentration of K^+ entering the proximal convoluted tubule (PCT) is similar to that of plasma. About 50–70% of the filtered load of K^+ is reabsorbed along the initial two thirds of the proximal tubule (PT). Reabsorption of K^+ along this segment closely follows that of Na^+ and water. Almost all K^+ reabsorption in the PCT is passive (Fig. 2) (12).

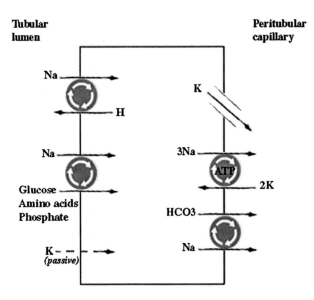

Fig. 2. Schematic illustration of a proximal tubular cell. At this site, there is only passive K^+ absorption following Na^+ and water reabsorption and plays only a minor role in the regulation of renal K^+ excretion. The tubular lumen contains glomerular filtrate with a K^+ concentration similar to the plasma. K^+ absorption is passive and follows Na^+ and water. ATP: adenosine triphosphate.

A number of apical K^+ channels have been identified in the PT. K^+ movement from the cell to the lumen through these channels contribute to the maintenance of the electrical driving force for Na^+-coupled transport (glucose and amino acids) in the PT.

The PT does not play a direct role in regulating net renal K^+ excretion. However, changes in Na^+ and Cl^- reabsorption in this nephron segment have considerable effects on distal tubular flow and distal tubular Na^+ delivery, with attendant effects on K^+ secretion and K^+ balance.

3.2. Thick Ascending Loop of Henle

The thick ascending loop of Henle (TALH) is an important site of K^+ reabsorption. Within the TALH, K^+ reabsorption is mediated, at least in part, by the apical bumetanide-sensitive $Na^+–K^+–2Cl^-$ cotransporter (NKCC2) *(13)*. Activity of this transporter is driven by the basolateral $Na^+–K^+$-ATPase *(13)*.

Apical secretory K^+ channels play a central role in K^+ secretion in the TALH, where it provides a pathway for K^+, taken up into the cell via the NKCC2, to recycle back into the lumen and thus sustain a lumen-positive potential difference *(10, 14)*. This provides the electrical driving force for paracellular K^+ as well as calcium (Ca^{2+}) and magnesium (Mg^{2+}) reabsorption (Fig. 3) *(10)*.

A considerable fraction of K^+ secreted by the cortical collecting duct (CCD) is reabsorbed by the medullary collecting ducts and then secreted into the late PT or descending thin limbs of long-looped nephrons (or both). Thus, there is a doubling of luminal K^+ in terminal thin descending limbs. This pathway consisting of secretion of K^+ in CCD, absorption in the outer medullary collecting duct (OMCD) and inner medullary

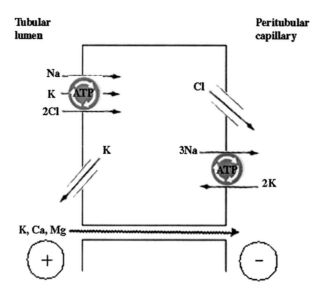

Fig. 3. Graphic illustration of a cell in the thick ascending loop of Henle (TALH). The apical Na^+–K^+–$2Cl^-$-cotransporter is the main channel for K^+ uptake in this section of the nephron. Cl^- exits the cell at the basolateral side leaving the intracellular space positively charged. This leads to part of the absorbed K^+ exiting back into the tubular lumen. In turn, the tubular lumen is positively charged, generating an electrochemical gradient to the peritubular capillary, which results in passive paracellular reabsorption of cations.

collecting duct (IMCD), and secretion in descending thin limb is called medullary K^+ recycling. It results in a marked increase in medullary interstitial K^+ *(14)*. This pathway can be interrupted by loop diuretics, which inhibit Na^+ absorption in the TALH (Fig. 4). This leads to an increase in interstitial K^+ and increased Na^+ delivery to the connecting tubule (CNT) and CCD, where Na^+ is then absorbed. The result is an enhanced lumen-negative potential difference in these tubules and increasing K^+ secretion *(14)*.

3.3. Distal Nephron

The late distal connecting tubule (DCT), CNT, and CCD in the distal nephron are considered to be the primary sites of K^+ secretion, contributing largely to urinary K^+ excretion. Up to 20% of the filtered K^+ load can be secreted in this nephron segment *(15)*. The DCT secretes a constant small amount of K^+ into the urinary space. Two morphological distinct cells, principal cells (PC), and intercalated cells (IC) are present in the CNT and CCD. PC and IC are responsible for K^+ secretion and for K^+ absorption, respectively *(10)*.

4. POTASSIUM SECRETION

The bulk of regulated secretion occurs in PC within the CNT and CCD *(10)*. K^+ secretion takes place by a two-step process: K^+ enters the cell via the basolateral Na^+–K^+-ATPase and is secreted into the lumen through apical K^+ channels along a favorable electrochemical gradient. Any factor that increases the electrochemical

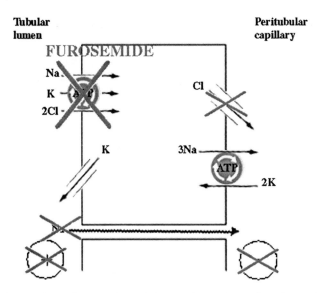

Fig. 4. Schematic illustration of the action of furosemide, a loop diuretic on the Na^+–K^+–$2Cl^-$-cotransporter (NKCC). By blocking the NKCC, the tubular lumen is less positively charged, which inhibits paracellular Na^+ reabsorption. Blocking of the NKCC also lowers the rate of Cl^- reabsorption. Decreased activity of the NKCC also leads to decreased K^+ absorption and passive loss of K^+ into the tubular lumen. As a consequence, there is increased K^+ loss in the urine.

gradient across the apical membrane or increases the apical K^+ permeability will promote K^+ secretion *(10)*.

In PC, apical Na^+ entry via the epithelial Na+ channel (ENaC) generates a lumen-negative potential difference, which drives passive K^+ exit through apical K^+ channels. Distal K^+ secretion is therefore dependent on delivery of adequate amounts of luminal Na^+ to the CNT and CCD. K^+ secretion essentially comes to a halt when luminal Na^+ drops <8 mEq/L *(10)*. In contrast, excess dietary Na^+ intake enhances K^+ secretion *(10)*.

4.1. Potassium Channels

There are two major subtypes of apical K^+ channels that mediate K^+ secretion: a low-conductance (renal outer medulla K, SK/ROMK) channel and a high-conductance, Ca^{2+}-activated (BK/maxi-K) channel *(16)*.

The SK/ROMK channel, restricted to the PC mediates baseline K^+ secretion. The BK/maxi-K channel is activated by cell depolarization, membrane stretch, and increases in intracellular Ca^{2+} concentration as occurs with increased tubular flow in volume expansion or diuretic therapy and mediates adaptive increases in K^+ secretion *(17)*.

SK/ROMK Channel. The SK/ROMK channel alone is capable of mediating the bulk of K^+ secretion in the CCD under baseline conditions. Loss of channel function prevents apical membrane K^+ recycling with secondary inhibition of Na^+–K^+–$2Cl^-$-cotransport in the TALH, resulting in a picture similar to diuretic therapy or Bartter's syndrome. SK/ROMK channels are pH-sensitive, and a decrease in cell pH from 7.4 to 7.0 completely inhibits channel activity *(18)*.

BK/Maxi-K Channel. The BK/maxi-K channel mediates flow-stimulated K$^+$ secretion in both the CNT and CCD and is activated by flow-induced increases in intracellular Ca^{2+} concentration. An increase in tubular flow, as elicited by extracellular fluid volume expansion or administration of diuretics, is a potent stimulus for K$^+$ secretion in the distal nephron *(19)*. Increases in tubular flow rate transduce mechanical signals (circumferential stretch, shear) into biochemical responses, including an increase in intracellular Ca^{2+} concentration, which in turn activate BK/maxi-K channels *(20)*. This channel assumes greater importance in regulating K$^+$ homeostasis under conditions where SK/ROMK channel-mediated K$^+$ secretion is limited.

Other Potassium Channels. A multitude of other K$^+$ channels are expressed in the distal nephron, including the K$^+$–Cl$^-$-co-transporter and the H$^+$–K$^+$-ATPase, which exist in two types: colonic H$^+$–K$^+$-ATPase and gastric H$^+$–K$^+$-ATPase. The colonic H$^+$–K$^+$-ATPase is mainly responsible for renal K$^+$ reabsorption and gastric H$^+$–K$^+$-ATPase is involved in mediating K$^+$-dependent H$^+$ secretion in the CCD *(21)*.

5. POTASSIUM ABSORPTION

In addition to K$^+$ secretion, the distal nephron is capable of considerable reabsorption, primarily during restriction of dietary K$^+$. IC reabsorb K$^+$ under conditions of K$^+$ depletion and metabolic acidosis via the H$^+$–K$^+$-ATPase that couples K$^+$ reabsorption to H$^+$ secretion *(21)*.

6. REGULATION OF DISTAL POTASSIUM TRANSPORT

Sodium Delivery and Absorption. K$^+$ secretion is dependent on the amount of Na$^+$ available in the CCD. If the tubular fluid Na$^+$ concentrations is <30 mEq/L, K$^+$ secretion falls sharply *(22)*. Extracellular volume expansion or administration of diuretics increases urinary excretion of both Na$^+$ and K$^+$. The kaliuresis is mediated not only by the increased delivery of Na$^+$ to the distal nephron, but also by the increased tubular fluid flow rate, which activates the BK/maxi-K channel. K$^+$-sparing diuretics, such as amiloride and triamterene, block distal Na$^+$ reabsorption, which reduces K$^+$ secretion (Fig. 5).

Na$^+$ delivered to the distal nephron is generally accompanied by Cl$^-$. Cl$^-$ reabsorption, which occurs predominantly via the paracellular pathway, tends to reduce the lumen-negative potential that would drive K$^+$ secretion (Fig. 6) *(3)*. When Na$^+$ is accompanied by an anion that is less reabsorbable than Cl$^-$, such as HCO$_3^-$ (as in proximal renal tubular acidosis [RTA]) or β-hydroxybutyrate (in diabetic ketoacidosis) luminal electronegativity is maintained, resulting in more K$^+$ secretion than occurs with a comparable Na$^+$ load delivered with Cl$^-$ *(3)*. These entities can result in hypokalemia. Penicillin-related antibiotics are associated with hypokalemia by delivering non-reabsorbable anions to the distal nephron *(23)*

Acid–Base Balance. Secretion of K$^+$ into the tubular lumen is affected by changes in acid–base homeostasis. In acute metabolic acidosis, the movement of H$^+$ into the cells from the extracellular space is concomitantly associated with the movement of K$^+$ out of the cells, causing hyperkalemia. Acidemia results in a reduction in intracellular

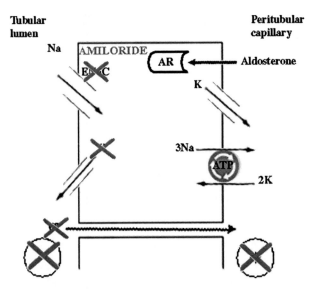

Fig. 5. Schematic illustration of the effect of amiloride, a K^+-sparing diuretic, on the epithelial Na^+ channel (ENaC) in the cortical collecting duct. By decreasing the negative electrical charge of the tubular lumen, it reduces K^+ secretion and paracellular absorption of Cl^-.

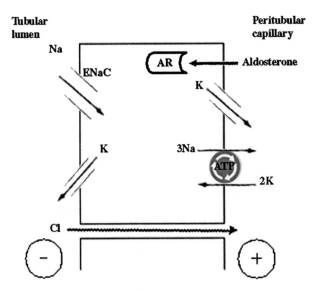

Fig. 6. Na^+ delivered to the distal nephron is accompanied by Cl^-. Cl^- reabsorption, which occurs predominantly via the paracellular pathway, tends to reduce the lumen-negative potential that would drive K^+ secretion. Hence, if more Na^+ is delivered to the distal tubule and reabsorbed via the epithelial Na^+ channel (ENaC), the lumen is progressively lumen-negative, driving urinary K^+ loss.

pH, which inhibits activity of the SK/ROMK channel and leads to a fall in urinary K^+ excretion *(24)*.

In acute metabolic and respiratory alkalosis, there is an increase in K^+ excretion *(12)*. The alkalosis-induced stimulation of K^+ secretion reflects two direct effects on PC: (1)

stimulation of basolateral K^+ uptake and (2) an increase in the permeability of the apical membrane to K^+ due to an increased activity of SK/ROMK channels (10).

Diet. Dietary K^+ intake plays a key role in the regulation of renal K^+ secretion in the CNT and CCD. The adult kidney responds to an increase in K^+ intake with an increase in urinary K^+ excretion within 1–2 days.

High Dietary Potassium Intake. High dietary K^+ intake stimulates aldosterone secretion, which increases activity of both Na^+–K^+-ATPase and ENaC (25). Both these effects ultimately stimulate K^+ secretion. High K^+ intake also significantly increases the activity of SK/ROMK and BK/maxi-K channels (25).

Low Dietary Potassium Intake. A reduction in dietary K^+ leads to a dramatic drop in urinary K^+ excretion within 24 h. K^+ restriction stimulates K^+ absorption through enhancing colonic H^+–K^+-ATPase activity, which results not only in K^+ retention, but also urinary acidification and metabolic alkalosis (25).

Vasopressin. Vasopressin has a stimulatory effect on K^+ secretion by the distal nephron (26). This effect serves to preserve K^+ secretion during dehydration and extracellular volume depletion, when tubular delivery of Na^+ and fluid is reduced. The stimulation of basolateral V2 receptors (via cAMP) results in an activation of ENaC, which increases the driving force for K^+ secretion. In addition, vasopressin activates SK/ROMK channels directly (26).

7. NEONATAL POTASSIUM REGULATION AND CHANGES IN THE MATURING KIDNEY

The developing kidney is uniquely adapted to meet the demands of the growing organism. The kidneys of infants and children are conserving K^+, because K^+ is essential for cell growth. During fetal life, K^+ is actively transported from mother to fetus. The fetal K^+ concentration is maintained at levels >5 mEq/L, even in the face of maternal K^+ deficiency (27).

In newborns, the renal K^+ clearance is low, even when corrected for their low glomerular filtration rate (GFR) (28). Healthy full-term newborns who are fed breast milk, which has a Na^+/K^+ ratio of about 0.5–0.6, excrete a urine, which has a Na^+/K^+ ratio of >1. This demonstrates their significant ability to retain K^+ (28). In contrast, following exogenous K^+ loading, infants can excrete K^+ at a rate that exceeds its filtration, indicating the renal capacity for tubular secretion. However, the rate of K^+ excretion in infants when adjusted to body weight is less than that observed in older children (29). This can place newborns at an increased risk for acute hyperkalemia. In sum, the limited K^+ excretory capacity of the immature kidney becomes clinically relevant only under conditions of K^+ excess.

To better highlight the developmental changes of the maturing kidney, nephron segments will be discussed individually.

Proximal Tubule (PT). K^+ handling in the PT does not undergo significant maturational changes given the passive nature of K^+ reabsorption in this segment.

Thick Ascending Loop of Henle (TALH). Postnatal maturation of the TALH is characterized by an increase in its capacity for K^+ reabsorption. While only ~65% of the filtered load of K^+ is reabsorbed in the TALH of the newborn, 90% of K^+ is reabsorbed across this segment in the adult *(10)*.

Cortical Collecting Duct (CCD). In the adult, regulated K^+ secretion by the distal tubule and the CCD contributes significantly to urinary K^+ excretion *(10)*. However, in the newborn kidney, the CCD has only a low K^+ secretory capacity. The maturational increase in the basal CCD K^+ secretory capacity is due to an increase in the number of SK/ROMK channels *(30)*.

The distal nephron of K^+-depleted adults may reabsorb K^+. This process is mediated by a H^+–K^+-ATPase that exchanges a single K^+ for a H^+. This channel is very active in newborns, suggesting that the collecting duct is poised to retain urinary K^+ early in life.

The appearance of flow-stimulated K^+ secretion is a later developmental event. It is mediated by the BK/maxi-K channel, which becomes active in the late newborn period *(30)*.

The neonatal CCD is relatively resistant to the effects of aldosterone. Therefore, plasma aldosterone levels in the newborn are high compared to those in the adult *(31)*.

8. CLINICAL ASSESSEMENT OF RENAL POTASSIUM EXCRETION

In the adult, a number of urinary indices can be utilized to assess renal response to disturbances in K^+ balance. The traditional approach to assess K^+ excretion is to measure the amount of K^+ in 24-h urine collections. However, in children or infants, the 24-h urine collection is inconvenient and is prone to errors due to inaccurate timing, incomplete collections, and/or calculation errors. More importantly, it is unwise to collect for 24 h during emergency situations and in states with an acute shift of K^+ into cells.

Spot urine K^+ concentrations alone might be misleading because K^+ depletion can cause polyuria and a relatively low K^+ concentration could still represent a large urinary K^+ loss.

In adults, a spot urine potassium-to-creatinine (K^+/Cr) ratio is useful to evaluate the basis of hypokalemia because of the near-constant rates of creatinine excretion. Adults normally excrete K^+ and Cr at rates close to 1 and 0.2 mEq/kg/day, respectively. Therefore the urine K^+/Cr ratio in mEq terms is approximately 5. The urine K^+/Cr ratio is usually <2 when hypokalemia is caused by low K^+ intake, increased transcellular shift of K^+, and extrarenal or former renal K^+ loss, whereas this ratio is >3 if renal K^+ wasting is ongoing *(32)*. Factors such as chronic kidney disease (CKD), low muscle mass, severe volume depletion, and marked rhabdomyolysis affect the rate of Cr excretion and thus the K^+/Cr ratio.

In children, the urine K^+/Cr is difficult to interpret due to the K^+-retaining state of the growing child and the gradual increase in plasma creatinine with increase in muscle mass.

Fractional excretion of K^+ (FEK) relates the quantity of excreted K^+ to the quantity of K^+ that was filtrated. This test is calculated as follows:

FEK (%) = (urine [K^+] × plasma [creatinine]) ÷ (plasma [K^+] × urine [creatinine]) × 100.

For an individual with normal kidney function with an average dietary K^+ intake, the FEK is ∼10%. When hypokalemia is due to extrarenal causes, the kidney conserves

K^+ maximally with an FEK < 7%. On the other hand, an FEK that is >7% suggests that there is renal K^+ wasting *(32)*. In patients with impaired renal function, there is reduced K^+ filtration and an adaptive increase in K^+ excretion per functioning nephron. Accordingly, one should utilize a nomogram to interpret the FEK in patients with renal function impairment.

The transtubular K^+ gradient (TTKG) is probably the most helpful tool in assessing the source of K^+ loss or retention in hypokalemic or hyperkalemic states, respectively. It is calculated as follows:

TTKG = {(urine [K^+] ÷ (urine osmolality/plasma osmolality)} ÷ plasma [K^+].

It is a semi-quantitative index that reflects the driving force for K^+ secretion in the CCD because it adjusts for the plasma K^+ concentration and for water reabsorption in the OMCD *(32)*. This formula is accurate as long as the urine osmolality exceeds that of the plasma and the urine Na^+ concentration is >25 mEq/L so that Na^+ delivery is not limiting *(32)*.

The TTKG in normal subjects on a regular diet is 8–9, and rises to >11 with a K^+ load. Thus, a value <7 and particularly <5 in a hyperkalemic patient is highly suggestive of decreased renal K^+ secretion, most likely due to hypoaldosteronism.

With the exception of advanced CKD, the other major cause of persistent hyper-kalemia is marked effective volume depletion. In this setting, the TTKG is >7. K^+ secretion in these disorders is limited primarily by the low urine flow not by the ability to secrete K^+ *(33)*.

The following sections will discuss disorders of K^+ homeostasis. The disorders with a common pathophysiologic denominator are grouped together. The groups are subdivided into common, uncommon, and rare causes.

9. HYPOKALEMIC DISORDERS

9.1. Definition and Pathophysiology

K^+ is a predominantly intracellular cation. Accurate assessment of total body K^+ stores cannot be done in the clinical setting. Generally, plasma K^+ measurements correlate with total body K^+ stores and are a more practical assessment tool. Hypokalemia is defined as a serum K^+ concentration < 3.5 mEq/L. Approximately each 1 mEq/L decrease in serum K^+ concentration below 3 mEq/L corresponds to a 200–400 mEq deficit in total body stores in the 70-kg adult *(34)*.

Hypokalemia is one of the most common findings in both outpatient and inpatient clinical practice settings. Hypokalemia is usually mild, with K^+ levels in the 3.0–3.5 mEq/L range, but in up to 25% it can be moderate to severe (<3.0 mEq/L) *(35)*.

9.2. Causes of Hypokalemia

9.2.1. DECREASED POTASSIUM INTAKE

The normal range of K^+ intake in children is about 1.5 mEq/kg/day. The kidney is able to lower K^+ excretion to a minimum of 5–25 mEq/day in the presence of K^+

depletion, but unable to produce K^+ free urine *(36)*. Decreased intake alone may cause hypokalemia, when the diet is limited to foods containing a high percentage of carbohydrate or refined sugar, by administration of K^+-free parenteral fluids, or when another problem is superimposed, such as diuretic therapy or the use of hypocaloric, liquid protein diets for rapid weight loss *(36)*.

9.2.2. REDISTRIBUTION OF POTASSIUM

9.2.2.1. Common Causes. *Spurious Hypokalemia.* Delayed sample analysis can cause increased cellular uptake of K^+. This commonly occurs if ambient temperature is increased *(37)*.

Sympathetic Activation. Transient hypokalemia can be caused in any setting in which there is stress-induced release of epinephrine, as with acute illness or vigorous exercise *(3)*. Occult sources of sympathomimetics such as pseudoephedrine in over-the-counter cold medicines are an overlooked cause of hypokalemia. Dietary caffeine in carbonated drinks also decrease K^+ levels *(38)*. Severe head trauma can cause profound hypokalemia, with reported serum K^+ levels of as low as 1.2 mEq/L *(39)*. This observation is related to a catecholamine effect, which occurs with trauma. Repeat serum K^+ levels are usually within normal limits.

Insulin Administration. Endogenous insulin is rarely a cause of hypokalemia. However, administered insulin is a frequent cause of iatrogenic hypokalemia. The plasma K^+ concentration can also be reduced by a carbohydrate load *(40)*.

9.2.2.2. Uncommon Causes. *Marked Increase in Blood Cell Production.* Patients with profound leukocytosis due to acute leukemia may present with artifactual hypokalemia caused by time-dependent uptake of K^+ by the large white cell mass *(3)*. In this setting, the measured plasma K^+ concentration may be <1 mEq/L without clinical symptoms or ECG changes.

Hypokalemic Periodic Paralysis. Hypokalemic periodic paralysis is a rare disorder, in which the sudden movement of K^+ into the cells can lower the plasma K^+ concentration to as low as 1.5 mEq/L. It is characterized by potentially fatal episodes of muscle weakness or paralysis, which can affect the limbs and the thorax *(3)*. Acute attacks are precipitated by exercise, stress, or a carbohydrate meal. The disorder may be autosomal dominant or may be acquired in patients with thyrotoxicosis. The oral administration of KCl aborts the attacks *(3)*.

9.2.2.3. Rare Causes. *Inhibition of Passive K^+ Efflux.* Barium is a potent inhibitor of K^+ channels and is found in rodenticides. Accidental or suicidal barium intoxication can cause hypokalemia by blocking the K^+ channels that normally allow cellular K^+ to diffuse into the extracellular fluid. Treatment of barium poisoning consists of K^+ supplementation and hemodialysis *(41)*.

Patients undergoing gastrointestinal or urological functional radiographic procedures using non-parenteral contrast are not at risk for this complication since the barium sulfate does not enter the systemic circulation.

Hypothermia. Accidental or induced hypothermia can drive K^+ into the cells and lower the plasma K^+ concentration to <3.0 mEq/L *(37)*.

9.2.3. Increased Gastrointestinal Losses

Loss of gastric or intestinal secretions from any cause (vomiting, diarrhea, or laxatives) is associated with K^+ losses *(3)*. The K^+ concentration in lower intestinal secretions is relatively high (20–50 mEq/L) compared to the concentration of K^+ in gastric secretions (5–10 mEq/L).

9.2.4. Increased Urinary Losses

Urinary K^+ excretion is primarily influenced by two factors: aldosterone and the distal delivery of Na^+ and water *(3)*. Increases in either aldosterone or distal flow, while the other parameter is at least normal or increased may lead to urinary K^+ wasting *(3)*.

9.2.4.1. Common Causes. *Diuretics.* Diuretics are an important cause of hypokalemia, due to their ability to increase distal flow rate and distal delivery of Na^+. Thiazides generally cause more hypokalemia than do loop diuretics, despite their lower natriuretic efficacy *(42)*. This is related to the hypercalciuria induced by loop diuretics. This increases the positive charge in the urinary lumen and as a consequence, the driving force for K^+ secretion diminishes.

Polyuria. Normal subjects can, in the presence of K^+ depletion, lower the urine K^+ concentration to a minimum of 5–10 mEq/L *(36)*. However, if the urine output is over 5–10 L/day, this regulatory mechanism is lost and then obligatory K^+ losses can exceed 50–100 mEq/day. This problem is most likely to occur in central or nephrogenic diabetes insipidus.

Metabolic Alkalosis. Vomiting induces an acute metabolic alkalosis, which leads to a shift of K^+ into cells in exchange for H^+. The alkalosis raises the plasma HCO_3^- concentration and ultimately, the filtered HCO_3^- load increases above its reabsorptive threshold leading to urinary K^+ losses. This effect is potentiated by a hypovolemia-induced increase in aldosterone, which also contributes to urinary K^+ losses.

Metabolic Acidosis. Metabolic derailments associated with acidemia, such as diabetic ketoacidosis (DKA), inborn errors of metabolism, or renal tubular acidosis (RTA) lead to increased urinary K^+ losses. However, the patient may seem to be hyperkalemic due to the tendency of acidemia to promote K^+ movement out of the cells. Correction of the underlying metabolic disorder may be complicated by profound hypokalemia.

Hyperaldosteronism. Increases in circulating aldosterone may be primary or secondary. Primary hyperaldosteronism may be genetic or acquired. Hypertension and hypokalemia are seen in patients with congenital adrenal hyperplasia (CAH) *(43)*. Patients typically present at an early age with hypertension. Aldosterone levels are modestly elevated. The patients are normokalemic, but may have a propensity to develop hypokalemia while on thiazide diuretics *(44)*. The diagnosis is confirmed by dexamethasone suppression test. Acquired causes of primary hyperaldosteronism include aldosterone-producing adenomas (APA) and hyperplastic adrenal glands, all of which are rare in children *(45)*.

In secondary hyperaldosteronism, increased levels of renin lead to increased angiotensin II (AII) and aldosterone, and can be associated with hypokalemia. Causes include renal artery stenosis and Page kidney (renal compression by a subcapsular mass or hematoma). The incidence of hypokalemia in renal artery stenosis is <20% *(46)*.

9.2.4.2. Uncommon Causes. *Amphotericin B.* Hypokalemia occurs in up to 50% of patients treated with amphotericin B for systemic fungal infections *(47)*. It leads to an increase in membrane permeability that promotes urinary K^+ loss. The hypokalemia is part of the nephrotoxic profile of amphotericin, which also includes decreased GFR, urinary loss of Mg^{2+}, renal tubular acidosis, loss of urine concentrating ability, and Fanconi's syndrome. Risk factors for amphotericin nephrotoxicity are mainly cumulative dosage and the combination of amphotericin with other nephrotoxic drugs. Mechanisms to prevent nephrotoxicity include the use of liposomal amphotericin B and volume repletion.

Magnesium Deficiency. Mg^{2+} deficiency results in refractory hypokalemia, particularly if the serum Mg^{2+} is <0.5 mg/dL. Hypomagnesemia has inhibitory effects on muscle Na^+–K^+-ATPase activity, resulting in significant K^+ efflux from muscle and secondary kaliuresis *(48)*. Hypomagnesemic patients are thus refractory to K^+ replacement in the absence of Mg^{2+} repletion. Mg^{2+} deficiency is commonly seen with hypokalemia, because many associated tubular disorders as in aminoglycoside nephrotoxicity, may cause both a kaliuresis and Mg^{2+} wasting. Serum Mg^{2+} must thus be checked on a routine basis in hypokalemic patients.

9.2.4.3. Rare Causes. *Syndrome of Apparent Mineralocorticoid Excess (AME).* In the classic form of AME, recessive loss-of-function mutations in the 11β-hydroxysteroid dehydrogenase-2 (11βHSD-2) gene cause a defect in the peripheral conversion of cortisol to the inactive glucocorticoid cortisone. The unregulated mineralocorticoid effect of glucocorticoids results in hypertension, hypokalemia, and metabolic alkalosis *(49)*.

Pharmacological inhibition of 11βHSD-2 is also associated with hypokalemia. The best known offender is licorice. The active ingredients (glycyrrhetinic/glycyrrhizinic acid and carbenoxolone) inhibit 11βHSD-2 and related enzymes *(50)*. Licorice intake remains high in Europe, mostly in Scandinavia. Glycyrrhizinic acid is also a component of Chinese herbal remedies prescribed for disorders such as for allergic rhinitis.

Bartter's Syndrome (BS). BS is an autosomal recessive disorder with mainly two major phenotypes and five genotypes. The estimated prevalence is approximately 1 per million. One group of patients present with antenatal BS, which is caused by defects in channels involved in the absorption of NaCl in the TALH. The defect reduces the lumen-positive transepithelial voltage, which impairs passive paracellular reabsorption of Ca^{2+} and Mg^{2+} in the TALH *(51)*. This leads to nephrocalcinosis. Because Cl^- absorption in the TALH is crucial for the generation of medullary hypertonicity, affected BS individuals lose their ability to concentrate urine. Thus, polyhydramnios in the absence of fetal anomalies and maternal diabetes should raise the suspicion for antenatal BS. Infants develop hyperkalemia and hyponatremia within the first 3 days of life with normalization by the end of the first postnatal week. Developmental delay is common and a mild dysmorphism has been described for some children (prominent forehead and eyes, large ears). In addition, there is markedly elevated renal prostaglandin (PG) production.

The second phenotype of BS has an insidious onset with failure to thrive and constipation in the first 2 years of life, hypokalemic alkalosis with high plasma renin and aldosterone and normal blood pressure. The patients have polyuria and polydipsia and developmental delay is also commonly present (52).

Thus far, five genotypes have been described: I, defect in the bumetanide-sensitive NKCC2; II, defect in the ROMK channel; III, defect in voltage-gated CLCNKB Cl⁻ channel; IV, defect in voltage-gated CLCNKB Cl⁻ channel; and V, defect in calcium-sensing receptor (51, 52). Type IV is a variant of antenatal BS and is associated with sensorineural deafness (53). Renal salt and water losses are more severe, requiring long-term parenteral fluid and electrolyte replacement. Hypercalciuria, and nephrocalcinosis are uncommon, but patients often show progression to CKD. Type V is associated with hypoparathyroidism due to gain-of-function mutations in the calcium-sensing receptor (CaSR) located both at the parathyroid gland and at the renal tubular basolateral membrane (54). This results in parathyroid hormone secretion, which is suppressed by lower than normal serum Ca^{2+} concentrations. Activation of the Ca^{2+}-sensing receptor inhibits the ROMK channel in the TALH (54). This form is distinguished from the classic form of BS by the presence of hypocalcemia, hypercalciuria, and hypomagnesemia. Hypercalciuria during hypocalcemia is an important feature, which is not seen in other variants of hypoparathyroidism.

There are acquired secondary forms of BS as well as pseudo-BS. Secondary BS is characterized by the presence of hypokalemic hypochloremic alkalosis, elevated plasma renin and aldosterone, and abnormally high levels of Cl⁻ in the urine. Typical examples are patients, who take loop diuretics for a long period of time. An acquired Bartter's-like syndrome occurring in association with gentamicin administration has been reported (55). Pseudo-BS have most, but not all clinical and biochemical abnormalities due to Cl⁻ deficit. Examples of this condition are cyclic vomiting and laxative abuse.

Gitelman's Syndrome (GS). GS presents in later childhood. The estimated prevalence is approximately 1 per 40,000. However, the prevalence of heterozygotes with mild clinical symptoms, who may be first-degree relatives of affected individuals and who are partially protected from hypertension through partial genetic loss of function of the thiazide-sensitive Na–Cl cotransporter (NCCT) (56) may be as high as 1%. GS is an autosomal recessive disease due to mutations in the gene encoding the NCCT in the distal tubule (57). A defect in this transporter can account for both Mg^{2+} wasting and decrease in Ca^{2+} excretion, which is similar to that induced by thiazide therapy.

The diagnosis is generally delayed, because the patients have milder symptoms. Hypokalemia and alkalosis are mild and the most typical findings are hypomagnesemia and hypocalciuria (<2 mg/kg/24 h). GS can be associated with serious clinical manifestations and may be mistaken for BS. Cramps, which may be severe, usually involve the arms and legs and are observed in most patients. They are due in part to hypokalemia and hypomagnesemia. About 10% of affected patients may also present with tetany, particularly in association with decreased intestinal absorption of Mg^{2+} (e.g., vomiting, diarrhea) (57). Severe fatigue and a lower than average blood pressure may be seen in some patients, consistent with salt wasting. Polyuria and nocturia are found in 50 and 80%, respectively. The polyuria may be accompanied by salt craving. However, concentrating ability is maintained, since function in the medullary TALH is intact. PG excretion is normal.

The diagnosis of the disorder is one of exclusion. Surreptitious vomiting and diuretic use are the two other major causes of unexplained hypokalemia and metabolic alkalosis in a normotensive patient. Patients with BS or GS have a urine Cl^- concentration > 40 mEq/L, while it is lower in patients who vomit *(58)*.

The treatment of BS consists of NaCl and K^+ supplementation as well as PG synthetase inhibitors. Patients with GS benefit from a K^+-sparing diuretic, such as spironolactone or amiloride, often in higher than usual doses to more completely block distal K^+ secretion. This treatment can raise the plasma K^+ concentration toward normal, largely reverse the metabolic alkalosis, and partially correct the hypomagnesemia *(59)*. Magnesium substitution is necessary in some patients *(57)* (Table 1).

Table 1

Table summarizing biochemical and clinical features of Gitelman's and Bartter's syndrome. TALH: thick ascending loop of Henle

Symptom/ pathophysiology	Gitelman's syndrome	Bartter's syndrome
Biochemical features in serum	Low K^+, low Mg^{2+}, alkalosis	Low K^+, alkalosis, high prostaglandins
Urinary findings	High Cl^-, low Ca^{2+}	High Cl^-, high K^+, high prostaglandins
Site of nephron	Distal tubule	TALH
Molecular defect	Na^+–Cl^- cotransporter	Na^+–K^+–$2Cl^-$ cotransporter BK/ROMK channel Cl^- channel
Blood pressure	Low	Low
Acts like	Thiazide diuretic	Loop diuretic
Salt-wasting	Yes	Yes
Concentrating defect	No	Yes
Polyhydramnios	No	Yes/possible
Time of presentation	Later in life	Birth or early infancy
Mental retardation	No	Yes/possible
Nephrocalcinosis	No	Yes
K-sparing diuretic useful	Yes	No
Required supplementation	NaCl, K^+, Mg^{2+}	NaCl, K^+
NSAIDs useful	No	Yes

Liddle's Syndrome: Liddle's syndrome constitutes an autosomal dominant gain-of-function mutation of ENaC, the amiloride-sensitive Na^+ channel of the CNT and CCD. It classically presents with the triad of hypertension, hypokalemia, and metabolic alkalosis in a relatively young patient. The consistent finding among such individuals is decreased urinary excretion of aldosterone *(60).*

The differential diagnosis includes congenital adrenal hyperplasia, familial cortisol resistance, the syndrome of apparent mineralocorticoid excess, and licorice ingestion. Sporadic cases also occur. Genetic testing is the most reliable test for diagnosis.

Therapy consists of potassium-sparing diuretics, which directly block the Na^+ channels. The mineralocorticoid antagonist spironolactone is ineffective, since the increase in Na^+ channel activity is not directly mediated by aldosterone in this disorder *(60).*

Chloride Deficiency. Dietary Cl^- deficiency can cause hypochloremic metabolic alkalosis, hypochloruria, and hypokalemia. This entity was described in babies fed chloride-deficient cow's milk formula due to a manufacturing error *(61).* The infants presented with anorexia, muscular weakness, lethargy, vomiting, and dehydration. The pathogenesis of the hypokalemia was related to volume contraction in the setting of Cl^--deficiency leading to secondary hyperaldosteronism, reduced formula intake, and alkalosis-induced shift of K^+ into cells.

9.2.5. INCREASED SWEAT LOSSES

Daily losses of K^+ in sweat are normally negligible, since the volume is low and the K^+ concentration is only 5–10 mEq/L. However, individuals exercising in a hot climate can produce 10 L or more of sweat per day, leading to K^+ depletion if these losses are not replaced *(62).* Significant loss of K^+ in sweat can also occur in cystic fibrosis, because of the high K^+ concentration *(63).*

9.2.6. DIALYSIS

Although patients with end-stage renal disease (ESRD) typically retain K^+ and tend to be hyperkalemic, hypokalemia can be induced in some patients by maintenance dialysis. Dialysis K^+ losses can be high in patients on chronic peritoneal dialysis. This can become clinically important if intake is reduced or if there are concurrent gastrointestinal losses *(64).* A different mechanism may be operative in patients treated with hemodialysis. In this setting, the metabolic acidosis induced by CKD can result in a relatively normal predialysis plasma K^+ concentration due to K^+ movement out of the cells. Hemodialysis not only removes K^+ rapidly, but it can also correct the acidemia, leading to K^+ entry into cells and a potentially large reduction in the plasma K^+ concentration.

Plasmapheresis may transiently lower K^+ concentrations if albumin is used as the replacement fluid. This problem can be avoided by adding 4 mEq/L of K^+ to the albumin solution.

9.3. Symptoms of Hypokalemia

Hypokalemia can cause palpitations, skeletal muscle weakness or cramping, paralysis or paresthesias, constipation, nausea or vomiting, abdominal cramping, polyuria, nocturia, or polydipsia, and even psychosis, delirium, hallucinations, or depression. Life-threatening symptoms are rhabdomyolysis, diaphragmatic paralysis, or cardiac arrhythmias. The latter complications can run the gamut from bradycardia, tachycardia, premature atrial or ventricular beats, to cardiac arrest. Changes on ECG include T-wave flattening or inverted T wave, prominent U wave that become more prominent with QT prolongation, ST-segment depression, ventricular arrhythmias, or atrial arrhythmias *(65)*.

During acute hypokalemia, the ability to appropriately conserve K^+ by both decreasing distal K^+ secretion and increasing active distal K^+ reabsorption is preserved. This response is important clinically, since it allows measurement of urinary K^+ excretion to distinguish between extrarenal and renal losses *(66)*.

The following renal abnormalities, most of which are reversible with K^+ repletion, can be induced by hypokalemia *(3)*:

Impaired Urinary Concentration. Nocturia, polyuria, and polydipsia, seen with chronic hypokalemia at plasma K^+ levels of ≤ 3.0 mEq/L, are due to diminished urinary concentrating ability. This is secondary to decreased collecting tubule responsiveness to vasopressin.

Increased Renal Ammonia Production and Net Acid Secretion. Hypokalemia increases the tubular production of ammonia (NH_3) and ammonium (NH_4^+), which enter both the tubular lumen and the peritubular capillary. K^+ then moves out of the cells to partially replete the extracellular stores, with electroneutrality being maintained by the entry of H^+ and Na^+ into the cells. The intracellular acidosis stimulates H^+ secretion and the production of NH_3 from glutamine. The increase in acid secretion, both as free H^+ ions and as NH_4^+ also promotes net HCO_3^- reabsorption *(67)*.

Altered Sodium Reabsorption. Mild to moderate hypokalemia can impair the ability to excrete a Na^+ load, at least in part by increasing proximal Na^+ reabsorption *(68)*. Some patients with severe hypokalemia may present with generalized edema secondary to this salt-retaining state.

Hypokalemic Nephropathy. Chronic K^+ depletion produces characteristic vacuolar lesions in the epithelial cells of the PT and occasionally the distal tubule. This abnormality requires at least 1 month to develop and is reversible if K^+ repletion is accomplished. However, with prolonged hypokalemia, lasting several years, more severe changes, including interstitial fibrosis, tubular atrophy, and cyst formation that is most prominent in the renal medulla can be seen. Correction of the hypokalemia can lead to a decrease in the number and size of cysts, but the tubulointerstitial lesions and associated renal insufficiency may be irreversible *(69)*.

9.4. Diagnosis of Hypokalemia

Urinary Response. The minimum urine K^+ concentration that can be achieved is 5–15 mEq/L *(38)*. Values above this level reflect at least a contribution from urinary K^+ wasting to the hypokalemia, unless the patient is markedly polyuric. Once urinary K^+ excretion is measured, the following diagnostic possibilities should be considered in the patient with hypokalemia of uncertain origin *(3)*:

Metabolic acidosis with a low rate of K^+ excretion is suggestive of lower gastrointestinal losses due to diarrhea *(70)*. Metabolic acidosis with K^+ wasting is most often due to diabetic ketoacidosis or to type 1 (distal) or type 2 (proximal) RTA. Metabolic alkalosis with a low rate of K^+ excretion can be due to vomiting, often seen in bulimia. Metabolic alkalosis with K^+ wasting and a low or normal blood pressure is most often due to vomiting or diuretic use or to Bartter's/Gitelman's syndrome. In this setting, measurement of the urine chloride concentration is often helpful, being low in vomiting when the excess HCO_3^- is excreted to maintain electroneutrality. The urine pH usually is >7.0.

9.5. Treatment

The goals of therapy in hypokalemia are to diagnose and correct the underlying cause, to prevent life-threatening conditions, and to replete any K^+ deficit. The urgency of therapy depends on the severity of hypokalemia, associated conditions and settings, and the rate of decline in serum K^+. A rapid drop to <2.5 mEq/L poses a high risk of cardiac arrhythmias and calls for urgent replacement *(71)*. Mg^{2+} levels should always be measured as well to expedite recognition of hypokalemia linked to hypomagnesemia.

Although replacement is usually limited to patients with a true deficit, it should be considered in patients with hypokalemia due to redistribution (e.g., hypokalemic periodic paralysis) when serious clinical complications such as cardiac arrhythmias are present or imminent *(71)*. Overcorrection or rebound hyperkalemia in hypokalemia caused by redistribution should be avoided because it may lead to fatal hyperkalemic arrhythmias.

K^+ replacement is the mainstay of therapy in hypokalemia. However, hypomagnesemic patients can be refractory to K^+ replacement alone, such that concomitant Mg^{2+} replacement is necessary to achieve correction of the serum K^+ concentration. The deficit and the rate of correction should be estimated as accurately as possible. The goal is to rapidly raise the serum K^+ to a safe range to avoid cardiac complications and then replace the remaining deficit at a slower rate over days to weeks *(40)*. In the absence of abnormal K^+ redistribution, the total deficit correlates with serum K^+ such that serum K^+ drops by approximately 0.27 mEq/L for every 100-mEq reduction in total body stores *(7)*.

Although the treatment of asymptomatic patients with borderline or low normal serum K^+ remains controversial, supplementation is recommended in patients with serum K^+ <3 mEq/L *(35)*. In asymptomatic patients with mild-to-moderate hypertension, an attempt should be made to maintain serum K^+ >4.0 mEq/L and K^+ supplementation should be considered when serum K^+ falls <3.5 mEq/L *(35)*.

The easiest and most straightforward method of oral K^+ supplementation is to increase dietary intake of K^+-rich foods (Table 2). Dietary K^+ is mainly available in the form of K^+ phosphate or K^+ citrate *(71)*. Salt substitutes are an inexpensive and potent source of KCl. Each gram contains 10–13 mEq of K^+ *(72)*. Medicinal K^+ is available in many oral forms, and KCl is the one used most frequently. In concurrent metabolic acidosis with hypokalemia, replacing Cl^- along with K^+ is essential in treating the alkalosis and preventing further kaliuresis.

Table 2
Short list of common food items with high K$^+$ content and low K$^+$ content in alphabetical order. (see for more details: http://www.kidney.org). Please note that juices made of fruits or vegetables with high K$^+$ content are also high in K$^+$

Food category	High potassium content	Low potassium content
Vegetables	Artichoke, bamboo shoots, beans, beets, broccoli, brussel sprouts, carrots, Chinese cabbage, lentils, mushrooms, parsnip, potato, seaweed, spinach, split peas, tomato and tomato products, squash	Alfalfa sprout, asparagus, iceberg lettuce, beans (green), cabbage (red or white), celery, corn, cucumber, eggplant, okra, onions, parsley, peas (green), radish, rhubarb, water chestnuts, watercress, yellow squash, zucchini squash
Fruit	Avocado, banana, cantaloupe, dried fruit (figs, dates, prunes), honeydew melon, kiwi, mango, nectarine, orange, papaya, pomegranate, prune, raisins	Apple, apricot, blackberries, blueberries, cherries, cranberries, grapes, grapefruit, mandarin, peach, pear, pineapple, plum, raspberries, strawberries, tangerine, watermelon
Meats/Fish	Beef, chicken, lamb, pork, veal; Cod, halibut	Eggs Tuna in water
Others	Bran and bran products, chocolate, granola, milk, molasses, nuts, peanut butter, salt-free broth, salt substitutes, seeds, wheat germ, yogurt	Bread and bread products except whole grain, cake (angel), coffee, cookies without nuts or chocolates, noodles, pasta, pies (without chocolate or high-K$^+$ fruits), rice, tea

The usual K$^+$ dose is 1–4 mEq/kg/day, divided in 2–4 doses. This dose is effective in maintaining serum K$^+$ in up to 90% of cases (73). In addition to K$^+$ supplementation, strategies to minimize K$^+$ losses should be considered. These measures may include minimizing the dose of non-K$^+$-sparing diuretics, restricting Na$^+$ intake, and using a combination of non-K$^+$-sparing and K$^+$-sparing medications, e.g., angiotensin-converting enzyme inhibitors, angiotensin receptor blockers, K$^+$-sparing diuretics, and β-blockers. The use of a K$^+$-sparing diuretic is of particular importance in hypokalemia resulting from primary hyperaldosteronism and related disorders, such as Liddle's syndrome (74). K$^+$ supplementation alone may be ineffective in these settings. In patients with hypokalemia due to loss through upper gastrointestinal secretion (continuous nasogastric tube suction, continuous or self-induced vomiting), proton-pump inhibitors are reportedly useful in helping to correct the metabolic alkalosis and reduce hypokalemia.

Parenteral (IV) K^+ administration should be limited to patients unable to utilize the enteral route or when the patient is experiencing associated signs and symptoms. The usual IV dose is 20–40 mEq of KCl/L. The rate is 0.5 mEq/kg/h over 1–2 h with ECG monitoring. As a general rule and to avoid venous pain, irritation, and sclerosis, concentrations of >40 mEq/L should not be given through a peripheral vein (71). Exceptions are feasible in patients with central lines and who are hospitalized in intensive care settings.

9.6. Hypokalemia Case Scenario

A 5-year-old boy presents to the pediatric emergency department complaining of pain in his legs. The mother states that over the past few days, the boy had a low-grade fever and occasional loose stools, but no vomiting. The boy is the product of a full-term uncomplicated pregnancy. His development has been unremarkable except for toilet training being achieved one year later than his older siblings. The mother also states that he likes to drink water and that he produces large amounts of urine. He also frequently craves salty foods. The boy is afebrile and has no dysmorphic features. The blood pressure is 85/53 mmHg and the pulse is 92 bpm. On examination of the lower extremities, both calf muscles are tense, but not hypertrophied. He denies perioral tingling. Laboratory tests reveal K^+ 2.5 mEq/L, bicarbonate 29 mEq/L and Mg^{2+} 1.0 mEq/L, with normal serum creatinine, calcium, and phosphorus levels. A urinalysis is negative for blood and protein with a specific gravity of 1.005. A spot urine calcium to creatinine ratio is 0.01 (normal range in this age group: 0.1–0.28).

Polyuria and polydipsia, as well as hypokalemia, metabolic alkalosis, hypomagnesemia, and hypocalciuria suggest Gitelman's syndrome. The patients do not have an intrinsic urinary concentrating defect, but due to renal salt wasting, they have concomitant water loss. These patients have renal K^+ and Mg^{2+} wasting due to a genetic mutation in a Na^+–Cl^- co-transporter in the distal tubule, resulting in a clinical picture similar to administration of hydrochlorothiazide. Intercurrent illnesses leading to increased loss of gastrointestinal secretions worsens the hypomagnesemia and hypokalemia and can provoke symptoms in otherwise well children. The finding of hypocalciuria distinguishes Gitelman's patients from those with Bartter's syndrome, who have marked hypercalciuria and nephrocalcinosis. The age of presentation for this boy is also typical of Gitelman's syndrome as opposed to patients with Bartter's syndrome who may present as early as in utero.

10. HYPERKALEMIC DISORDERS

Hyperkalemia is extremely rare in normal individuals, because cellular and renal adaptive mechanisms do not permit significant elevations of serum K^+ levels. Gradual increase in K^+ intake leads to so-called K^+ adaptation. This mechanism leads to more rapid elimination of K^+ in the urine and enhanced extrarenal disposal of K^+ (3).

10.1. Definition and Pathophysiology

Hyperkalemia is usually defined as a K^+ level of 5.5 mEq/L or higher *(75)*. Hyperkalemia has been reported in 1–10% of all hospitalized patients, with ~1% of patients having significant hyperkalemia ($\geq$6.0 mEq/L) *(75)*. Hyperkalemia is associated with a higher mortality rate (14–41%). In most hospitalized patients, the pathophysiology of hyperkalemia is multifactorial, with reduced renal function and medications being the most common contributing factors *(75)*. In patients with ESRD, the prevalence of hyperkalemia is 5–10% *(76)*. Hyperkalemia is a significant factor in 2–5% of deaths among patients with ESRD and it is the reason for emergency hemodialysis in 24% of patients with ESRD. CKD is the most common cause of hyperkalemia diagnosed in the emergency room *(76)*.

10.2. Consequences of Hyperkalemia

10.2.1. EXCITABLE TISSUES: MUSCLE AND HEART

Hyperkalemia constitutes a medical emergency, primarily due to its effect on the heart.

Cardiac Conduction Abnormality. Hyperkalemia has no premonitory clinical manifestations. Classically, a tall peaked T wave with shortened QT interval is the first change seen on the ECG in a patient with hyperkalemia. This is followed by progressive lengthening of the PR interval and QRS duration. The P wave may disappear, and ultimately the QRS widens further to a "sine wave." Ventricular standstill with a flat line on the ECG ensues. Ventricular fibrillation or standstill are the most severe consequences. There is large variability in the actual K^+ level leading to progression of ECG changes with worsening hyperkalemia. The severity of the electrophysiological abnormalities may be related to the presence or absence of concomitant hypocalcemia, acidemia, or hyponatremia *(77)*. Thus, measuring serum electrolytes and pH and monitoring of the ECG are essential *(3)*.

Hyperkalemia potentiates the blocking effect of lidocaine on the cardiac Na^+ channel, such that use of this agent may precipitate asystole or ventricular fibrillation in this setting.

Severe Muscle Weakness Or Paralysis. Muscle weakness usually begins with the lower extremities and progresses to the trunk and upper extremities. If severe, it can progress to flaccid paralysis and can mimic Guillain–Barré syndrome *(78)*. It is rare to have respiratory muscle weakness, and patients usually have normal cranial nerve examination. Weakness resolves with correction of the hyperkalemia.

10.2.2. RENAL CONSEQUENCES

Hyperkalemia has a significant effect on the ability to excrete an acidic urine, due to interference with the urinary excretion of ammonium (NH_4^+). The NH_4^+ produced by the PT in response to acidosis is reabsorbed across the TALH, concentrated in the medullary interstitium, and secreted in the collecting duct. Hyperkalemia inhibits renal acid excretion by competing with NH_4^+ for reabsorption by the TALH. This may be a major factor in the acidosis associated with various defects in K^+ excretion *(79)*.

10.3. Diagnosis

There are very few symptoms or signs of hyperkalemia and they generally occur at plasma K^+ concentration >7.0 mEq/L, unless the rise in K^+ concentration is very rapid *(3)*.

The differential diagnosis of persistent hyperkalemia consists of those disorders in which urinary K^+ excretion is impaired. The most common causes of this problem are advanced CKD and marked effective volume depletion.

In addition to measurement of plasma renin and aldosterone levels, calculation of the TTKG can help in the diagnosis of the cause of hyperkalemia *(3)*. Hyperkalemic patients, in whom all of these tests are normal and in whom renal function is not markedly impaired, probably have a selective K^+ secretory defect or the hyperkalemic form of type 1 renal tubular acidosis *(3)*.

10.4. Causes of Hyperkalemia

10.4.1. REDISTRIBUTION OF POTASSIUM

10.4.1.1. Common Causes. *Pseudohyperkalemia:* Factitious or pseudohyperkalemia is an artifactual increase in serum K^+ due to the release of K^+ during or after venipuncture.

There are also hereditary forms of pseudohyperkalemia, caused by increase in passive K^+ permeability of erythrocytes *(80)*.

Tissue Necrosis: Tissue necrosis is an important cause of hyperkalemia, which commonly occurs with rhabdomyolysis, due to the large store of K^+ in muscle. In many cases, volume depletion, medications (statins in particular), and metabolic predisposition contribute to the genesis of rhabdomyolysis *(81)*.

10.4.1.2. Uncommon Causes. *Tumor Lysis Syndrome.* Massive release of K^+ and other intracellular contents may occur as a result of acute tumor lysis *(82)*. This is a well-known side-effect of chemotherapy and preventive measures such as aggressive parenteral hydration have reduced the incidence of this entity.

Hypertonicity of Serum. Increases in serum K^+ due to hypertonic mannitol or hypertonic saline are due to a "solvent drag" effect, as water moves out of cells in response to the osmotic gradient *(3)*. The use of hypertonic IV contrast dye in patients with CKD may also lead to considerable increases in serum K^+ *(83)*.

10.4.1.3. Rare Causes. *Bufadienolide Intoxication.* The skin and venom gland of the cane toad Bufo marinus contains high concentrations of bufadienolide, a glycoside similar to digoxin. The direct ingestion of such toads or of toad extracts can result in fatal hyperkalemia *(84)*. Certain herbal aphrodisiac pills contain appreciable amounts of toad venom. Treatment with digoxin-specific Fab fragment may be effective and life-saving in bufadienolide toxicity.

Fluoride. Fluoride ions inhibit Na^+–K^+-ATPase, such that fluoride poisoning is typically associated with hyperkalemia.

Succinylcholine. Succinylcholine depolarizes muscle cells, resulting in the efflux of K^+ and a rapid, but transient hyperkalemia. The use of this agent is contraindicated in patients who have sustained thermal trauma, neuromuscular injury, or muscular dystrophy, disuse atrophy, or prolonged immobilization in an ICU setting, because the efflux of K^+ is enhanced in these patients and can result in significant hyperkalemia *(85)*.

10.4.2. INCREASED POTASSIUM INTAKE

Increased intake of K^+ be it iatrogenic or due to intake of dietary sources rich in K^+, may provoke hyperkalemia in patients in CKD. However, there are situations, in which patients with normal renal function may be at risk for hyperkalemia as well.

10.4.2.1. Common Causes. *Transfusions.* Red blood cell transfusions are a well-described cause of hyperkalemia in children *(86)*. Risk factors for transfusion-related hyperkalemia include rate and volume of the transfusion, the use of a central venous infusion and/or pressure pumping, the use of irradiated blood, and the age of the blood infused.

10.4.2.2. Uncommon Causes. *KCl Supplementation.* Sustained-release KCl tablets can cause hyperkalemia in suicidal overdoses. Such pills are radio-opaque, and may be seen on radiographs. Whole bowel irrigation is indicated for gastrointestinal decontamination *(87)*.

10.4.2.3. Rare Causes. *Sports Beverages.* Marked intake of K^+, for example in sports beverages, may provoke severe hyperkalemia in individuals free of predisposing factors *(88)*.

Hidden Sources. Occult sources of K^+ must also be considered, including alternative medicines and alternative diets *(89)*.

Pica. Geophagia with ingestion of K^+-rich clay, and cautopyreiophagia (ingestion of burnt matchsticks), are two forms of pica that have been reported to cause hyperkalemia in dialysis patients *(90)*.

10.4.3. REDUCED RENAL POTASSIUM EXCRETION

10.4.3.1. Common Causes. *Nonsteroidal Antiinflammatory Drugs (NSAIDs).* PGs produced in the kidney partially mediate renin secretion. NSAIDs lower renal renin secretion and consequently increase serum K^+ levels *(91)*. Hyperkalemia is a well-recognized complication of NSAIDs. NSAIDs also cause hyperkalemia by decreasing GFR and increasing Na^+ retention. The flow-activated apical BK/maxi-K channel is also activated by PGs; hence NSAIDs will reduce its activity and the flow-dependent component of K^+ excretion *(92)*. They also blunt the adrenal response to hyperkalemia, which is at least partially dependent on PGs.

ACE-Inhibitors (ACEIs). ACEIs diminish aldosterone release *(93)* Thus, an ACEI may decrease both ATII- and K^+-mediated aldosterone release *(93)*. Renin is increased with ACEIs. ACEIs usually raise the plasma K^+ concentration by less than 0.5 mEq/L in patients with relatively normal renal and cardiac function. ARBs appear to have a lesser effect on plasma K^+ in patients with renal insufficiency. The patients at risk for the development of hyperkalemia in response to drugs that target the RAAS axis, singly or in combination therapy, are those in whom the ability of kidneys to excrete the potassium load is markedly diminished due to one or a combination of the following: (1) decreased delivery of Na^+ to the cortical collecting duct, (2) decreased circulating aldosterone,

(3) inhibition of amiloride-sensitive Na^+ channels in the CNT and CCD, (4) chronic tubulointerstitial disease, and (5) increased K^+ intake.

Potassium-sparing Diuretics. K^+-sparing diuretics are probably the most common cause of hyperkalemia related to aldosterone deficiency. These drugs antagonize the action of aldosterone on the collecting tubule cells. Spironolactone competes for the aldosterone receptor and amiloride and triamterene act to close the Na^+ channels in the luminal membrane *(9)*. Inhibition of apical ENaC activity in the distal nephron by amiloride and other K^+-sparing diuretics predictably results in hyperkalemia.

Trimethoprim (TMP) and Pentamidine. TMP and pentamidine can cause hyperkalemia by closing Na^+ channels (ENaC) due to their structural similarity with amiloride *(94)*. TMP-induced hyperkalemia is dose-dependent. Originally, this complication was seen primarily when very high doses were used in patients with pneumocystis pneumonia in the setting of AIDS. However, TMP can raise serum K^+ levels at conventional doses as well *(94)*. The peak effect is after 4–5 days of therapy. Patients with mild CKD may be at risk for more severe hyperkalemia.

Heparin. Aldosterone synthesis is selectively reduced by heparin, with a 7% incidence of hyperkalemia associated with heparin therapy *(95)*. Heparin has a direct toxic effect on the adrenal zona glomerulosa cells *(3)*. Heparin reduces the adrenal aldosterone response to both ATII and hyperkalemia, resulting in hyperreninemic hyperaldosteronism (Table 3). Both unfractionated and low-molecular weight heparin can cause hyperkalemia *(95)*. Even low-dose heparin can lead to a substantial reduction in plasma aldosterone levels.

Table 3
Aldosterone and renin levels in various hyperkalemic states

Entity	Aldosterone	Renin
Pseudohyperkalemia	Normal	Normal
High K intake	Normal or slightly elevated	Normal or low
Congenital adrenal hyperplasia	Low	High
Pseudohypoaldosteronism Type I	High	Low
Pseudohypoaldosteronism Type II (Gordon's syndrome)	Low	Low
Hypoaldosteronism	Low	High
Hyporeninemic hypoaldosteronism	Low	Low
NSAIDs	Low	Low
ACE-inhibitors	Low	High
Cyclosporine, Tacrolimus	Low	Low
Primary adrenal insufficiency	Low	High
Potassium-sparing diuretics	Low	High
Heparin	High	High
Severe illness	Low	Low

Cacineurin Inhibitors. Cyclosporine A (CsA) and tacrolimus cause hyperkalemia. CsA leads to hyperkalemia in 15–25% of renal transplant recipients, due in part to diminished secretion of, as well as responsiveness to, aldosterone *(96)*. The risk of sustained hyperkalemia may be higher in renal transplant patients on tacrolimus than in those on CsA. CsA causes hyporeninemic hypoaldosteronism and inhibits the SK/ROMK channel in the CCD in addition to the basolateral $Na^+-K^+-APTase$ *(96)*. CsA causes redistribution of K^+ and hyperkalemia, particularly when used in combination with β-blockers.

10.4.3.2. Uncommon Causes. *Congenital Adrenal Hyperplasia (CAH).* Hypoaldosteronism can result from a deficiency of enzymes required for aldosterone synthesis, which may or may not be associated with concurrent abnormalities in cortisol and androgen production. The clinical presentation is typical of aldosterone deficiency: affected infants have recurrent dehydration, salt wasting, and failure to thrive. The usual defect in this disorder is in the activity of the terminal enzyme in the aldosterone biosynthetic pathway, aldosterone synthase *(97)*. Children have low serum aldosterone concentration, normal cortisol concentration, and a high plasma renin activity (PRA). The diagnosis is usually made based on the newborn screen, but genetic testing is now available.

10.4.3.3. Rare Causes. *Pseudohypoaldosteronism (PHA) Type I.* PHA type I is a rare hereditary disorder, which is associated with a decreased response to aldosterone effects, leading to hyperkalemia and metabolic acidosis. Two different modes of inheritance have been described *(98)*. The milder autosomal dominant form is due, at least in some patients, to mineralocorticoid receptor mutations. This form may improve with age. Loss-of-function mutations in the ENaC Na^+ channel cause the autosomal recessive variant of type I PHA, which is more severe and affects aldosterone action in many organs, including sweat glands, salivary glands, the respiratory tract, the gut, and the kidney. Hyperkalemia persists after birth and is always associated with metabolic acidosis. The affected individuals present in infancy with Na^+ wasting, hypovolemia, and hyperkalemia. Plasma aldosterone levels are markedly elevated *(99)*. Impairment of extrarenal Na^+ channel activity often leads to frequent lower respiratory tract infections and, together with increases in sweat NaCl concentrations, may result in a clinical picture mimicking cystic fibrosis *(98)*.

Initial therapy of PHA type I consists of a high salt diet, which prevents volume depletion and, by enhancing Na^+ delivery to the K^+ secretory site in the collecting tubules, increases K^+ excretion and lowers the plasma K^+ concentration. Most patients require use of K^+ binding resins. High dose fludrocortisone can be added if a high salt intake is ineffective or not well tolerated *(100)*.

PHA Type II. PHA type II is also rare and is known as Gordon's syndrome. It has been described in patients who present with hypertension, hyperkalemia, metabolic acidosis, hypercalciuria, and low bone density, but normal renal function, and low or low-normal PRA and aldosterone concentrations, making it in many respects the mirror image of Gitelman's syndrome *(98)*. The defect is transmitted as an autosomal dominant trait. PHA type II behaves like a gain-of-function in the thiazide-sensitive Na^+-Cl^- cotransporter NCC, and treatment with thiazides results in resolution of the entire clinical picture *(101)*.

Hypoaldosteronism. Aldosterone release from the adrenal most often is reduced due to autoimmune diseases, infections, or medications. Primary hypoaldosteronism may be genetic or acquired *(102)*.

Infection with the human immunodeficiency virus (HIV) is the most important infectious cause of adrenal insufficiency. The most common cause of adrenalitis in HIV disease is cytomegalovirus or mycobacterium avium intracellulare *(103)*. Although the adrenal involvement in HIV is usually subclinical, adrenal insufficiency may be precipitated by stress or drugs such as ketoconazole that inhibit steroidogenesis. Administration of pentamidine, heparin, or trimethoprim–sulfamethoxazole may also contribute to hyperkalemia in HIV-infected patients.

Patients with adrenal insufficiency should receive replacement therapy with fludrocortisone and hydrocortisone or prednisone as clinically indicated.

Severe Illness. Hypoaldosteronism due to decreased adrenal production can occur in critically ill patients. Volume expansion may play a contributory role in some patients.

Distal Renal Tubular Acidosis (RTA). Unlike hyporeninemic hypoaldosteronism, hyperkalemic distal RTA is associated with a normal or increased aldosterone level and/or PRA. Urine pH in these patients is >5.5 and they are unable to increase acid or K^+ excretion. The development of overt hyperkalemia is most common in patients with other risk factors that further impair the efficiency of K^+ excretion, such as renal insufficiency, reduced renal perfusion, or the administration of drugs that interfere with K^+ handling such as ACEIs, ARBs, or renin inhibitors. The hyperkalemia is associated with a mild metabolic acidosis with a normal anion gap (i.e., hyperchloremic acidosis) unless there is concurrent renal insufficiency. Classic causes include SLE and sickle cell anemia *(104)*.

Hyporeninemic Hypoaldosteronism. The syndrome of hyporeninemic hypoaldosteronism is characterized by decreased angiotensin II production and an intraadrenal defect, both of which contribute to the decline in aldosterone secretion *(3)*. This disorder is most common in children with volume expansion due to acute glomerulonephritis (GN), such as postinfectious GN or in SLE, and is also seen in diabetes mellitus, and renal insufficiency *(105)*. The hyperkalemia responds to mineralocorticoid replacement. Recovery of renal function within 1–2 weeks is associated with restoration of normal K^+ balance *(105)*. About 50% of patients have an associated acidosis, with a reduced renal excretion of NH_4^+, a positive urinary anion gap, and urine pH <5.5. Many patients will respond to either NaCl restriction or furosemide with an increase in PRA meaning that renin is secondarily rather than pathologically suppressed *(106)*.

10.4.3.4. Other Causes. *Prematurity.* Non-oliguric hyperkalemia is a common and potentially life-threatening complication in preterm neonates in the intensive care setting. Hyperkalemia affects up to 50% of very low birth weight (<1000 g) premature infants *(107)*. It often causes cardiac arrhythmias and can lead to periventricular leukomalacia and death. This hyperkalemia has been shown to be unrelated to leakage of intracellular K^+ following cell membrane disruption associated with bruising, intracranial hemorrhage, hemolysis, perinatal asphyxia, or acidosis *(107)*. It is defined as a serum K^+ concentration of >6.5 mEq/L resulting in shifting of K^+ from the intracellular to the extracellular compartment *(108)*. The higher cut-off used to define hyperkalemia in premature babies is due to the higher baseline K^+ levels in these babies.

The immature kidney, the relative resistance to aldosterone, and the need to preserve K^+ for cellular growth result in serum K^+ levels of up to 5.8 mEq/L to still be considered normal. Non-oliguric hyperkalemia is transient, because gradually the activity of the Na^+–K^+-ATPase increases in all body cells. Administration of steroids prenatally can prevent nonoliguric hyperkalemia by upregulating the enzyme activity in the fetus *(109)*.

Insulin and dextrose have been successfully used to lower serum K^+ levels. Treatment with ion exchange resins can have a mortality rate of up to 80%, due to complications including impaction and/or rectal perforation *(110)*.

10.5. Treatment of Hyperkalemia

The first priority in the management of hyperkalemia is to assess the need for emergency treatment based on ECG changes and $K^+ \geq 6.0$ mEq/L. This should be followed by a comprehensive workup to determine the cause. Initial laboratory tests should include electrolytes, BUN, creatinine, serum osmolality, Mg^{2+}, and Ca^{2+}, a complete blood count, and urinary pH, osmolality, creatinine, and electrolytes. Careful monitoring of the ECG and muscle strength is indicated to assess the functional consequences of the hyperkalemia. Patients with a value <6 mEq/L can often be treated with a low K^+ diet and diuretics. Any extra source of K^+ intake should be eliminated and any potentiating drugs should be discontinued. An asymptomatic patient with a plasma K^+ concentration of 6.5 mEq/L whose ECG does not manifest signs of hyperkalemia can be treated with a cation exchange resin alone. At a plasma $K^+ > 7.0$ mEq/L, severe muscle weakness, or marked ECG changes are potentially life threatening and require immediate treatment. If these complications are noted, urgent treatment is warranted, regardless of the degree of hyperkalemia *(111)*.

Treatment of hyperkalemia is threefold: (1) antagonizing the membrane effects of K^+, (2) driving extracellular K^+ into the cell, and (3) removing excess K^+ from the body *(3)*.

10.5.1. ANTAGONISM OF MEMBRANE EFFECTS OF POTASSIUM

Calcium. Ca^{2+} directly antagonizes the membrane actions of hyperkalemia. It antagonizes the depolarizing membrane effect of hyperkalemia *(112)*. The protective effect of Ca^{2+} begins within minutes, but is relatively short-lived. Therefore, Ca^{2+} infusions are indicated for severe hyperkalemia like widening of the QRS complex or loss of P waves, but not peaked T waves alone. Such ECG changes indicate that it is potentially dangerous to wait the 30–60 min needed for more long-lasting measures to lower K^+ to start acting. Ca^{2+} can be given as either Ca^{2+}-gluconate or $CaCl_2$. $CaCl_2$ contains three times the concentration of elemental Ca^{2+} compared to Ca^{2+}-gluconate. Ca^{2+} gluconate is infused slowly over 2–3 min, with constant cardiac monitoring. The dose of either formulation can be repeated after 5 min if the ECG changes persist.

10.5.2. Shift of Potassium to Intracellular Space

Insulin and Glucose. Insulin and glucose lower the plasma K^+ concentration by driving K^+ into the cells. Effective therapy usually leads to a 0.5–1.5 mEq/L fall in the plasma K^+ concentration, an effect that begins in 15 min, peaks at 60 min, and wears off by 1–3 h *(8)*.

NaCO₃. The use of $NaHCO_3$ is controversial in the management of hyperkalemia. The only setting, in which the authors make use of this measure, is in patients who have advanced CKD with severe hyperkalemia and acidosis. However, $NaHCO_3$ has generally produced little acute reduction in the plasma K^+ concentration and may even delay life-saving interventions *(8)*. Controlled studies are required to show a beneficial role for $NaHCO_3$ in the management of hyperkalemia. Until then, the authors do not recommend its use in this setting.

β₂-Adrenergic Agonists. β_2-agonists like epinephrine drive K^+ into the cells by increasing $Na–K^+$-ATPase activity. These drugs can be effectively used in the acute treatment of hyperkalemia, lowering the plasma K^+ concentration by 0.5–1.5 mEq/L. The peak effect is seen within 30 min with IV infusion, and at 90 min with nebulization *(113)*.

10.5.3. Removal of Excess Potassium

The above modalities only transiently lower the plasma K^+ concentration. Therapy is required to remove K^+ from the body. This can be achieved in normal subjects with loop or thiazide diuretics.

Loop or Thiazide Diuretics. Diuretics have a relatively modest effect on urinary K^+ excretion in patients with CKD, particularly in an acute setting. However, these medications are useful in correcting hyperkalemia in patients with the syndrome of hyporeninemic hypoaldosteronism, and selective renal K^+ secretory problems that occur after transplantation or administration of TMP *(114)*.

In patients with impaired renal function, use of the following agents is recommended: (1) oral diuretics with the highest bioavailability (e.g., torsemide) and the least renal metabolism (e.g., torsemide, bumetanide) in order to minimize the chance of accumulation and toxicity, (2) IV agents (short-term treatment) with the least hepatic metabolism (e.g., furosemide rather than bumetanide), (3) combinations of loop and thiazide-like diuretics for better efficacy, and (4) use of the maximal effective dose *(114)*.

Cation Exchange Resin. The major available cation exchange resin is sodium polystyrene sulfonate (SPS). In the gut, this resin takes up K^+ and releases Na^+. Each gram of resin may bind as much as 1 mEq of K^+ and releases 1–2 mEq of Na^+. Thus, a potential side effect is exacerbation of edema due to Na^+ retention. The discrepancy is caused in part by the binding of small amounts of other cations (Ca^{2+} and Mg^{2+}) *(115)*. Studies demonstrating efficacy with SPS have documented a K^+-lowering effect after multiple doses were given over 1–5 days. In patients with advanced CKD, use of SPS in sorbitol is reasonable as a temporizing maneuver during preparation of the patient for hemodialysis. Ischemic colitis and colonic necrosis are the most serious complications of SPS *(116)*. Although data are limited, SPS in sorbitol should not be used in patients in a perioperative setting. SPS can be given either orally or as a retention enema (needs to stay 30–60 min, preferably 2–4 h). The oral dose is usually 1 g/kg/dose. The dose can be repeated every 4–6 h as necessary. SPS is generally well tolerated and can be given one to three times per day to control chronic mild hyperkalemia in patients with renal insufficiency. Its effect on K^+ is slow, and the full effect may take between 4 and 24 h *(3)*. Thus it should be used only in conjunction with other measures in the management of acute hyperkalemia.

Dialysis. Dialysis can be used if the conservative measures are ineffective, if the hyperkalemia is severe, or if the patient has marked tissue breakdown and is releasing large amounts of K^+ from the injured cells *(3)*. All modes of acute renal replacement therapies are effective in removing K^+. Continuous hemodiafiltration is increasingly used in the management of critically ill and hemodynamically unstable patients. Hemodialysis is the preferred mode when rapid correction of a hyperkalemic episode is desired. In most patients, the greatest decline in serum K^+ and the largest amount of K^+ removed occur during the first hour; the serum K^+ usually reaches its nadir at about 3 h. The amount of K^+ removed depends primarily on the type and surface area of the dialyzer used, blood flow rate, dialysate flow rate, dialysis duration, and serum to dialysate K^+ gradient. The acute induction of hypokalemia can cause potentially life-threatening arrhythmias *(117)*.

10.5.4. PREVENTION OF HYPERKALEMIA

Most patients with persistent hyperkalemia have advanced CKD. There are several measures that can help prevent hyperkalemia in patients with CKD. These include (1) use of a low K^+ diet and (2) avoiding the use of drugs that raise the plasma K^+ concentration such as ACEIs or ARBs and nonselective β-blockers *(118)*. $β_1$-selective blockers are much less likely to cause hyperkalemia.

10.6. Hyperkalemia Case Scenario

A 1-week-old boy is brought in to the pediatrician's office with a 2-day history of inconsolable crying and irritability. The mother states that he is being breast fed, but that she has to supplement the feeds with formula, because he seems to be very hungry, and most of the feeds are followed by non-projectile vomiting. The mother has one older boy who is healthy and she says that compared to the sibling, the boy is producing significantly more wet diapers. The boy was born full-term and his birth weight was 3.3 kg. In the office, he weighs 2.8 kg and the physical exam is notable for dry mucus membranes. The blood pressure cannot be obtained, because of the baby's constant movements and shrill crying. He is making tears as he cries and he has no facial dysmorphism. The remainder of the physical exam is remarkable for loss of subcutaneous fat. There is no organomegaly or rash. A CBC is normal; Na^+ 123, K^+ 7.8 mEq/L, and there is metabolic acidosis with a bicarbonate level of 15 mEq/L on a venous blood gas. Analysis of the newborn screen is consistent with congenital adrenal hyperplasia (CAH). Genetic testing confirms a mutation in the gene encoding CYP21. All symptoms resolve once supplementation with NaCl, fludrocortisone, and hydrocortisone are initiated. On a follow-up visit 2 weeks later the baby weighs 3.2 kg and sleeps peacefully throughout the office visit.

This baby presented with the classic salt-wasting form of CAH. The onset of symptoms occurs typically in the first week of life, when the baby presents with vomiting and progressive weight loss. Renal salt wasting leads to increased urine volume and worsening dehydration. Aldosterone levels are low in these patients, leading to hyperkalemia. Typically, renin levels are elevated. Supplementation with salt and hormones leads to immediate improvement of the clinical picture and allows the child to thrive normally. However, special care has to be given to these children with intercurrent illnesses because they may require hospitalization and intravenous substitution of salt and hormones, if they do not tolerate oral intake.

REFERENCES

1. Edelman IS, Leibman J. Anatomy of body water and electrolytes. Am J Med 1959;27:256–277.
2. Clausen T, Everts ME. Regulation of the Na,K-pump in skeletal muscle. Kidney Int 1989;35:1–13.
3. Rose BD, Post TW. Clinical Physiology of Acid–Base and Electrolyte Disorders. 5th edition, McGraw-Hill, New York, 2001, pp. 333–344, 383–396, 836–856, 860–866, 888–930.
4. Clausen T, Flatman JA. Effects of insulin and epinephrine on Na+–K+ and glucose transport in soleus muscle. Am J Physiol 1987;252:E492–E499.
5. DeFronzo RA, Lee R, Jones A, et al. Effect of insulinopenia and adrenal hormone deficiency on acute potassium tolerance. Kidney Int 1980;17:586–594.
6. Ewart HS, Klip A. Hormonal regulation of the Na(+)–K(+)-ATPase: mechanisms underlying rapid and sustained changes in pump activity. Am J Physiol 1995;269:C295–C311.
7. Sterns RH, Cox M, Feig PU, et al. Internal potassium balance and the control of the plasma potassium concentration. Medicine 1981;60:339–354.
8. Daut J, Maier-Rudolph W, von Beckerath N, et al. Hypoxic dilation of coronary arteries is mediated by ATP-sensitive potassium channels. Science 1990;247:1341–1344.
9. Adrogue HJ, Madias NE. Changes in plasma potassium concentration during acute acid–base disturbances. Am J Med 1981;71:456–467.
10. Giebisch G. Renal potassium transport: Mechanisms and regulation. Am J Physiol 1998;274: F817–F833.
11. Conte G, Dal Canton A, Imperatore P, et al. Acute increase in plasma osmolality as a cause of hyperkalemia in patients with renal failure. Kidney Int 1990;38:301–307.
12. Wilson RW, Wareing M, Green R. The role of active transport in potassium reabsorption in the proximal convoluted tubule of the anaesthetized rat. J Physiol 1997;500:155–164.
13. Gimenez I. Molecular mechanisms and regulation of furosemide-sensitive Na–K–Cl cotransporters. Curr Opin Nephrol Hyperten 2006;15:517–523.
14. Stokes JB. Consequences of potassium recycling in the renal medulla. Effects of ion transport by the medullary thick ascending limb of Henle's loop. J Clin Invest 1982;70:219–229.
15. Imai M, Nakamura R. Function of distal convoluted and connecting tubules studied by isolated nephron fragments. Kidney Int 1982;22:465–472.
16. Frindt G, Palmer LG. Apical potassium channels in the rat connecting tubule. Am J Physiol Renal Physiol 2004;287:F1030–F1037.
17. Taniguchi J, Imai M. Flow-dependent activation of maxi-K+ channels in apical membrane of rabbit connecting tubule. J Membr Biol 1998;164:35–45.
18. Choe H, Zhou H, Palmer LG, et al. A conserved cytoplasmic region of ROMK modulates pH sensitivity, conductance, and gating. Am J Physiol 1997;273:F516–F529.
19. Morimoto T, Liu W, Woda C, et al. Mechanism underlying flow stimulation of sodium absorption in the mammalian collecting duct. Am J Physiol Renal Physiol 2006;291:F663–F669.
20. Liu W, Xu S, Woda C, et al. Effect of flow and stretch on the $[Ca2+]_i$ response of principal and intercalated cells in cortical collecting duct. Am J Physiol 2003;285:F998–F1012.

21. Kone BC. Renal H,K-ATPase: structure, function and regulation. Miner Electrolyte Metab 1996;22:349–365.

22. Good DW, Wright FS. Luminal influences on potassium secretion: Sodium concentration and fluid flow rate. Am J Physiol 1979;236:F192–205.

23. Johnson DW, Kay TD, Hawley CM: Severe hypokalaemia secondary to dicloxacillin. Intern Med J 2002;32:357–358.

24. Stanton BA, Giebisch G: Effects of pH on potassium transport by renal distal tubule. Am J Physiol 1982;242:F544–551.

25. Wang WH. Regulation of Renal K transport by dietary K intake. Annu Rev Physiol 2004;66: 547–569.

26. Cassola AC, Giebisch G, Wang W. Vasopressin increases density of apical low-conductance K+ channels in rat CCD. Am J Physiol 1993;264:F502–F509.

27. Dancis J, Springer D. Fetal homeostasis in maternal malnutrition: potassium and sodium deficiency in rats. Pediatr Res 1970;4:345–351.

28. Satlin LM. Regulation of potassium transport in the maturing kidney. Semin Nephrol 1999;19: 155–165.

29. McCance RA, Widdowson EM. The response of the newborn piglet to an excess potassium. J Physiol 1958;141:88–96.

30. Woda CB, Miyawaki N, Ramalakshmi S, et al. Ontogeny of flow-stimulated potassium secretion in rabbit cortical collecting duct: Functional and molecular aspects. Am J Physiol Renal Physiol 2003;285:F629–639.

31. Van Acker KJ, Scharpe SL, Deprettere AJ, et al. Renin–angiotensin–aldosterone system in the healthy infant and child. Kidney Int 1979;16:196–203.

32. West ML, Marsden PA, Richardson RM, et al. New clinical approach to evaluate disorders of potassium excretion. Miner Electrolyte Metab 1986;12:234–238.

33. Ethier JH, Kamel KS, Magner PO, et al. The transtubular potassium concentration in patients with hypokalemia and hyperkalemia. Am J Kidney Dis 1990;15:309–315.

34. Schwartz GJ. Potassium. In: Pediatric Nephrology 5th Edition, Avner ED, Harmon WE, Niaudet P, Eds. Lippincott, Williams, and Wilkins, Philadelphia, 2004, 147–188.

35. Cohn JN, Kowey PR, Whelton PK, et al. New guidelines for potassium replacement in clinical practice: A contemporary review by the National Council on Potassium in Clinical Practice. Arch Intern Med 2000;160:2429–2436.

36. Squires RD, Huth EJ. Experimental potassium depletion in normal human subjects. I. Relation of ionic intakes to the renal conservation of potassium. J Clin Invest 1959;38:1134–1148.

37. Ulahannan TJ, McVittie J, Keenan J. Ambient temperatures and potassium concentrations. Lancet 1998;352:1680–1681.

38. Wong KM, Chak WL, Cheung CY, et al. Hypokalemic metabolic acidosis attributed to cough mixture abuse. Am J Kidney Dis 2001;38:390–394.

39. Schaefer M, Link J, Hannemann L, et al. Excessive hypokalemia and hyperkalemia following head injury. Intensive Care Med 1995;21:235–237.

40. Kunin AS, Surawicz B, Sims EA. Decrease in serum potassium concentrations and appearance of cardiac arrhythmias during infusion of potassium with glucose in potassium-depleted patients. N Engl J Med 1962;266:228–233.

41. Wells JA, Wood KE. Acute barium poisoning treated with hemodialysis. Am J Emerg Med 2001;19:175–177.

42. Clausen T. Clinical and therapeutic significance of the Na+,K+ pump. Clin Sci (Lond) 1998;95:3–17.

43. White PC. Steroid 11 beta-hydroxylase deficiency and related disorders. Endocrinol Metab Clin North Am 2001;30:61–79

44. Litchfield WR, Coolidge C, Silva P, et al: Impaired potassium-stimulated aldosterone production: A possible explanation for normokalemic glucocorticoid-remediable aldosteronism. J Clin Endocrinol Metab 1997;82:1507–1510.

45. Blumenfeld JD, Sealey JE, Schlussel Y, et al. Diagnosis and treatment of primary hyperaldosteronism. Ann Intern Med 1994;121:877–885.

46. Bunchman TE, Sinaiko AR. Renovascular hypertension presenting with hypokalemic metabolic alkalosis. Pediatr Nephrol 1990;4:169–170.

47. Douglas JB, Healy JK. Nephrotoxic effects of amphotericin B, including renal tubular acidosis. Am J Med 1969;46:154–162.

48. Dorup I, Clausen T. Correlation between magnesium and potassium contents in muscle: Role of Na(+)-K+ pump. Am J Physiol 1993;264:C457–C463.

49. White PC, Mune T, Agarwal AK. 11 beta-Hydroxysteroid dehydrogenase and the syndrome of apparent mineralocorticoid excess. Endocr Rev 1997;18:135–156.

50. Borst JGG, Ten Holt SP, de Vries LA, et al. Synergistic action of liquorice and cortisone in Addison's and Simmond's disease. Lancet 1953;1:657–663.

51. Jeck N, Derst C, Wischmeyer E, et al. Functional heterogeneity of ROMK mutations linked to hyperprostaglandin E syndrome. Kidney Int 2001;59:1803–1811.

52. Stein JH. The pathogenetic spectrum of Bartter's syndrome. Kidney Int 1985;28:85–93.

53. Birkenhager R, Otto E, Schurmann MJ, et al. Mutation of BSND causes Bartter syndrome with sensorineural deafness and kidney failure. Nat Genet 2001;29:310–314.

54. Hebert SC. Extracellular calcium-sensing receptor: Implications for calcium and magnesium handling in the kidney. Kidney Int 1996;50:2129–2139.

55. Chou CL, Chen YH, Chau T, et al. Acquired Bartter-like syndrome associated with gentamicin administration. Am J Med Sci 2005;329:144–149.

56. Fava C, Montagnana M, Rosberg L, et al. Subjects heterozygous for genetic loss of function of the thiazide-sensitive cotransporter have reduced blood pressure. Hum Mol Genet. 2008;17:413–418.

57. Simon DB, Nelson-Williams C, Bia MJ, et al. Gitelman's variant of Bartter's syndrome, inherited hypokalemic alkalosis, is caused by mutations in the thiazide-sensitive sodium-chloride cotransporter. Nat Genet 1996;12:24–30.

58. Veldhuis JD, Bardin CW, Demers LM. Metabolic mimicry of Bartter's syndrome by covert vomiting: Utility of urinary chloride determinations. Am J Med 1979;66:361–363.

59. Vinci JM, Gill JR, Bowden RE, et al. The kallikrein–kinin system in Bartter's syndrome and its response to prostaglandin synthetase inhibition. J Clin Invest 1978;61:1671–1682.

60. Botero-Velez M, Curtis JJ, Warnock DG. Brief report: Liddle's syndrome revisited: A disorder of sodium reabsorption in the distal tubule. N Engl J Med 1994;330:178–181.

61. Roy S III, Arant BS Jr. Alkalosis from chloride-deficient Neo-Mull-Soy. N Engl J Med 1979; 301:615.

62. Godek SF, Godek JJ, Bartolozzi AR. Hydration status in college football players during consecutive days of twice-a-day preseason practices. Am J Sports Med 2005;33:843–851.

63. Dave S, Honney S, Raymond J, Flume PA. An unusual presentation of cystic fibrosis in an adult. Am J Kidney Dis 2005;45:e41–e44.

64. Rostand SG. Profound hypokalemia in continuous ambulatory peritoneal dialysis. Arch Intern Med 1983;143:377–378.

65. ECC Committee, Subcommittees and Task Forces of the American Heart Association. 2005 American Heart Association Guidelines for Cardiopulmonary Resuscitation and Emergency Cardiovascular Care. Circulation 2005;112:IV1–203.

66. Rubini M. Water excretion in potassium deficient man. J Clin Invest 1961;40:2215–2224.

67. Tizianello A, Garibotto G, Robaudo C, et al. Renal ammoniagenesis in humans with chronic potassium depletion. Kidney Int 1991;40:772–778.

68. Garella S, Chazan JA, Cohen JJ. Saline-resistant metabolic alkalosis or "chloride-wasting nephropathy". Ann Intern Med 1970;73:31–38.

69. Torres VE, Young WF Jr, Offord KP, et al. Association of hypokalemia, aldosteronism, and renal cysts. N Engl J Med 1990;322:345–351.

70. Schwartz WB. Relman AS. Metabolic and renal studies in chronic potassium depletion resulting from overuse of laxatives. J Clin Invest 1953;32:258–271.

71. Kone BC. In: DuBose Jr. TD, Hamm LL, eds. Hypokalemia in Acid–base and Electrolyte Disorders: A companion to Brenner, Rector's the Kidney, WB Saunders, Philadelphia, 2002, 381–394.

72. Sopko JA, Freeman RM. Salt substitutes as a source of potassium. JAMA 1977;238:608–610.

73. Gennari FJ. Hypokalemia. N Engl J Med 1998;339:451–458.
74. Griffing GT, Cole AG, Aurecchia AJ, et al. Amiloride in primary hyperaldosteronism. Clin Pharmacol Ther 1982;31:56–61.
75. Moore ML, Bailey RR. Hyperkalaemia in patients in hospital. N Z Med J 1989;102:557–558.
76. Ahmed J, Weisberg LS. Hyperkalemia in dialysis patients. Semin Dial 2001;14:348–356.
77. Montague, BT, Ouellette, JR, Buller, GK. Retrospective review of the frequency of ECG changes in hyperkalemia. Clin J Am Soc Nephrol 2008;3:324–330.
78. Livingstone, IR, Cumming, WJ. Hyperkalaemic paralysis resembling Guillain–Barre syndrome. Lancet 1979;2:963–964.
79. DuBose TD. Hyperkalemic hyperchloremic metabolic acidosis: Pathophysiologic insights. Kidney Int 1997;51:591–602.
80. Carella M, D'Adamo AP, Grootenboer-Mignot S, et al. A second locus mapping to 2q35–36 for familial pseudohyperkalaemia. Eur J Hum Genet 2004;12:1073–1076.
81. Rosenberg H, Davis M, James D, et al. Malignant hyperthermia. Orphanet J Rare Dis. 2007;2:21.
82. Arrambide K, Toto RD. Tumor lysis syndrome. Semin Nephrol 1993;13:273–280.
83. Sirken G, Raja R, Garces J, et al. Contrast-induced translocational hyponatremia and hyperkalemia in advanced kidney disease. Am J Kidney Dis 2004;43:e31–e35.
84. Chi HT, Hung DZ, Hu WH, et al. Prognostic implications of hyperkalemia in toad toxin intoxication. Hum Exp Toxicol 1998;17:343–346.
85. Martyn JA, Richtsfeld M. Succinylcholine-induced hyperkalemia in acquired pathologic states: Etiologic factors and molecular mechanisms. Anesthesiology 2006;104:158–169.
86. Smith HM, Farrow SJ, Ackerman JD, et al. Cardiac arrests associated with hyperkalemia during red blood cell transfusion: a case series. Anesth Analg 2008;106:1062–1069.
87. Su M, Stork C, Ravuri S, et al. Sustained-release potassium chloride overdose. J Toxicol Clin Toxicol 2001;39:641–648.
88. Parisi A, Alabiso A, Sacchetti M, et al. Complex ventricular arrhythmia induced by overuse of potassium supplementation in a young male football player. Case report. J Sports Med Phys Fitness 2002;42:214–216.
89. Nagasaki A, Takamine W, Takasu N. Severe hyperkalemia associated with "alternative" nutritional cancer therapy. Clin Nutr 2005;24:864–865.
90. Gelfand MC, Zarate A, Knepshield JH. Geophagia A cause of life-threatening hyperkalemia in patients with chronic renal failure. JAMA 1975;234:738–740.
91. Oates, JA, FitzGerald, GA, Branch, RA, et al. Clinical implications of prostaglandin and thromboxane A2 formation. N Engl J Med 1988;319:761–767.
92. Ling BN, Webster CL, Eaton DC. Eicosanoids modulate apical $Ca(2+)$-dependent $K+$ channels in cultured rabbit principal cells. Am J Physiol 1992;263:F116–F126.
93. Kifor, I, Moore, TJ, Fallo, F, et al. Potassium-stimulated angiotensin release from superfused adrenal capsules and enzymatically digested cells of the zona glomerulosa. Endocrinology 1991;129:823–831.
94. Velazquez H, Perazella M, Wright FS, Ellison DH. Renal mechanism of trimethoprim-induced hyperkalemia. Ann Intern Med 1993;119:296–301.
95. Oster JR, Singer I, Fishman LM. Heparin-induced aldosterone suppression and hyperkalemia. Am J Med 1995;98:575–586.
96. Bantle JP, Nath KA, Sutherland DE, et al. Effects of cyclosporine on the renin–angiotensin-system and potassium excretion in renal transplant recipients. Arch Intern Med 1985;145:505–508.
97. White PC. Aldosterone synthase deficiency and related disorders. Mol Cell Endocrinol 2004;217:81–87.
98. Bonny O, Rossier BC. Disturbances of Na/K balance: Pseudohypoaldosteronism revisited. J Am Soc Nephrol 2002;13:2399–2414.
99. Chang SS, Grunder S, Hanukoglu A, et al. Mutations in the subunits of the epithelial sodium channel cause salt wasting with hyperkalaemic acidosis, pseudohypoaldosteronism type 1. Nat Genet 1996;12:248–253.

100. Arai K, Tsigos C, Suzuki Y, et al. Physiological and molecular aspects of mineralocorticoid action in pseudohypoaldosteronism: A responsiveness test and therapy. J Clin Endocrinol Metab 1994;79:1019–1023.
101. Mayan H, Vered I, Mouallem M, et al. Pseudohypoaldosteronism type II: Marked sensitivity to thiazides, hypercalciuria, normomagnesemia, and low bone mineral density. J Clin Endocrinol Metab 2002;87:3248–3254.
102. Fujieda K, Tajima T: Molecular basis of adrenal insufficiency. Pediatr Res 2005; 57:62R–69R.
103. Mayo J, Collazos J, Martinez E, Ibarra S. Adrenal function in the human immunodeficiency virus-infected patient. Arch Intern Med 2002;162:1095–1098.
104. DeFronzo RA, Cooke CR, Goldberg M, et al. Impaired renal tubular potassium secretion in systemic lupus erythematosus. Ann Intern Med 1977;86:268–271.
105. Don BR, Schambelan M. Hyperkalemia in acute glomerulonephritis due to transient hyporeninemic hypoaldosteronism. Kidney Int 1990;38:1159–1163.
106. Chan R, Sealey JE, Michelis MF, et al. Renin–aldosterone system can respond to furosemide in patients with hyperkalemic hyporeninism. J Lab Clin Med 1998;132:229–235.
107. Gruskay J, Costarino AT, Polin RA, et al. Nonoliguric hyperkalaemia in the premature infant weighing less than 1000 grams. J Pediatr 1988;113:381–386.
108. Sato K, Kondo T, Iwao H, et al. Internal potassium shift in premature infants: cause of nonoliguric hyperkalemia. J Pediatr 1995;126:109–113.
109. Omar SA, DeCristofaro JD, Agarwal BI, et al. Effect of prenatal steroids on potassium balance in extremely low birth weight neonates. Pediatr 2000;106:561–567.
110. Ohlsson A, Hosking M. Complications following oral administration of exchange resins in extremely low birth weight infants. Eur J Pediatr 1987;146:571–574.
111. Esposito C, Bellotti N, Fasoli G, et al. Hyperkalemia-induced ECG abnormalities in patients with reduced renal function. Clin Nephrol 2004;62:465–468.
112. Greenberg A. Hyperkalemia: Treatment options. Semin Nephrol 1998;18:46–57.
113. Allon M. Hyperkalemia in end-stage renal disease: Mechanisms and management. J Am Soc Nephrol 1995;6:1134–1142.
114. Suki WN. Use of diuretics in chronic renal failure. Kidney Int 1997;59:S33–S35.
115. Scherr L, Ogden DA, Mead AW. Management of hyperkalemia with cation-exchange resin. N Engl J Med 1961;264:115–119.
116. Dardik A, Moesinger RC, Efron G, et al. Acute abdomen with colonic necrosis induced by Kayexalate-sorbitol. South Med J 2000;93:511–513.
117. Allon M, Shanklin N. Effect of albuterol treatment on subsequent dialytic potassium removal. Am J Kidney Dis 1995;26:607–613.
118. Knoll GA, Sahgal A, Nair RC, et al. Renin–angiotensin system blockade and the risk of hyperkalemia in chronic hemodialysis patients. Am J Med 2002;112:110–111.

II — Disorders of Calcium, Magnesium and Phosphorus Homeostasis

4 Disorders of Calcium Metabolism

Charles P. McKay

Key Points

1. Three organ systems are involved in the transport of calcium into the extracellular fluid: gastrointestinal, renal, and bone.
2. Two interdependent endocrine systems are responsible for the control of the concentration of extracellular calcium: parathyroid and vitamin D axis.
3. For disorders of extracellular calcium concentrations in complicated patients, measure ionized calcium rather than relying on "corrected" calcium measurements.
4. 25(OH)vitamin D and not 1,25(OH)$_2$vitamin D concentration is the best measure of vitamin D deficiency.
5. In refractory hypocalcemia, especially in infants, hypomagnesemia should be considered as a possible cause.
6. Hypercalcemia generally results from increased absorption from the gastrointestinal tract, decreased excretion by the kidneys, or an imbalance of bone mineralization and resorption.
7. In contrast to adults where primary hyperparathyroidism and hypercalcemia of malignancy account for the vast majority of cases of hypercalcemia, these conditions are relatively rare in childhood.

Key Words: Calcium; hypercalcemia; hypocalcemia; parathyroid hormone; bisphosphonates; vitamin D

1. INTRODUCTION

Calcium plays several very diverse roles in the body. In the skeleton where 99% of the calcium lies, calcium crystals provides structural integrity, in the extracellular fluid ionized calcium modulates enzymatic processes and acts as an important intracellular second messenger. To provide these functions, its concentration in the extracellular and intracellular fluids must be tightly regulated and calcium balance must be maintained to assure skeletal integrity. Calcium balance is achieved by transport across three organ systems: the intestine, the kidney, and bone. Two hormones are primarily responsible for regulation of the control of the calcium fluxes across the membranes of these organs: parathyroid hormone (PTH) and 1,25-dihydroxyvitamin D (1,25(OH)$_2$D).

From: *Nutrition and Health: Fluid and Electrolytes in Pediatrics*
Edited by: L. G. Feld, F. J. Kaskel, DOI 10.1007/978-1-60327-225-4_4,
© Humana Press, a part of Springer Science+Business Media, LLC 2010

2. DISTRIBUTION OF CALCIUM IN THE BODY

The total amount of calcium in the body increases from 30 g at birth to about 1300 g in adulthood *(1)*. It is the most abundant electrolyte in the body but 99% is in the mineral phase of bone where the majority exists in crystalline form as hydroxyapatite $[Ca_{10}(PO4)_6(OH)_2]$. The other 1% is in the teeth, soft tissues and extracellular space. It is the 1 g of calcium in the plasma and extravascular space that is responsible for the control of multiple biologic systems and is regulated by PTH and vitamin D *(2, 3)*.

2.1. Serum Calcium

Normal serum calcium concentrations range from 9.0 to 10.5 mg/dL, although normal values vary by age and from laboratory to laboratory *(4, 5)*. About 50% of the total calcium exists in the ionized form (Ca^{2+}), 40% is bound to protein, and 10% complexed with phosphate, citrate, bicarbonate, and lactate. The ionized and complexed fractions together make up the ultrafilterable calcium, which can cross membranes such as the glomerular basement membrane. Ionized calcium is the physiologically important moiety. It can freely exchangeable across membranes, is responsible for regulation of cellular processes, and is highly regulated by PTH and vitamin D.

The percentage of Ca^{2+} can be altered by a number of factors including the concentration of albumin, the complexing anions, and blood pH. The most important variation in the fraction of ionized calcium occurs with changes in the concentration of albumin, which accounts for 75–90% of the protein bound calcium. Protein bound calcium acts as a rapidly available reserve pool during periods of rapid change in total calcium. Each gram of albumin binds approximately 0.8 mg of calcium. In hypoproteinemic states such as nephrotic syndrome, total calcium may be low but the concentration of Ca^{2+} remains in the normal range. Since calcium binding to albumin is pH dependent, changes in serum pH will affect the concentration of ionized calcium without altering the level of total calcium. During alkalosis, binding to albumin increases so the concentration of ionized calcium can drop resulting in physiologic changes such as tetany while measurements of total calcium remain in the normal range. The levels of the complexing anions are less commonly associated with physiologically important changes in the ionized calcium but there are rare circumstances such as with "citrate lock" where very high levels of citrate are associated with high total serum calcium but low ionized calcium. In general changes in total calcium are equally distributed across all three fractions. Since only about 10–15% of the albumin binding sites for calcium are occupied, albumin has the capacity to bind extra calcium in hypercalcemic states.

2.2. Distribution Across Cellular Membranes

In contrast to extracellular fluids where Ca^{2+} is 10^{-3} M, the concentration of cytosolic calcium is 10^{-6} M *(2)*. The level of Ca^{2+} is maintained by a series of pumps and transporters that extrude calcium from the cell, intracellular organelles which sequester calcium and by the binding of calcium to organic and inorganic compounds in the cytosol. The two major mechanisms responsible for the transport across the cell membrane or into the organelles are the Na^+–Ca^{2+} exchanger (NCX) and Ca^{2+}-ATPase (PMCA).

These cellular processes must protect the level of intracellular Ca^{2+} despite a 1000-fold gradient of calcium across the plasma membrane and a 50-mV electrical gradient that also favors entry of calcium into the cell. The mitochondria and the endoplasmic reticulum can also sequester calcium. There is a Ca-uniporter in mitochondria that can trap calcium in the form of amorphous tricalcium phosphate and help maintain cytosolic Ca^{2+}. Without proper functioning of these processes, toxic levels of calcium would enter the cell and lead to cell death. Inside the cell, calcium also performs important intracellular signaling function by the opening of Ca^{2+} channels by the second messenger IP_3.

2.3. Calcium Distribution During Neonatal Period

The fetus accumulates 120–150 mg of calcium per kilogram body weight from across the placenta during the third trimester resulting in approximately a whole body calcium content of 30 g in the normal full term infant (1, 6). The concentration of serum total and ionized calcium falls after birth. The normal total calcium in cord blood from term infants starts above 10 mg/dL and falls to a nadir at 24 h whereas in preterm infants the concentration starts slightly lower but falls to a much lower nadir at 48 h of life and may not return to the baseline concentration until the 5th day of life (Table 1). A rise in the concentration of phosphorus and bicarbonate also may cause a physiologically significant fall in ionized calcium as the proportion of complexed calcium increases.

Table 1
Mean Serum Calcium Concentrations (mg/dL) in Term and Preterm Infants Over First 5 Days of Life

Age	Term	Preterm
Birth (Cord Blood)	10.2	8.96
Day 1	9.0	7.76
Day 2	9.56	7.4
Day 5	9.84	8.88

3. HOMEOSTASIS

After birth, calcium enters the body from absorption of dietary calcium in the intestine (7). The calcium can be excreted by the kidneys through the processes of filtration and reabsorption or it can enter the skeleton, which is the largest repository of calcium. Calcium fluxes in and out of bone through the processes of bone mineralization and bone resorption but there is also a significant rapidly exchangeable calcium pool. During development, the body must protect the concentration of calcium in the serum and extracellular fluid while maintaining sufficient calcium intestinal absorption and retention by the kidneys to allow skeletal growth. The body must adjust for variability of dietary calcium and factors that affect renal calcium handling. The adaptations to these challenges are mediated largely by PTH and $1,25(OH)_2D$ although there is also a role for growth hormone and the sex steroids.

3.1. Systemic Transport of Calcium

3.1.1. INTESTINE

The intestine is the only organ system by which calcium enters the body *(7)*. The net amount of calcium absorbed normally equals the amount deposited in bone and lost in the urine and sweat. The net absorption of calcium is approximately 30% of the normal dietary intake with variation from 20 to 60% depending on the intake and the age of the individual with net absorption in the normal newborn approaching the upper range. The balance of calcium must also account for the 100–200 mg/day of calcium secreted from pancreatic and biliary juices and mucosal secretion. Intestinal absorption occurs by both passive and active transport and at low intakes the active transport is stimulated by 1,25(OH)$_2$D increasing net absorption.

Active transport across the intestinal mucosa is transcellular and occurs in the duodenum and upper jejunum, which are normally responsible for 90% of the calcium absorption *(8)*. The duodenum is the segment most responsive to stimulation of active transport by 1,25(OH)$_2$D. The cellular processes of active transport involve transport of calcium across the apical membrane, movement across the cytoplasm and then extrusion across the basolateral membrane into the interstitial fluid. Influx of calcium into the cell is mediated by the calcium transport protein 1 (TRPV6). Calcium then is transported along the microvillar stalk by calmodulin/myosin to the glycocalyx where it is then bound to vesicles containing the calcium binding protein calbindin 9K. This compound is involved in the transport of calcium across the cytosol while protecting the cell from potential toxic effects of concentrations of calcium. On the basolateral surface, calcium is extruded from the cell by low-affinity, high capacity Na$^+$–Ca^{2+} exchanger and energy-dependent, high affinity, limited capacity Ca^{2+}-ATPase. To move calcium across the intestinal cell requires a "pump" action that is provided by Ca^{2+}-ATPase.

In contrast to the active transport, passive absorption occurs by diffusion from the lumen to the blood by diffusion via a paracellular pathway. This pathway becomes more significant as calcium intakes increase in part due to inhibition of 1,25(OH)$_2$D levels. Factors that increase calcium absorption include the young age, low calcium and phosphorus intake, vitamin D, and PTH through activation of 1,25(OH)$_2$D formation. Glucocorticoids can also decrease calcium absorption.

Calcium absorption in preterm infants fed human milk has been measured to be as high as 60–70% with formula fed infants absorbing 35–60% *(1, 6, 9)*. Net retention of calcium though is limited by phosphorus content and other mediators of solubility. In preterm infants the fatty acid content of most preterm formulas may limit calcium absorption, a problem that is ameliorated with fat blends that do not result in calcium soap formation. Even with optimal feeding, the preterm infant cannot match the accretion of calcium achieved during the last trimester of pregnancy with calcium transport across the placenta.

3.1.2. KIDNEY

Renal calcium handling is the product of filtration at the glomerulus and reabsorption by the renal tubule *(2, 3)*. The ionized and complexed fractions of calcium combined make up the "ultrafilterable" portion and this fraction that is equal to about 60% of the total calcium, which is freely filtered. Approximately 8 g of calcium are filtered daily in the adult, which exceeds by about 10-fold the calcium content of the non-skeletal calcium. After filtration, about 98% of the filtered load is normally reabsorbed resulting in the adult of 150–200 mg of calcium appearing in the urine. By matching the amount of calcium absorbed by the intestine, renal excretion in the adult keeps calcium in balance. In contrast, in the growing child, calcium excretion is less than net intestinal absorption, which results in net retention of calcium and accretion by the skeleton.

Calcium is reabsorbed by the different segments in the renal tubule in the following proportions: 65% proximal tubule, 20% thick ascending limb, 10% distal tubule, and 2% collecting duct. The proximal convoluted tubule (PCT) is responsible for the majority of the reabsorption of calcium. The mechanisms responsible include solvent drag, increased tubular concentration of calcium as result of sodium and water reabsorption and as result of the transepithelial potential difference. Whereas the majority of the reabsorption is passive and paracellular, there is also evidence of an active transcellular component as well. In the proximal straight tubule, which includes the parts of the S_2 and S_3 segments, the reabsorption is passive in S_2 and active in S_3. Ca^{2+}-ATPase (PMCA) appears to play the predominant role in straight portion of the proximal tubule with there being involvement of the Na^+–Ca^{2+} exchanger (NCX).

The thick ascending limb of the loop of Henle is very important for calcium reabsorption and its control (10). This segment, which accounts for about 20% of calcium reabsorption, is the site of regulation of calcium excretion by PTH and calcitonin. There appears to be both active transcellular and passive paracellular mechanisms. The reabsorption is coupled to sodium reabsorption and is inhibited by the loop diuretics: furosemide, bumetanide, and ethacrynic acid. The calcium sensing receptor, CaSR, has also been linked to the control of calcium as well as sodium and magnesium reabsorption in this segment of the renal tubule. Finally, recent studies have shown that the epithelial tight junction protein paracellin-1 (PCLN1) also plays an important role in both calcium and magnesium reabsorption. Under resting conditions, calcium transport across the thick ascending limb is driven by the transepithelial potential difference with the lumen being positive as generated by sodium reabsorption by the Na–K–2Cl transporter. Decreased activity of this transporter by the loop diuretics lowers the potential difference and calcium reabsorption. Paracellin-1 allows selective permeability for calcium and magnesium while otherwise establishing a tight junction for the passage of other ions.

Calcium reabsorption in the distal convoluted tubule is interesting for a number of reasons including its disassociation from sodium reabsorption in certain circumstances. The epithelial transport is all transcellular and is against the electrochemical gradient. Entry of calcium into the cells from the apical membrane involves the calcium channel (TRPV6) and has been suggested to be the rate-limiting step for calcium transport in this segment. The insertion of these calcium channels into the membrane is increased by agents such as PTH and calcitonin that stimulate calcium reabsorption. Calcium diffuses across the cytosol while being bound by the vitamin D stimulated calcium binding protein, calbindin D_{28K}. At the basolateral surface, calcium is extruded from the cell by PMCA, possibly with the involvement of the calcium binding protein, calbindin D_{9K}. The presence of the CaSR in the basolateral membrane of the DCT cells suggests a possible role in this segment as well. One of the interesting features of calcium transport across the distal tubule is the stimulation by thiazide diuretics. These agents, which inhibit the entry of sodium across the apical membrane by the Na^+–Cl^- cotransporter, have been shown to activate apical calcium entry through calcium channels and extrusion of calcium across the basolateral surface by a Na^+–Ca^{2+} exchange.

There is further transport in the connecting tubule and collecting duct accounting for about 1–2% of total calcium reabsorption. This transport is stimulated by amiloride, which inhibits the apical sodium channel suggesting a mechanism involving a sodium calcium exchange that drives calcium exit across the basolateral membrane. Other mechanisms described in the distal nephron include active transport involving either the Na^+–Ca^{2+} exchanger (NCX) or Ca^{2+}-ATPase (PMCA).

3.1.3. BONE

Bone is the repository of more than 99% of the total body calcium *(7)*. Skeletal calcium exists in both a rapidly exchangeable pool as well as a much more slowly exchangeable pool. The latter refers to calcium in the form of hydroxyapatite that is deposited with collagen fibers whereas the rapidly exchangeable pool is much more poorly characterized but includes calcium at the site of active bone formation. The processes of bone formation and bone resorption are generally well coordinated or "coupled." Due to the large amount of calcium constantly entering and leaving bone, disease states that disturb the coupling of bone resorption and mineralization can overwhelm other physiologic systems in the body to maintain calcium homeostasis.

Osteoblasts, the cells responsible for bone mineralization, arise from bone marrow derived osteoprogenitor cells and are also responsible for activation of osteoclasts *(11)*. Osteoblasts activated by PTH (Section 3.2.1) express the ligand (RANKL) for a receptor on osteoclasts and their precursors termed "receptor for activation of nuclear factor kappa B" or RANK *(12)*. PTH also increases the production of macrophage-colony stimulating factor (M-CSF), which is also required for osteoclastic differentiation. The activity of RANK is also normally suppressed by a decoy receptor for RANKL called osteoprotegerin (OPG), which is formed by osteoblasts and whose secretion is also decreased by PTH. Osteoblasts therefore in response to PTH stimulate osteoclasts to differentiate and to resorb bone by expressing RANKL, secreting M-CSF, and decreasing levels of the inhibitor OPG. This coupling between osteoblasts and osteoclasts is responsible for the increases and decreases in mineralization and bone resorption that occurs during skeletal remodeling.

3.1.4. PLACENTA

Transport of calcium across the placenta is an active process for transfer of calcium from the mother to the fetus *(6, 13)*. The mechanism is active transport by a calcium pump in the basal membrane of the placental cells that normally maintains a positive fetal–maternal gradient. This process is regulated by parathyroid hormone related protein (PTHrP), which appears to be produced in the placenta as well as the fetal parathyroid glands. Fetal PTH otherwise controls the level of serum calcium in the fetus and is involved in bone mineralization. During the third trimester of pregnancy, 120–150 mg calcium/kg fetal weight is transported daily across the placenta. This movement of calcium is critical for normal fetal bone accretion and cannot be matched in the extremely preterm infant through other routes. This very large influx of calcium into the exchangeable pool of calcium is lost at the time of birth and homeostatic mechanisms must be in play to avoid the development of severe hypocalcemia.

3.2. Regulation of Calcium Metabolism

3.2.1. PARATHYROID

The parathyroid gland plays the central role in the control of calcium metabolism through the secretion of parathyroid hormone (PTH) *(14)*. The primary regulator of serum PTH levels is serum calcium, which inhibits PTH secretion through activation of the calcium-sensing receptor (CaSR). CaSR is a G-protein coupled receptor on the surface of parathyroid cells that responds to changes in extracellular calcium by actions on a series of effects depending on duration of effect *(15)*. There is an increase in the secretion of preformed PTH in seconds to minutes, an increase PTH gene expression over several hours to a few days then finally an increase in the number of parathyroid cells through cell proliferation in a time period taking days or longer. There have been described activating and inactivating defects of the CaSR gene, which lead to states of hypo- and hyperparathyroidism. The CaSR is also the target of a class of medications called "calcimimetics" or "calcilytics," which suppress or activate PTH secretion, respectively.

Other regulators of PTH secretion include $1,25(OH)_2D$ and extracellular phosphate, both of which inhibit secretion. The mechanism for suppression of PTH by vitamin D is through the vitamin D receptor, which acts as a nuclear transcription factor. The effects of vitamin D and phosphate on PTH secretion are more long-term than calcium and predominantly affect PTH gene expression and cell proliferation.

The actions of PTH in the body are mediated by through the PTH/PTHrP receptor (PTH1R), which is a G-protein coupled receptor that then activates adenylate cyclase or phospholipase C *(3)*. Many tissues express PTH1R but the kidney and bone have the greatest physiologic relevance for mineral homeostasis. Defects in the $G\alpha_s$ peptide as found in pseudohypoparathyroidism type 1, result in hypocalcemia, hyperphosphatemia, and a variety of bone defects. In bone, osteoblasts and their precursors are directly activated by PTH where they stimulate the differentiation and activation of osteoclasts through activation of RANK (Section 3.1.3). In response to PTH, there is release of calcium from the rapidly exchangeable pool at the surface of bone in minutes and from a more slowly exchangeable pool within hours. As osteoclasts are stimulated to resorb bone, phosphate and collagen degradation products are released into bloodstream.

In the kidney, PTH receptors are found along the renal tubule where it activates PTH1R leading to a variety of actions. PTH regulates mineral metabolism in the kidney by stimulating calcium reabsorption, phosphate excretion, and $1,25(OH)_2D$ formation. PTH stimulates calcium reabsorption by activating paracellular mechanisms in the thick ascending limb and transcellular processes in the distal convoluted tubule (Section 3.1.2). Despite the fact that PTH stimulates calcium reabsorption, in hyperparathyroid states with hypercalcemia, calcium excretion is elevated as result of the increased filtered load resulting from calcium released from bone and absorbed from the intestine.

In response to hypocalcemic stresses, PTH stimulates both calcium and phosphorus release from bone (directly) and absorption from the intestine (indirectly through $1,25(OH)_2D$ formation *(3)*. To maintain serum calcium, the excess phosphate must be excreted and PTH stimulates phosphaturia by blocking the sodium-dependent phosphate in the proximal renal tubule through inhibition of expression of the phosphate transporter NPT-2a. In hyperparathyroid states, hypophosphatemia is the result. PTH increases calcium by stimulating the synthesis of 25-hydroxyvitamin D_3-1-α-hydroxylase found in mitochondria of the proximal renal tubule. This process over hours increases the formation of $1,25(OH)_2D$ that stimulates calcium absorption in the intestine and calcium release from bone.

3.2.2. VITAMIN D AXIS

Vitamin D through its biologically active form $1,25(OH)_2D$ plays a central role in calcium homeostasis *(14)*. $1,25(OH)_2D$ stimulates absorption of dietary calcium and recruits stem cells in bone to form osteoclasts, which can then release calcium from the skeleton. $1,25(OH)_2D$ acts as a hormone in the body whose formation in the kidney is highly regulated by PTH, calcium, phosphate and other factors. There are now well-described non-calcemic functions for vitamin D where local formation of $1,25(OH)_2D$ leads to autocrine and paracrine effects.

Vitamin D can either be formed in the skin or be absorbed in the diet but the latter pathway usually requires supplementation because of the paucity of natural sources. Formation in the skin involves the transformation of 7-dehydroxycholesterol (provitamin D_3) by sunlight to previtamin D_3, which is rapidly isomerized to vitamin D_3 (cholecalciferol). Continued or excessive sunlight leads to the conversion of vitamin D_3 to inert products, which prevents toxic amounts of vitamin D from resulting from sun exposure. Many factors can modulate the cutaneous formation of vitamin D_3 including the amount of melanin in the skin, the intensity of the suns rays, the age of the patient, and the use of sunscreens. The vitamin D_3 that is formed is then bound to vitamin D-binding protein in the blood. Dietary vitamin D usually comes from certain foods such as oily fish but more commonly comes from either supplements or fortified foods. Fortified foods such as milk usually contain vitamin D_2 (ergocalciferol) but supplements can contain either vitamin D_3 or vitamin D_2. Whereas in the past, these two forms were thought to be biologically equal, more recent evidence suggests that vitamin D_3 may be 2–3 times more potent.

To become biologically active, vitamin D must undergo two hydroxylation steps *(16)*. The first occurs in the liver where one of several cytochrome P_{450}-vitamin D-25-hydroxylases converts vitamin D to $25(OH)D$ in substrate dependent, non-regulated process. This compound is then transported in the blood to the kidney and other tissues where it can undergo further metabolism. In the proximal renal tubule, where it is bound to $25(OH)D$-DBP and taken in to the cell where the cytochrome P_{450}-mono-oxygenase, $25(OH)$-1-α-hydroxylase (CYP27B1) converts it to $1,25(OH)_2D$.

The conversion from 25(OH)- to 1,25(OH)$_2$D is stimulated by PTH, low serum phosphate and low calcium. Other regulators include fibroblast growth factor-23 (FGF-23) that lowers 1,25(OH)$_2$D formation and IGF-1 that increases it. Another important determinant of 1,25(OH)$_2$D concentration is metabolism by the renal 24-hydroxylase (CYP24), which can act on both 25(OH)D and 1,25(OH)$_2$D to form 24,25(OH)$_2$D and 1,24,25(OH)$_3$D, respectively.

1,25(OH)$_2$D works to maintain serum calcium by its affects on the intestine and bone. This steroid hormone binds to the vitamin D receptor (VDR) in the cytoplasm in its target tissues after it translocates to the nucleus and forms a heterodimeric complex with RXR. This complex then is able to bind to chromosomal VDR response element (VDRE) where after binding other initiation factors, and the transcription of vitamin D responsive genes are either enhanced or inhibited. In the intestine, such genes as the TRPV6, calbindin 9 K, and other proteins promote calcium transport across the intestinal epithelial cell. In bone, the proteins induced by activation of VDR by 1,25(OH)$_2$D in osteoblasts include RANKL, alkaline phosphatase, osteocalcin, and osteoprotegerin. The stimulation of bone mineralization by vitamin D is through its ability to maintain adequate levels of calcium and phosphorus rather than by direct effects on bone.

3.2.3. OTHER

Calcitonin is a peptide hormone secreted by the C cells in the thyroid in response to elevated levels of serum calcium (17). It can inhibit osteoclasts although the exact physiologic significance in human mineral metabolism is unclear. There are reports of elevated calcitonin in certain hypocalcemic conditions. Parathyroid hormone-related protein (PTHrP), which is part of the PTH gene family and can activate a common receptor (PTH1R), functions primarily in the fetus where formation of the cartilaginous growth plate, transport of calcium across the placenta, and development of the teeth. Postnatally, the most important function for PTHrP appears to be the development of the mammary gland and transport of calcium into breast milk. Clinically though, PTHrP is important as the most common mediator of hypercalcemia of malignancy.

4. CLINICAL ASSESSMENT OF CALCIUM DISORDERS – INTRODUCTION

Evaluation of calcium disorders requires proper measurement and interpretation of the divalent ions, calcium, phosphorus, and magnesium. Secondly the evaluation of the calcium regulating hormones, parathyroid hormone (PTH), vitamin D metabolites and in hypercalcemia, parathyroid hormone-related protein (PTHrP) is essential to evaluate their role in or response to changes in serum calcium. Studies of renal calcium handling may be helpful but is a less useful tool than the previous mentioned studies. Finally radiologic studies of the skeleton may help pinpoint certain diagnoses. Markers of bone turnover, bone density measurements, and bone biopsy are important in the evaluation of skeletal health but do not add significantly to the evaluation of disorders of calcium metabolism.

5. MEASUREMENT OF DIVALENT IONS

5.1. Serum Calcium

Serum calcium is made up by three fractions: protein-bound, complexed, and ionized. The ionized portion, representing about 50% of the total, is the only one that is physiologically important (7). Ionized calcium helps maintain normal blood coagulation, membrane stability, bone mineralization, and other process and is the only portion that is regulated by PTH and 1,25-dihydroxyvitamin D (1,25(OH$_2$)D). Disorders of serum calcium are often expressed by deviation of total calcium from normal although it is the level of ionized calcium that is clinically relevant. Therefore changes in ionized calcium are the product of the total serum calcium and relative distribution between the three fractions.

Total serum calcium is measured by most laboratories using automated spectrophotometric analysis using dyes such as o-cresolphthalein as an indicator (4). In most clinical use in the United States, the calcium concentration is expressed as mg/dL. With an atomic weight of 40.08 and valence of 2, this value can be easily converted to mmol/L (mM) and mEq/L by dividing by 4 and 2, respectively. The normal value for total calcium ranges from about 9–10.4 but can vary by age with greater values in infants and young children (Table 2). Total calcium should be measured either in serum or heparinized plasma whereas plasma from samples using citrate, oxalate, or EDTA that form complexes with calcium should be avoided. Hemolysis, icterus, and lipemic samples can also interfere with the normal spectrophotometric analysis.

Table 2
Total (mg/dL) and Ionized (mM) Calcium Serum Concentrations in Childhood

Age (years)	Total calcium	Ionized calcium
Infants 0.25–1	8.8–11.3	1.22–1.4
Young child 1–5	9.4–10.8	1.22–1.32
Older child 6–12	9.4–10.3	1.15–1.32
Adolescents	9–10.2	1.12–1.3

Total calcium measurements also display both postural and circadian increases of up to 0.5 mg/dL during midday when an upright position leads to increased albumin concentrations, which accounts for up to 90% of protein bound calcium (18). Improper tourniquet technique causing venous stasis can also increase albumin and total calcium (19). The proportion of total calcium that is protein-bound to albumin is also altered by changes in pH that changes the conformation of albumin. An increase in pH of 0.1 will increase the protein-bound form of calcium by about 1.2 mg/dL resulting in the lowering of the physiologically and clinically relevant ionized portion of 0.05 mM (20). The shifting of calcium to the protein-bound fraction with alkalosis is a common cause of hypocalcemia and tetany in the patent with a borderline ionized calcium level. Disease states that are associated with low levels of serum albumin such as nephrotic syndrome or liver cirrhosis characteristically have low total calcium but normal ionized calcium levels.

To better evaluate the clinically relevant ionized portion of the total serum calcium a number of formulas have been suggested to "correct" the serum calcium for changes in albumin including: corrected serum calcium (mg/dL) = total calcium (mg/dL) + 0.8 (4) – serum albumin (g/dL) (2). It has been found that these "corrected" values poorly predict the changes in ionized calcium in many individuals. Changes in pH, the complexing anions citrate, and phosphate, and other factors can all alter ionized calcium in ways not appreciated with "corrected" values. With the availability of semi-automated instruments using ion-specific electrodes to measure ionized calcium, it is now recommended to directly measure ionized calcium in the sick and hospitalized patients (21). Routine use of total calcium measurements in relatively well outpatients is usually adequate. The normal levels of ionized calcium do vary by age but not to the extent as total calcium (Table 2). There are minor circadian effects on ionized calcium and samples should be collected anaerobically to avoid pH effects. Heparinized plasma samples for rapid analysis are best collected with either 50 IU/ml of calcium-titrated heparin or 15 U/ml of lithium heparin and the tubes completely filled to avoid dilutional and heparin effects.

5.2. Serum Phosphate

The measurement of serum phosphate is covered more comprehensively in later chapters but is considered briefly here because of its importance in evaluation of calcium disorders. It is the inorganic phosphorus in the form of phosphate in blood that is measured and is expressed as phosphate (4, 18). Again serum is preferred but heparinized samples can be used but the values are 0.2–0.3 mg/dL lower. Citrate, oxalate, and EDTA that interfere with the analysis method should be avoided. Serum or plasma should be rapidly separated from red blood cells that contain greater amounts of phosphorus and can artifactual increases. Phosphorus levels are usually expressed in mg/dL or with its atomic weight of 30.98, in mM by dividing by 3.1. To express in mEq/L, the value is pH dependent since there is a mixture of monovalent and divalent ions with a composite valence of 1.8 at pH 7.4. Therefore at normal pH, the mEq of phosphorus can be calculated by multiplying the mM by 1.8.

There is both a significant circadian rhythm to serum phosphate levels as well as a dietary effect that can increase phosphorus levels by 1.2 mg/dL. The optimal time to measure phosphate is a morning, fasting sample. Factors that can redistribute phosphorus into cells such as insulin, glucose, and other carbohydrate loads, respiratory alkalosis and epinephrine, all can acutely lower phosphorus levels as much as 2 mg/dL. Much more than calcium, there is strong role of age in phosphorus levels. Normal phosphorus levels fall from a normal range of 4.8–7.4 mg/dL in infants to 4.5–6.2 mg/dL young children to a range of 3.5–5.5 mg/dL in older children till late adolescence.

5.3. Serum Magnesium

Serum magnesium has three fractions as calcium but in different proportions (see also Section 5, Chapter 8, Clinical Assessment of Magnesium Metabolism in Infants and Children). The protein-bound portion of magnesium is only 30%, complexed portion makes up 15%, and the ionized portion represents 55% of total serum magnesium *(4)*. Like calcium, it is the ionized portion that is physiologically and clinically important since it involved in neuromuscular and cardiovascular function. Unlike calcium, the measurement of ionized magnesium is not measured in clinical situations. The normal serum concentration of magnesium is 1.6–2.4 mg/dL and does not vary significantly with age. With a molecular weight of 24.31 and valence of 2, to convert the concentration of magnesium from mg/dL to mM, the value is divided by 2.4 and by 1.2 to derive the concentration in mEq/L *(19)*.

6. MEASUREMENT OF CALCIOTROPIC HORMONES

6.1. Parathyroid Hormone

The normal inverse relationship between serum calcium and PTH secretion makes measurement of PTH an invaluable tool in the evaluation of disorders of serum calcium. If control of PTH secretion is intact and not part of the primary cause of the disturbance in serum calcium, PTH levels should be suppressed in hypercalcemia and elevated in hypercalcemia. PTH is now routinely measured by 2-site assays that recognize the "intact" PTH molecules and not fragments as were recognized by older "mid-region" and "carboxy-terminal" assays *(21)*. There are both immunoradiometric assays (IRMA) that use radioactive tracers and immunochemiluminometric assays (ICMA) that have the advantage of not needing radioactivity. The normal ranges for each assay are laboratory specific but the normal adult range are usually about 10–65 pg/ml. Over the last few years, "third generation" PTH assays that measure "whole molecule" has been promoted for use with renal failure, but there is no current indication for their use with hypo- and hypercalcemic disorders.

PTH as measured by the intact PTH assays has a very short half-life (2–4 min) and has been shown to demonstrate pulsatile secretion *(22)*. Because of the inverse relationship between calcium and PTH secretion, PTH levels should be performed with simultaneous calcium levels. In the presence of non-parathyroid hypercalcemia, PTH values are below the normal range in 70–80% of patients and below 25 pg/ml in the rest. In patients with primary hyperparathyroidism, 90% will have elevated PTH levels by the intact assay with the rest having PTH levels inappropriately elevated for the degree of hypercalcemia. In patients with hypocalcemia and hypoparathyroidism, PTH levels are usually below the normal range or inappropriately low for the level of calcium in contrast to non-parathyroid causes of hypocalcemia where secondary hyperparathyroidism with high PTH levels are expected.

6.2. Vitamin D

The two vitamin D metabolites with assays available for measurement are 25-hydroxyvitamin D (25(OH)D) and 1,25(OH$_2$)D. 25(OH)D is the major circulating form of vitamin D and reflects vitamin D nutrition including cutaneous formation *(16)*. In contrast, the levels of biologically active 1,25(OH$_2$)D normally reflect the highly regulated renal formation that is stimulated by high PTH and low phosphorus and calcium levels. 25(OH)D is measured most often by a competitive protein-binding assay after chromatography over a C-18 silica column *(23)*. The normal values are 10–80 ng/ml (25–200 nmol/L) but can vary seasonally with higher levels in summer and fall after sun exposure *(20)*. Lower levels are often seen in people with greater skin pigmentation or who live at higher latitudes. $1,25(OH_2)D$ normally circulates in concentrations of 20–60 pg/ml (50–150 pmol/l) and where it is not affected by season, there are higher levels recorded in infants and children. Vitamin D exists in two forms: cholecalciferol (vitamin D_3) and ergocalciferol (vitamin D_2). Cholecalciferol is naturally formed in the skin whereas ergocalciferol is artificially derived from yeast. Despite the ability of certain assays to differentiate between vitamin D_2 and D_3, in general for both 25(OH)D and $1,25(OH_2)D$, both D_2 and D_3 are measured because the total is most clinically relevant.

Measurement of 25(OH)D is useful in determining the presence of vitamin D deficiency or excess in hypocalcemia and hypercalcemia, respectively *(20, 23)*. In vitamin D deficiency, serum 25(OH)D levels are less than 8 ng/ml whereas in hypercalcemia due to vitamin D intoxication, levels greater than 200 ng/ml are required. In contrast to 25(OH)D, $1,25(OH_2)D$ is usually normal in vitamin D deficiency and its measurement is only useful in selective clinical situations. Levels can be high in the presence of hypercalcemia due to extrarenal production of $1,25(OH_2)D$ by certain lymphomas and granulomatous disorders such as sarcoidosis. Levels are characteristically low in patients with vitamin D dependent rickets type 1 who lack the renal 25(OH)-1-α-hydroxylase and very high in vitamin D dependent rickets type 2 in which there is the lack of the vitamin D receptor leading to hypocalcemia, secondary hyperparathyroidism, and stimulation of $1,25(OH_2)D$ formation. For the most part, measurement of $1,25(OH_2)D$ in disorders of serum calcium is inappropriate and not cost-effective.

6.3. Parathyroid Hormone-Related Protein

Parathyroid hormone-related protein (PTHrP) plays a number of important roles in the fetus and in the postnatal period, but after birth it is measurable only in certain rare disease states *(24)*. It is most associated with certain cancers and the syndrome of humoral hypercalcemia of malignancy, which is characterized, by severe hypercalcemia, low serum phosphate, suppressed PTH, and elevated PTHrP. The most common assay is an immunoradiometric assay (IRMA) with an antibody directed against the N-terminal, which shares homology with PTH as well as mid-region that recognizes an area distinct from PTH so the assay can distinguish between PTH and PTHrP *(25)*. Whereas normal individual have levels of <1 pmol/L but most humoral hypercalcemia of malignancy (HHM) patients have levels >5 pmol/L. PTHrP is a very labile molecule and proper handling of the sample is required.

7. CLINICAL EVALUATION OF RENAL DIVALENT HANDLING

The assessment of renal function in patients with disorders of renal handling is three fold. First, is the proper assessment of glomerular filtration rate (GFR) since renal failure may be a cause of hypocalcemia or acute and chronic renal failure may be the result of calcium disorders especially hypercalcemia? For most clinical purposes, serum creatinine is an adequate measure of GFR and normally rises from 0.3 mg/dL after a few weeks of age to adult levels of about 0.8–1 mg/dL by early adolescence. Secondly, assessment of renal calcium excretion gives valuable information about calcium balance and may point to the etiology of hypo- and hypercalcemia as well as the possible role of the kidney. Renal calcium excretion is equal to gastrointestinal calcium absorption minus skeletal calcium balance. In normal healthy children, calcium excretion is less than the calcium absorbed in the GI tract. Conditions associated with low calcium absorption are very low calcium intake, vitamin D deficiency, malabsorption (states possibly associated with hypocalcemia), and familial benign hypocalciuric hypercalcemia where the kidney contributes to the hypercalcemia. In contrast hypercalciuria is usually present in vitamin D induced hypercalcemia, hyperparathyroidism and immobilization and humoral hypercalcemia of malignancy. Under these conditions, hypercalcemia occurs when the kidney can no longer excrete calcium released from bone or absorbed from the GI tract.

Normal calcium excretion can be expressed in relation to body weight with the normal values being less than 4 mg calcium/kg body weight/day. Simultaneous measurement of creatinine should be performed to assess the completeness of the collection and should equal 15–25 mg/kg/day (20). Alternatively, calcium excretion can be expressed as a ratio of creatinine excretion but these results are age dependent (Table 3). Finally, since calcium excretion is dependent on the filtered calcium load, a useful measure of calcium handling is the ratio of calcium clearance to creatinine clearance, which can be calculated in a spot urine sample where the urine volumes cancel out to equal: $Ca_{cl}/Cr_{cl} = (Ca_u \times Cr_s)/(Cr_u \times Ca_s)$. This index is especially helpful in evaluation of familial hypocalciuric hypercalcemia where the index is typically less than 0.01 (26).

Table 3
Calcium Excretion by Age

Age (years)	Ca/cr (mg/mg) 95th percentiles
0.5–1.0	<0.81
1–2	<0.56
2–3	<0.5
4–5	<0.41
5–7	<0.3
7–17	<0.25

8. HYPOCALCEMIA – INTRODUCTION

Hypocalcemia in infants and children is a relatively common disorder especially in the neonate. Hypocalcemia is the result when the influx of calcium in the extracellular fluid does not keep pace with calcium efflux into bone, excretion into the urine or less commonly as deposits into the soft tissue. The level of intravascular calcium is regulated and protected by the parathyroid and vitamin D systems and their effects on bone resorption, renal excretion, and gastrointestinal absorption of calcium. Acute hypocalcemia can cause life-threatening events especially through disordered neuromuscular and cardiovascular physiology.

CASE SCENARIOS

Case Scenario 1: Hypocalcemia in a school aged child.

An 8-year-old boy has been admitted with cramping of his hands and feet that began with a recent illness. He has been healthy except for a chronic infection of his skin and nails for which he sees a dermatologist. Your physical exam of this normal appearing boy includes Chvostek's and Trousseau's signs, both of which are positive. Labs come back with a normal CBC, normal renal function, and electrolytes but a total serum calcium of 7.2 mg/dL, phosphorus of 7.9 mg/dL, and an albumin of 3.9 g/dL.

What is the most likely diagnosis and what studies would you like to perform next? What should your initial treatment be? What other illnesses do you need to be monitoring?

Case Scenario 2: Infant with new onset seizures and heart disease.

An 8-day-old full-term infant with the diagnosis of congenital heart disease from a VSD is found to have a creatinine of 1.4 mg/dL, calcium 6.9 mg/dL, and a phosphorus of 10.2 mg/dL. He is just starting to feed and has been on a standard infant formula. The mother is healthy and is on no medications. On physical exam he has an unusual facies and is extremely jittery. EKG shows an abnormal QT interval.

What is the most likely diagnosis and what studies would you like to order? What would your initial treatment be?

9. DEFINITION OF HYPOCALCEMIA

The lower limits of normal for total serum calcium in children range from 8.8 mg/dL in infants to 9.4 mg/dL in pre-adolescents and dropping back to 9 mg/dL in adolescents (Table 2) *(18)*. The most important fraction – ionized calcium – does not exactly follow total calcium with lower limits of normal of 1.22 mM or 4.9 mg/dL until age 6 years and then it drops slightly to 1.15 in older children and 1.12 in young adults. Some of the variation with age is due to changes protein-bound and complexed fractions of calcium. The latter occurs when serum concentrations of lactate, sulfate, and citrate are elevated. Measurement of total calcium is adequate in most stable out-patients but variations of low serum albumin are an important cause of "pseudohypocalcemia" in which total serum calcium is low but ionized calcium is normal *(27)*. In contrast, changes in pH or excessive levels of citrate can give a picture of normal or even high total calcium in the presence of significant drops in ionized calcium. Total serum calcium can be "corrected" for alterations in serum albumin and pH although in ill or complex patients or in those patients known to have changes in albumin, pH, or one of the complexing anions, ionized calcium should be measured directly.

10. CLINICAL FEATURES

The clinical symptoms related to hypocalcemia are mainly related to affects on the cardiac and neuromuscular systems (Table 4) *(28)*. Some signs and symptoms such as abnormal calcification may be more common in states of abnormal PTH function. The two classic signs are those of Chvostek and Trousseau *(27)*. Chvostek's sign is elicited

Table 4
Clinical Manifestations of Hypocalcemia

Cardiovascular
    Prolonged QT interval on EKG
    Heart failure
Neuromuscular
    Parasthesias, perioral tingling
    Muscle cramps, tetany
    Laryngospasm
    Trousseau's sign
    Chvostek's sign
    Seizures (all types)
    Irritability, abnormal mental function
    Basal ganglion calcifications
Other
    Cataracts, papilledema
    Coarse skin, brittle nails

by tapping with three fingers over the facial nerve anterior to the ear. A positive sign can be arranged from twitching of the lip at the angle of the mouth to twitching of nasolabial fold, lateral angle of the eye or finally all of the facial muscles on that side. The mildest response can be seen in 8% of normocalcemic individuals but more dramatic twitching is specific for hypocalcemia. Trousseau's sign is elicited by pumping a sphygmomanometer cuff 20 mmHg above the systolic BP for 5 min to produce ischemia of the ulnar nerve. A positive sign is when the metacarpophalangeal joints flex, interphalangeal joints extend, and the thumb adducts. Neither of these signs are 100% sensitive.

11. CAUSES OF HYPOCALCEMIA

Normally the body is protected from hypocalcemia by the actions of parathyroid hormone (PTH) and $1,25(OH)_2$vitamin D ($1,25(OH)_2D$). Hypocalcemia results when there abnormal secretion of these two hormones or the body cannot adequately respond to them either because of congenital or acquired conditions (29). PTH acts to lower phosphorus by its actions on the kidney and $1,25(OH)_2D$ increases it by its action on bone and the GI tract. The level of phosphorus therefore is a useful clue to the cause of hypocalcemia because it is elevated in abnormal parathyroid states and low in vitamin D dysfunction (28). Other hypocalcemic conditions can be the result of hyperphosphatemia from endogenous and exogenous sources or be associated with hypophosphatemia as calcium and phosphorus are being deposited in bone (Table 5).

11.1. Hypoparathyroidism

Hypoparathyroidism is characterized by hypocalcemia, hyperphosphatemia, and inappropriately low PTH levels for the calcium level (30, 31). There are transient hypoparathyroid states that are common in young infants and which will be covered

Table 5
Causes of Hypocalcemia

Hyperphosphatemia

Hypoparathyroidism
   Congenital hypoparathyroidism
      DiGeorge and related syndromes
      Maternal hyperparathyroidism
      Calcium receptor activating mutations
   Acquired hypoparathyroidism
      Autoimmune
      Surgical removal or damage
      Hypomagnesemia
PTH resistance
   Pseudohypoparathyroidism
   Hypomagnesemia
Phosphorus loads
   Endogenous
      Tumor lysis, rhabdomyolysis
      Renal failure
   Exogenous
      Phosphorus containing enemas
      High phosphorous formulas

Hypophosphatemia

Vitamin D deficiency
   Lack of sun and dietary
   Malabsorption
   Renal failure
   Increased metabolism
   Vitamin D Dependent Rickets (VDDR) Type I
Resistance to vitamin D – VDDR Type II
Deposition of Ca and P into tissues
   Hungry bone syndrome

Other

Sepsis and other critical illness
Drugs
Pancreatitis
Altered bound calcium-citrate

---

under Neonatal Causes (Section 11.5). The major categories of hypoparathyroidism are agenesis as in DiGeorge syndrome, destruction by surgery, radiation, infiltrative disease, or autoimmune processes and functional such as with severe hypomagnesemia. The causes of hypoparathyroidism can be often be recognized by history and associated findings. With acute surgical hypoparathyroidism, a sudden drop in the PTH level can lead to a condition called "hungry bone syndrome" can develop as result of interrupted bone resorption in the presence of continued bone mineralization. In "hungry bone syndrome" there can be hypophosphatemia in addition to hypocalcemia, which is unusual for other hypoparathyroid states.

There are a number of syndromes associated with agenesis or hypoplasia of the parathyroid glands (Table 6) that usually present in the first week of life with hypocalcemia and tetany *(32)*. The most common is DiGeorge syndrome, which can occur in 1:500 live births. DiGeorge syndrome is due to abnormal development of the 3rd and 4th branchial pouches and can include hypoparathyroidism, immunodeficiency, congenital cardiac defects, and a distinctive facies. In greater than 90% of cases it is due to a microdeletion of chromosomal band 22q11.2 and has been termed "CATCH 22" to refer to the Cardiac, Abnormal facies, Thymic aplasia, Cleft palate, Hypocalcemia with 22q deletion *(33)*. The clinical spectrum may include a Shprintzen (velocardiofacial) syndrome or conotruncal anomaly face syndrome. Genetic diagnosis can be made in most cases with cytogenetic analysis for the 22q11.2 using fluorescence in situ hybridization (FISH). Other chromosomal abnormalities have been associated with a DiGeorge syndrome including deletions of 10p. The degree of the defects can vary in patients with DiGeorge syndrome including normocalcemic infants with normal PTH levels but who cannot respond adequately to a hypocalcemic stress with increased PTH secretion. Other syndromes associated with congenital hypoparathyroidism include Kenny–Caffey (skeletal dysplasia and dwarfism), Kearns–Sayre (mitochondrial myopathy, cardiac conduction defects, and ocular abnormalities), Barakat (nephrosis and sensorineural deafness), and Sanjad–Sakati (IUGR, dysmorphic facies, skeletal defects, and developmental delay) *(30)*.

An autosomal dominant form of hypoparathyroidism results from activating of the gene for the calcium receptor, CaSR. This disorder is the mirror image of familial hypocalciuric hypercalcemia (FHH) and is characterized by hypocalcemia, hypercalciuria, and hypoparathyroidism *(34)*. Recognition of the condition is important to avoid hypercalciuria and nephrocalcinosis with treatment. Another familial hypoparathyroid disorder that can present in either an autosomal dominant or recessive form is due to a PTH gene defect resulting in decreased secretion of normal PTH.

Table 6
Syndromes with Parathyroid Dysgenesis*

DiGeorge syndrome
    Chromosomal – del(10p), del(22q)
    Monogenetic – autosomal dominant, autosomal recessive,
    "Catch 22 syndrome"
Isolated hypoparathyroidism (11p15)
X-linked hypoparathyroidism
Kenny–Caffey syndrome
Barakat syndrome
Kearns-Sayre syndrome (mitochondrial)
MELAS (mitochondrial)

---

*chromosomal defect shown if known

In adults, relatively common causes of acquired hypoparathyroidism are due to damage after thyroid or parathyroid surgery, radiation to the neck or infiltration of the parathyroid by cancer, heavy metals, or granulomatous disease. In children, destruction by autoimmune disease is more common especially in a condition variably referred to as HAM (hypoparathyroidism, Addison's disease, monilial infection), APS1 (autoimmune polyendocrinopathy syndrome, type 1), or PGA (polyglandular autoimmune) disease, type 1 *(35)*. PGA type 1 is an autosomal recessive disorder caused by abnormalities of the AIRE-1 gene on chromosome 21q22.3 that regulates autoimmunity. Many endocrine and non-endocrine tissues can be affected but the classic triad is chronic mucocutaneous candidiasis followed by hypoparathyroidism followed by Addison's disease. It occurs equally in males and females and its incidence varies in different populations but has been reported to be as high as 1:25,000 among the Finnish and 1:9000 in Iranian Jews. The age of onset of the hypoparathyroidism is usually between 6 and 9 years and about 4 years after the onset of candidiasis. For those affected with Addison's disease, its onset is typically about 5 years after the hypoparathyroidism. In the classic study by Blizzard et al, in 32 patients with idiopathic hypoparathyroidism, 66% had candidiasis and 56% had Addison's disease. Other less common features of the syndrome include diabetes mellitus, gonadal failure, hypothyroidism, pernicious anemia, dermal abnormalities, and autoimmune hepatitis. The management of these patients includes careful surveillance for signs of other organ involvement. The manifestations of hypoparathyroidism are greatly influenced by those of untreated Addison's disease but with glucocorticoid replacement, hypocalcemia may become severe and life threatening.

An important cause of refractory hypocalcemia is that due to hypomagnesemia, which will be described in more detail in Chapter 8. Hypomagnesemia causes hypocalcemia by the dual mechanisms of inhibiting PTH secretion as well as blocking the action of PTH on bone and kidney *(27)*. Whereas mild decreases in the divalent cation magnesium stimulate PTH secretion in a similar fashion as calcium by decreasing the inhibition of secretion by the CaSR, severe hypomagnesemia (Mg < 1.0 mg/dL) blocks the ability of the parathyroid cell to secrete PTH. Hypomagnesemic hypocalcemia can be demonstrated in neonates such as in infants of diabetic mothers as well as in children such as in those with celiac disease and malabsorption. Treatment of hypocalcemia in these patients must begin with at least partial correction of the hypomagnesemia or other measures are likely to prove ineffective.

11.2. Parathyroid Resistance

Resistance to PTH can occur with severe hypomagnesemia or hypovitaminosis D but is usually associated with the genetic disorder pseudohypoparathyroidism (PHP). PHP is a disease in which abnormal components of the G protein-coupled receptors such as the PTH/PTHrP receptor for PTH prevent normal formation of second messengers such as cAMP *(36)*. In PHP Type 1a, deficiency of G_s is responsible for preventing the formation of the second messenger cAMP in response to activation of the PTH1 receptor by PTH as well as other G-protein-coupled receptors including those for TSH, gonadotropins, and glucagon. The chromosomal defect is on chromosomal fragment

20q13.3. Recent studies show that the tissue specificity is the result suppression of the paternal gene and expression only of the maternal gene due to imprinting in the affected tissues. Patients with PHP Type 1a also demonstrate a characteristic phenotype known as Albright's hereditary osteodystrophy (AHO), which includes a round face, short stature, obesity, mental retardation, subcutaneous calcifications, and brachydactyly. The latter is due to short metacarpals and metatarsals that result in the knuckle dimple sign when these individuals make a fist. In some kindreds with PHP Type 1a, there are individuals who express the AHO phenotype but have normal PTH responsiveness, a condition referred to as pseudo-pseudohypoparathyroidism. There are other types of PHP due to other genetic defects. PHP Type 1b lacks the features of AHO and whereas there is resistant to PTH in the kidneys, there is responsiveness in bone leading to osseous changes of hyperparathyroidism. PHP Type 1c is not due to a defect in G_s or G_i but there remains resistance to PTH. Finally, in PHP Type 2, there is normal cAMP excretion but no phosphaturia in response to PTH.

Biochemically, the affected individuals with PHP have hypocalcemia, hyperphosphatemia as in hypoparathyroidism but in contrast display elevated PTH levels. Magnesium and 25(OH)D levels should be measured to rule out these conditions as possible causes of PTH resistance. Formerly, tests for cAMP production by PTH were performed using the Ellsworth–Howard test but now for PHP Type 1a, genetic testing is now available.

11.3. Vitamin D Disorders

Hypocalcemia secondary to abnormalities of vitamin D are the result of the precursors of active 1,25(OH)$_2$D as result of nutritional or metabolic reasons or two rare genetic disorders termed vitamin D dependent rickets (37). The features of hypovitaminosis D are typically hypophosphatemia, secondary hyperparathyroidism, elevated alkaline phosphatase and variably hypocalcemia. The reason for the latter is that secondary hyperparathyroidism is often able to compensate for deficiency of the precursors of 1,25(OH)$_2$D. Once thought to be a condition of the past, classic vitamin D deficiency is reemerging due to the combination inadequate sun exposure and inadequate vitamin D in the diet, especially breast milk. Low vitamin D can be seen in a variety of GI disorders including Crohn's disease, celiac disease, pancreatic insufficiency, cystic fibrosis, and hepatobiliary disease. The etiology of hypovitaminosis D in these conditions is fat malabsorption or interruption of the enterohepatic circulation. In addition to malabsorption, vitamin D levels may be low due to increased metabolism to inactive metabolites by hepatic microsomal P-450 oxidases that can be induced by phenobarbital, Dilantin, and other agents. In each of these disorders, the diagnostic test of choice to evaluate vitamin D stores is that of circulating 25(OH)D and not the level of 1,25(OH)$_2$D. Disorders affecting the renal proximal renal tubule including acute and chronic renal failure and Fanconi syndrome can cause decreased formation of 1,25(OH)$_2$D and contribute to hypocalcemia by this mechanism.

Two rare inherited disorders of vitamin D are so called vitamin D-dependent rickets type 1 (pseudo-vitamin D-deficiency) and vitamin D-dependent rickets type 2. The former is an autosomal recessive disorder the enzyme responsible for formation of 1,25(OH)$_2$D: 25-hydroxyvitamin D 1α hydroxylase. In this illness, there is low circulating 1,25(OH)$_2$D and the patient can be cured by physiologic doses of 1,25(OH)$_2$D. In vitamin D-dependent rickets type 2, there is an abnormality of the vitamin D receptor leading to an end-organ resistance. The management of hypocalcemia in some of these patients with mild defects is with large doses of oral 1,25(OH)$_2$D and calcium but the most severely affected require parenteral calcium.

11.4. Critical Illnesses and Other Causes

Hypocalcemia is a common complication in a variety of severe illnesses including sepsis and toxic shock syndrome (27, 38). Hypoalbuminemia is common in severe acute and chronic disease so pseudohypocalcemia with normal ionized calcium must be ruled out. Massive tissue breakdown as seen in tumor lysis syndrome and rhabdomyolysis releases intracellular phosphate which through precipitation of calcium in soft tissues and other mechanisms can cause hypocalcemia. Acute pancreatitis can cause hypocalcemia by several proposed mechanisms including fat necrosis and calcium soap formation as well as decreased PTH secretion. In all of these conditions, hypocalcemia is a bad prognostic sign.

Certain medications can lead to hypocalcemia (38, 39). Phosphate containing enemas can lead to severe hypocalcemia and hyperphosphatemia, especially if there is concurrent renal failure. Citrate given parenterally as an anticoagulant with massive transfusions or during extracorporeal procedures like ECMO can cause an unusual situation in which the total calcium is elevated but the ionized calcium is low. This is because of an increase in the complexed fraction of calcium. Bisphosphonates are a useful class of drugs for the treatment of hypercalcemia but there may be an overshoot with the development of hypocalcemia. This is particularly true in the presence of other factors such as vitamin D deficiency.

11.5. Neonatal Causes

Neonates can suffer from hypocalcemia from many of the causes described above but there are also a group of disorders described under the term "neonatal hypocalcemia" (40– 42). These conditions are largely due to abnormalities in the transition from fetal to postnatal life when the placenta that supplies the fetus with calcium is suddenly removed. The fetus goes from being hypercalcemic to a physiologic period of mild hypocalcemia in the first 2 days of life and returns to normal levels over the next several days. Premature infants often demonstrate a greater fall than term infants. Neonates who are sick, preterm, asphyxiated or are infants of diabetic mothers are at greatest risk for hypocalcemia. Due to a fall in serum albumin after birth as well, measurement of ionized calcium is important in the diagnosis of true hypocalcemia. A total calcium level less than 8 mg/dL in term infants and less than 7 mg/dL in preterm infants is considered abnormal but an ionized calcium less than 1.0 mM or 4 mg/dL in both is considered low. The symptoms of hypocalcemia in the neonate are similar to those in older children (Table 1) but also include apnea, cyanosis, tachypnea, tachycardia, and vomiting.

Table 7
Causes of Neonatal Hypocalcemia

Early (Days 1–4 of life)
    Prematurity
    Perinatal distress/asphyxia
    Infants of diabetic mothers
    Intrauterine growth restriction
Late (Days 5–10 of life)
    High phosphate load
    Transient hypoparathyroidism
    Other hypoparathyroid conditions
        Maternal hyperparathyroidism
    Transient PTH resistance
    Hypomagnesemia
        RTA Type 1
        Primary hypomagnesemia
        Maternal hypomagnesemia
    Maternal vitamin D deficiency
Late-Late hypocalcemia (2–4 mo of age if premature)
Other-low ionized calcium, normal total calcium
    Alkalosis
    Citrate from blood transfusions

Neonatal hypocalcemia has usually been described by time of onset (Table 7). Early hypocalcemia occurs in the first 3–4 days of life and is an exaggeration of the normal transition period. It occurs typically under 3 conditions: prematurity, infant of diabetic mothers (IDM), and intrauterine growth restriction (IUGR). The mechanism is usually a lack of response by the immature kidney to respond to PTH but lack of feeding, rise in calcitonin, renal failure, and hyperphosphatemia all may contribute. With IDM, an exaggerated physiologic drop is often seen with maternal and resultant neonatal hypomagnesemia play a causative role (Chapter 8). Hypocalcemia in IDM correlates with severity of maternal diabetes and can be particularly severe in preterm IDM with IUGR. Late neonatal hypocalcemia is defined as occurring after 4 days of age and is usually due to high dietary phosphate intake and an inadequate parathyroid response that may be transient or be the presentation of one of the disorders described in Section 11.1. Hypoparathyroidism at this point may also be the result of maternal hypercalcemia as seen with maternal hyperparathyroidism. Maternal hypercalcemia can lead to fetal hypercalcemia and fetal hypoparathyroidism that may take weeks to resolve after birth. Hypomagnesemia may be the result of IDM or of one of the conditions described in Chapter 8. Maternal vitamin D deficiency as a result of lack of sunlight or vitamin D intake is an important cause of neonatal hypocalcemia. Finally, hypocalcemia can be seen in infants, especially prematures, as a result of many other causes including sepsis, pancreatitis, and citrate administration with blood transfusions, or ECMO.

12. HYPOCALCEMIA – DIAGNOSTIC EVALUATION

The first step in the evaluation of a child with hypocalcemia is to confirm that they truly have the condition. We recommend direct measurement of ionized calcium in any patient who is acutely or chronically ill or is likely to have abnormalities of serum albumin or pH. The initial diagnostic studies should include electrolytes, magnesium, BUN, creatinine, and phosphorus. If associated clinical conditions do not point to the likely diagnosis then the laboratory studies can be helpful in narrowing down the diagnosis. Hypomagnesemia and renal failure are important diagnoses that should be recognized immediately. It must be remembered that mild decreases in serum magnesium stimulate PTH secretion but hypocalcemia is more likely associated with levels less than 1 mg/dL. Serum phosphorus can be used in a diagnostic strategy to narrow the diagnosis (Table 5). High phosphorus levels in the absence of renal failure suggest abnormal PTH function (decreased secretion or decreased action) or endogenous or exogenous phosphorus load. Low serum phosphorus suggests abnormalities of vitamin D action or movement of calcium and phosphorus into bone or the soft tissues.

The second level of testing includes PTH and 25(OH)D levels (Table 8). PTH levels are low or inappropriately normal in states of decreased secretion and are elevated with resistance to its action (pseudohypoparathyroidism) as well as most other states where its secretion is being stimulated. To investigate for vitamin D deficiency whether due to decreased intake, malabsorption or increased metabolism, 25(OH)D levels and not $1,25(OH)_2D$ levels are the test of choice to evaluate for vitamin D deficiency. $1,25(OH)_2D$ levels are usually in the normal range with classic rickets but inappropriately low in light of the hypocalcemia, hypophosphatemia, and secondary hyperparathyroidism that are usually present. Rarely in states of decreased proximal renal tubular function or even more rare vitamin D-dependent rickets type 1 are $1,25(OH)_2D$ diagnostic.

Table 8
Laboratory Features of Hypocalcemic Syndromes

Condition	PO4	PTH	Vitamin D
Hypoparathyroidism	⇑	⇓	$1,25(OH)_2D$ nl to ⇓
Pseudohypoparathyroidism	⇑	⇑	$1,25(OH)_2D$ nl to ⇓
Tumor lysis syndrome	⇑	⇑	⇔
Vitamin D deficiency	⇓	⇑	25(OH) D ⇓
Vitamin D dep. rickets type 1	⇓	⇑	$1,25(OH)_2D$ ⇓
Vitamin D dep. rickets type 2	⇓	⇑	$1,25(OH)_2D$ ⇑
Hypomagnesemia	nl to ⇑	⇓	$1,25(OH)_2D$ nl to ⇓

13. MANAGEMENT OF HYPOCALCEMIA

In children with severe, symptomatic hypocalcemia, emergency treatment with intravenous calcium is indicated (Table 9) *(40, 43)*. In older children and adults, 10–20 ml of

Table 9
Treatment of Hypocalcemia in Children-Common Forms of Calcium, Magnesium,
Vitamin D

Agent	Concentration	Dose	Comment
Calcium carbonate*	100 mg/ml suspension	50–75 mg/kg/day÷q6 h	Oral-liquid
	200, 300, 400, 500 mg		Oral-tabs
Calcium glubionate*	115 mg/5 ml	50–75 mg/kg/day÷q6 h	Oral-syrup
Calcium citrate*	53.5, 200 mg	50–75 mg/kg/day÷q6 h	Oral tabs-use with achlorhydria
Calcium gluconate*	100 mg/ml injection	10–20 mg/kg/dose	IV
Magnesium sulfate^	500 mg/ml injection	50–100 mg/kg/dose	IV
Ergocalciferol	8000 IU/ml	800–8,000 IU/day	Oral-liquid
	50,000 IU	50,000 IU/2–4 weak	Oral-tablet
Cholecalciferol	1000, 2000 IU	1000–8000 IU/day	Oral-tabs (OTC)
1,25(OH)$_2$D	0.25, 0.5 mcg	0.25–1 mcg/day	Oral-capsules
	1 mcg/ml		Oral-liquid
1,25(OH)$_2$D	1.0 mcg/ml	0.25–1 mcg/day	IV

* elemental calcium; ^ elemental magnesium

10% calcium gluconate (10 ml ampules) over 10–15 min is often sufficient to stop the acute manifestations including seizures. In younger children and neonates, the dose is 10–20 mg/kg or 1–2 ml/kg or 10% calcium gluconate at a rate no greater than 1 ml/min using constant cardiac monitoring. Hypomagnesemic hypocalcemia will be refractory to this treatment and should be treated with 0.1–0.2 ml/kg of 50% magnesium sulfate (50–100 mg/kg) IV over a 10-min period, a dose that can be repeated every 12–24 h. Calcium infusions can be given for persistent hypocalcemia in children by mixing ten 10 ml calcium gluconate ampules in 1 L D5W and given at a rate of 50–75 mg/kg/day (44). It is imperative that it is only given in a well-functioning IV to avoid chemical burns with calcium extravasation into the tissues and with continuous cardiac monitoring to avoid bradycardia. Calcium can be given on the chronic basis orally at a dose 1–4 g of elemental calcium daily depending on the body size. The form of oral calcium generally is not clinically relevant except for states achlorhydria in the stomach where calcium carbonate does not dissolve and calcium citrate in preferable.

For infants with late hypocalcemia and hyperphosphatemia, low phosphorus feeding such as breast milk or Similac PM 60/40^{TM} is important (41). With severe acute hyperphosphatemia as with tumor lysis especially with renal failure, hemodialysis or other renal replacement therapy may be necessary. In vitamin D deficiency states, ergocalciferol (vitamin D$_2$) or cholecalciferol (vitamin D$_3$) can be given at a dose of 800–8000 units daily. In young infants the dose should be no more than 2000 units daily. Calcium, phosphorus, and 25(OH)D levels are useful guides to therapy in hypocalcemia patients with severe hypovitaminosis D. In the presence of renal failure, hypoparathyroidism, active 1,25(OH)$_2$D can be given orally or by IV at a dose of 20–40 ng/kg/day or in older patients 0.25–1 μg/kg/day. In hypoparathyroidism, especially that due to CaSR disorders, hypercalciuria may develop with normalization of serum calcium. In those states, the minimal amount of calcium to keep the serum calcium in the low normal range should be give to avoid nephrocalcinosis or renal stones. Thiazide diuretics (1 mg/kg) can be given cautiously to increase calcium reabsorption and support the serum calcium in hypoparathyroidism.

CASE SCENARIO DISCUSSIONS

Case Scenario 1: Hypocalcemia in a school aged child. This child has symptomatic hypocalcemia with a low serum calcium and high serum phosphorus. The high phosphorus points to likely dysfunction of PTH secretion or function but the normal body habitus suggests that he does not have Albright's Hereditary Osteodystrophy (AHO) as with pseudohypoparathyroidism. He does not have renal failure and the normal CBC makes tumor lysis less likely. You look for hypomagnesemia that could cause this picture but the magnesium level is normal and an EKG shows prolonged QT interval. Other studies that are sent off with the initial labs are PTH and 25(OH)D levels. Because he is not having serious manifestations like seizures or tetany, you choose to start treatment with oral calcium to both raise the serum calcium and to act as a phosphate binder. You choose a dose of 500 mg of elemental calcium four times daily as calcium carbonate and you place the patient on a low phosphate diet of 800 mg/day or less. As soon as the phosphorus level starts to come down you start active 1,25(OH)$_2$D at a "physiologic" dose of 0.5 mcg daily. The PTH level comes back in the low normal range, which is inappropriate for the level of calcium consistent with hypocalcemia and the 25(OH)D level is normal. The rash turns out to be chronic Candida infection and the diagnosis of polyglandular autoimmune syndrome (PGA) type 1 is strongly suggested. Since a high percentage of PGA type 1 patients will go on to develop Addison's disease, you must carefully monitor for this potentially life-threatening condition, which can present with electrolyte abnormalities such as hyponatremia, hypokalemia, and acidosis. A random cortisol of less than 18 μg/dL is suggestive of adrenal insufficiency but a cortisol stimulation test may be required. In addition to Addison's disease, other disorders associated with PGA 1 should be suspected if other clinical abnormalities develop.

Case Scenario 2: Infant with new onset seizures and heart disease. This infant presents as a "late" neonatal hypocalcemia with a heart defect and an abnormal facies. The possibility of "late" neonatal hypocalcemia includes high-phosphate dietary load, maternal vitamin D, or magnesium deficiency, and maternal parathyroid disease do not appear to be present. Initial studies should include magnesium, ionized calcium, CBC with differential and PTH. In this case, the magnesium is normal but the ionized calcium confirms the hypocalcemia and the PTH comes back just above the lower limit of 10 pg/ml suggesting hypoparathyroidism with an inappropriate response to the hypocalcemia. The diagnosis of DiGeorge Syndrome should be considered even though the VSD is not one of the classic aortic arch or cardiac outflow lesions usually described with this syndrome. Karyotypes with fluorescence in situ hybridization (FISH) studies should be sent to look for microdeletions in the 22q11.2 (CATCH-22) and 10p regions (HDR). The initial treatment was with 10 ml/kg of calcium gluconate (parenteral), which improved the serum calcium and the neuromuscular symptoms. This child also had renal failure with a normal renal ultrasound (pointing away from the renal dysplasia of Barakat syndrome), which improved as the hypocalcemia was corrected suggesting a prerenal (or decreased perfusion) etiology related to heart failure. Long term management is with oral calcium (up to 1000 mg/day in divided doses), low phosphorus diet (breast milk or Similac PM 60/40^{TM}), and possibly $1,25(OH)_2D$ (0.04–0.08 mg/kg/day).

14. HYPERCALCEMIA – INTRODUCTION

Hypercalcemia is a relatively uncommon disorder in children. The diagnosis is most commonly made with the incidental finding of elevated serum calcium on routine measurement of serum electrolytes. Clinical sign and symptoms of hypercalcemia are usually vague and non-specific but their recognition can be important in certain clinical settings. The determination of the etiology of the hypercalcemia requires investigation of the mechanisms that regulate the level of serum calcium and the known causes that disrupt these mechanisms. Treatment should include both non-specific measures to lower the level of serum calcium as well as specific therapies to address the primary cause.

CASE SCENARIOS

Case Scenario 1: Hypercalcemia in a healthy adolescent

You have consulted psychiatry on a 16-year-old male who is depressed and lethargic while in the hospital for an injury of his leg. He is very tearful about being kept in the hospital and not being able to go home to his friends and family. He is not eating and has not had a bowel movement in 3 days. This formerly athletic male had been admitted 4 weeks prior after being thrown from a four-wheeler and suffering a displaced femur fracture with soft tissue injury. He is in traction and on antibiotics for infection of the wound. He has a poor appetite and is constipated and has lost 8 kg since admission. His vital signs show a pulse of 110/min, BP of 140/95, temperature of 37.5, and normal respiratory weight. On examination, he appears somewhat cachectic despite the history of being on the football team prior to his injury. Routine labs which show a normal CBC are sent but the chemistry panel shows a BUN 22 mg/dL, creatinine 1.4 mg/dL, and a serum calcium 15.2 mg/dL, phosphorus 4.2 mg/dL, albumen 4.8 g/dL. Urinalysis shows a specific gravity of 1.005 and small blood on the dipstick.

What are the signs and symptoms that suggested the patient had hypercalcemia? What is the basic etiology of his hypercalcemia and what are the contributing factors in its development? What studies would you order? How would you treat him?

Case Scenario 2: Neonatal hypercalcemia

Thirty-four-week gestation SGA infant develops mild respiratory distress requiring oxygen on day 2 of life. Chest X-ray shows evidence of abnormal, washed out clavicles, and ribs. Skeletal survey shows diffuse demineralization of the long bones with no rachitic changes at the metaphyses and the skull shows no evidence of wormian bones.

Chemistry profile: sodium 135 mEq/L, potassium 4.8 mEq/L, bicarbonate 19 mEq/L, chloride 98 mEq/L, BUN 5 mg/dL, creatinine 0.9 mg/dL, calcium 12.5 mg/dL, phosphorus 3.8 mg/dL, albumen 2.9 g/dL.

What are the studies that you want to order? What is the most likely direct cause of the hypercalcemia? How would you manage this patient?

15. DEFINITION OF HYPERCALCEMIA

Hypercalcemia can be defined as a total serum calcium level in a child greater than 10.3 mg/dL but as has been explained in Sections 2.1 and 5.1, it is the ionized calcium that is physiologically and clinically significant (18, 34). Total serum calcium may not reflect the level of ionized calcium in states that alter either the protein-bound fraction with changes in the serum albumin level or the complexed fractions with changes in the concentrations of either serum phosphate or citrate. Methods to "correct" total serum calcium are too often inaccurate in the sick hospitalized patient and so it is recommended to at least initially directly measure serum ionized calcium and levels > 1.35 mmol/(5.5 mg/dL) in the child or >1.4 mmol/L (5.6 mg/dL) in the neonate can be considered elevated. The degree of hypercalcemia has diagnostic, prognostic and therapeutic significance with more severe hypercalcemia requiring more aggressive diagnosis and treatment. In terms of total calcium (mg/dL), hypercalcemia can therefore be classified as mild (10.5–11.2), moderate (11.3–13.5) and severe (>13.5).

16. HYPERCALCEMIA – CLINICAL FEATURES

The signs and symptoms of hypercalcemia are typically vague and non-specific but do relate to the severity of the hypercalcemia with the patient with more severe hypercalcemia (calcium > 14 mg/dL) being more likely to be symptomatic (45, 46). The symptoms are listed in Table 10 and can be broken down into cardiovascular, gastrointestinal, neuromuscular, renal, and general. By increasing cardiac repolarization, high calcium can cause a shortened Q–T interval, which can be a classic sign. The gastrointestinal symptoms are a very common presentation but are totally non-specific as are the neuromuscular symptoms. The renal manifestations of polyuria, polydipsia, and nocturia are not so significant for their prominence but the ensuing dehydration can lead to increasing inability of the kidney to excrete calcium leading to a vicious cycle of worsening hypercalcemia and renal dysfunction. This sequence can be especially important in the presence of poor oral intake that can exacerbate the dehydration. Prolonged severe hypercalcemia can cause renal calcification in the form of stones and nephrocalcinosis. In young children unlike adults, a common presentation of chronic hypercalcemia is poor growth and failure to thrive.

17. CAUSES OF HYPERCALCEMIA

17.1. Parathyroid Disorders

There are two disorders whose pathophysiology is an inappropriately elevated secretion of PTH for the level of serum calcium, which is due to the loss of the normal

Table 10
Clinical Manifestations of Hypercalcemia

Cardiovascular
  Shortened QT interval on EKG
  Hypertension
  Bradycardia
Gastrointestinal
  Nausea and vomiting
  Constipation
  Peptic ulcer
  Pancreatitis
Neuromuscular
  Lethargy
  Depression
  Stupor
  Confusion
  Muscle weakness
Renal
  Polyuria and polydipsia
  Decreased concentrating ability
  Hypercalciuria
  Nephrocalcinosis
  Nephrolithiasis
General
  Weakness
  Metastatic calcifications
  Failure to thrive

feedback by calcium on PTH secretion (Table 11). The first is primary hyperparathy-roidism (HPT), one of the two most common causes of hypercalcemia in adults but a fairly rare cause of hypercalcemia in children. The second condition is famil-ial hypocalciuric hypercalcemia (FHH), a generally benign disorder of the calcium receptor CaSR with the exception being when it presents in the neonatal period (see Section 17.6.1).

17.1.1. PRIMARY HYPERPARATHYROIDISM

The incidence of HPT in children is 2–5 per 100,000, which is only about 1% of that in adults (47, 48). This may contribute to the fact that there is often a delay in the diagnosis of HPT in children who present with non-specific symptoms (Table 1) as compared to adults. As a result, almost 79% of the children were symptomatic in one study and 44% had some sort of end-organ involvement, which is different from adults who most often have asymptomatic hypercalcemia. Also in children, only 65% of children are found to have an adenoma of a single parathyroid gland versus 80% in adults leaving about 30% children with four-gland hyperplasia (49). The reason is the

Table 11
Infections and Granulomatous Causes of
1,25(OH) Mediated Hypercalcemia

Infectious
    Tuberculosis
    Coccidiomycosis
    Cat-scratch disease
    Histoplasmosis
    Candidiasis
Inflammatory
    Sarcoidosis
    Wegener's granulomatosis
    Crohn's disease
    Silicone-induced granulomatosis
    Subcutaneous fat necrosis
Lymphoproliferative
    B-cell lymphoma
    Hodgkin's disease

relatively higher incidence of familial HPT in children that accounts for over 50% of the children with four-gland hyperplasia. In contrast to other causes of hypercalcemia, children with HPT are more likely to present with kidney stones or bone involvement including fractures.

Primary HPT can present as one of several familial disorders *(50)* including the multiple endocrine neoplasia Types 1 (MEN1) and 2A (MEN2A), hyperparathyroidism-jaw tumor syndrome (HPT-JT), familial isolated hyperparathyroidism, and fore-mentioned neonatal severe HPT (NSHPT), which will be discussed below. MEN1 is a rare autosomal dominant disorder in which there is an inactivating germ-line mutation of the tumor suppressor gene *MEN1* on chromosome 11q13 leading to the development of tumors of the parathyroid, anterior pituitary, pancreatic islets as well as other tissues. HPT in this condition can begin as young as 8 years of age, often with symptomatic hypercalcemia. MEN 2A is more associated with medullary thyroid carcinoma (90%) but can also have HPT (20%) and pheochromocytoma (40%). This autosomal dominant disorder arises from a germ-line mutation of the *RET* proto-oncogene and is more likely to be associated with asymptomatic HPT. HPT-SJ, a is a very rare syndrome in which there may be ossifying fibromas of the mandible or maxilla as well as possibly renal cysts, hamartomas or even Wilm's tumor. The mutation in this condition is on chromosome 1q.

The diagnosis of HPT is based on the presence of an elevated PTH level in the presence of hypercalcemia *(47)*. The standard test for PTH is measurement of intact PTH by IRMA or ICMA (see Section 6.1). About 15% of children with HPT may have PTH values in the upper range of normal and high serum calcium levels, which should be associated with PTH levels below the mean. Other associated laboratory findings include low or low normal serum phosphorus; elevated markers of bone formation and bone resorption such as serum alkaline phosphatase and urinary N-telopeptide/creatinine, respectively, and increased urinary calcium excretion as result of increased circulating $1,25(OH)_2$vitamin D ($1,25(OH)_2D$). Measurement of serum phosphate and urinary calcium is clinically useful, measurement of markers of bone turnover and $1,25(OH)_2D$ are not since they do not distinguish between other causes of hypercalcemia (see Section 5). Other studies in HPT may include X-rays for bone involvement but these are not cost effective and do not add to the direct measurement of PTH.

Treatment of HPT includes the non-specific management of hypercalcemia (Section 19) but in children should include surgical removal of the abnormal parathyroid tissue *(32, 48)*. Controversy remains over the role of pre-operative imaging of the parathyroid, which can include ultrasound, CT, MRI, and scintigraphy with technetium-99m-sestamibi. The latter is the most common study because of its ability to localize a single adenoma but it can be combined with adjunctive modalities such as single photon emission computed tomography (SPECT) to more precisely localize the parathyroid tissue. An axiom of parathyroid surgery has been that the most important factor is to have an experienced surgeon perform the exploration because of the great variability in location of the parathyroids, which can include the mediastinum or multiple locations in the neck. The surgical procedure of choice is to remove any adenomas, a procedure that should be accompanied by a drop of PTH levels intraoperatively by 50%. If the drop in PTH levels is less, there is likely to be more hyperplastic parathyroid glands, especially in children. In multiglandular disease the choice is to mark and leave a small piece of parathyroid tissue in situ or to remove all of the parathyroid tissue and autotransplant a portion in the non-dominant forearm. After surgery a brief period of hypocalcemia is expected requiring either oral or intravenous calcium or possibly $1,25(OH)_2D$. If both severe, prolonged hypocalcemia and hypophosphatemia develop post-operatively, this is a likely sign of "hungry bone" syndrome in which there is a transient high turnover of bone. After surgery bone resorption is suppressed with the loss of PTH stimulation but activated bone mineralization continues for a period of time.

17.1.2. FAMILIAL HYPOCALCIURIC HYPERCALCEMIA

Familial hypocalciuric hypercalcemia (FHH), which is also know as familial benign hypercalcemia, is an autosomal dominant loss of function abnormality of the calcium receptor (CaSR) *(51)*. The majority of cases have abnormalities of the CaSR locus on chromosome 3q. Most patients who have a heterozygous CaSR defect in the parathyroid and the renal tubule require a higher serum calcium levels to suppress PTH secretion (increased set point) and demonstrate increased tubular reabsorption of calcium. The latter defect helps maintain serum calcium levels at a higher level even in the absence of PTH but is also responsible for the relative hypocalciuria in this condition. Homozygous CaSR defects result in the massive, life-threatening neonatal severe primary hyperparathyroidism covered under "Hypercalcemia in Infants" (Section 17.6.1).

Children with FHH present with mild asymptomatic hypercalcemia with serum magnesium levels in the high normal range and phosphorus levels in the low range. Characteristically, calcium excretion is low for the level of serum calcium and can be measured by the ratio of calcium clearance to creatinine clearance. Similarly, magnesium excretion is also increased, leading to the mild hypermagnesemia. The diagnosis of FHH can usually be made in the presence of autosomal dominant inheritance of hypercalcemia, hypocalciuria and normal PTH levels. Currently genetic testing for FHH is only able to detect 70% of affected kindreds so false negatives remain a possibility. The management for most cases of FHH is to avoid parathyroidectomy except for the neonatal form covered below and rare cases with serum calcium greater than 14 mg/dL. There is a possible future role for calcimimetics that has yet to be determined.

17.2. Vitamin D Mediated

Vitamin D can cause hypercalcemia by stimulating calcium absorption from the GI tract and resorption from bone (52, 53). Toxicity can result from intoxication by vitamin D or one of its active analogues can result from endogenous formation of active $1,25(OH)_2D$ in a variety of disease states. Characteristically, both serum calcium and phosphorus will be elevated since the actions of vitamin D elevate both minerals, and serum PTH levels should be suppressed. Another effect is increased excretion of calcium, which may precede hypercalcemia, but other factors such as thiazide diuretic use may trigger frank hypercalcemia by limiting the ability of the kidneys to excrete the excess calcium. The measurement of vitamin D metabolites may be helpful in these disorders. In states of intoxication by regular vitamin D_2 or D_3, the level of 25(OH)D but not $1,25(OH)_2D$ is high, whereas in other vitamin D disorders described below, the formation and serum levels of $1,25(OH)_2D$ are elevated.

17.2.1. VITAMIN D INTOXICATION

Hypercalcemia from vitamin D supplements is a fairly rare disorder (54). Despite recommended upper limits of intake of 2000 IU/day, intakes of 10,000 IU/day are well tolerated in adults. Most reported cases are due to consumption of vitamin D in amounts greater than 100,000 units daily for a period of time as a result of an error in the production of supplemented products or a bizarre intake of huge amount of vitamin D. In these cases, it is the level of 25(OH)D but not $1,25(OH)_2D$ that is elevated, and recent expert opinion suggests that levels greater than 100 ng/ml are necessary for toxicity. The mechanism is unclear but likely includes competition for the vitamin D receptor, elevated free $1,25(OH)_2D$, interference with vitamin D metabolism and upregulation of the vitamin D receptor. The half-life of $25(OH)D_3$ is 7–30 days and so the duration of the hypercalcemia may be for weeks. In cases where the parent compound, vitamin D2 or vitamin D3 is elevated, the duration of hypercalcemia can last as long as 18 months due to large stores of fat soluble vitamin in adipose tissue. Treatment for severe cases can include the use of corticosteroids and low calcium diet. More commonly, hypercalcemia from vitamin D intoxication is the result of administration of active forms of vitamin D in renal failure or other metabolic conditions. In these cases, $1,25(OH)_2D$ or another active metabolite are the culprits. Due to their short half lives of more like 24 h, resolution of the hypercalcemia will occur in days after discontinuation of the medication and is usually all that is required in the treatment.

17.2.2. GRANULOMATOUS DISORDERS

Hypercalcemia has been long associated with certain infectious and granulomatous disorders with sarcoidosis as the classic example *(55)*. The enzyme responsible for formation of $1,25(OH)_2D$, $25(OH)D-1\alpha$-hydroxylase is known to be expressed in many extra-renal tissues including monocytes and macrophages. In these tissues, formation of $1,25(OH)_2D$ is not stimulated by PTH, low calcium and low phosphorus as in the kidney rather by immune mediators and cytokines such as IL-2 and γ-interferon. In a number of these states (Table 11), increased levels of $1,25(OH)_2D$ appear to be the cause of the hypercalcemia and its measurement can be diagnostic. Hypercalcemia in certain lymphoproliferative diseases and subcutaneous fat necrosis in infants appear to have a similar pathogenesis. The malignancies most often associated with increased $1,25(OH)_2D$ formation are Hodgkin's and non-Hodgkin's lymphomas. Treatment of $1,25(OH)_2D$ mediated hypercalcemia includes control of the primary disease or reduction of $1,25(OH)_2D$ production by the macrophages/monocytes by glucocorticoids or in refractory cases by chloroquine, hydroxychloroquine, and ketoconazole.

17.3. Bone-Related

Release of calcium from bone is associated with most hypercalcemic disorders but under certain conditions this is not secondary to increases in PTH or vitamin D. Increased resorption of bone by osteoclasts combined with the suppression of mineralization by osteoblasts (uncoupling) can lead to massive release of calcium from bone, which can overwhelm the homeostatic mechanisms to maintain normal serum calcium.

17.3.1. HYPERCALCEMIA OF MALIGNANCY

Hypercalcemia associated with malignancy is much less common in children than adults where it is one of the two most common causes of hypercalcemia *(56)*. Malignancy associated hypercalcemia is often severe (total calcium >14 mg/dL) and can be life threatening. Unlike adults where 30-day survival is only about 50% with this condition, the prognosis in children appears to be better which is related to the kind of associated cancers in children *(57)*. There are several described mechanisms, including $1,25(OH)_2D$ formation described with certain lymphomas (Section 3.2.2). Local osteolytic hypercalcemia (LOH), typified by breast cancer with extensive metastatic disease to bone, is caused by local production by the cancer cells of cytokines and PTHrP, which activate local resorption of bone by osteoclasts. Leukemias, including ALL, which cause hypercalcemia, may have a similar mechanism. The biochemical features of LOH are hypercalcemia, normal to high serum phosphorus, low PTH, hypercalciuria, and suppressed $1,25(OH)_2D$ levels.

The second syndrome is "humoral hypercalcemia of malignancy" in which there is little evidence of direct skeletal metastases. Once thought due to ectopic secretion of PT, it was found in the majority of cases to be due to PTHrP. The majority of tumors associated with PTHrP such as squamous cell carcinoma of the lung, esophagus, head and neck, and cervix, are rare in the pediatric age group but there are still many reported cases of cancer in children due to PTHrP. Whereas PTH and PTHrP act through similar receptors, patients with HHM share with those with HPT of having hypercalcemia, and hypophosphatemia but differ in that $1,25(OH)_2D$ formation is not elevated and that bone formation by osteoblasts is suppressed by PTHrP in contrast to PTH.

There are some non-malignant illnesses that have been associated with PTHrP and hypercalcemia including SLE, HIV, lymphedema, massive mammary hyperplasia, and certain benign tumors including pheochromocytoma.

17.3.2. IMMOBILIZATION

Hypercalcemia in children who have been immobilized is a relatively common and is the result of the sudden suppression of osteoblastic bone mineralization simultaneous with a striking increase in osteoclastic bone resorption *(58)*. With a growing child or adolescent who is physically active, this uncoupling of bone mineralization and resorption in a skeleton that is rapidly turning over can lead to hypercalciuria in a few days and hypercalcemia in a few weeks. The immobilization may be the result of spinal cord injury, femur fractures, or other acute injury. Symptoms of nausea, loss of appetite, lethargy, and depression caused by the hypercalcemia are often attributed to the circumstances and missed as a sign of hypercalcemia. The laboratory evaluation should show hypercalcemia, hypercalciuria along with a suppressed PTH level. The treatment is remobilization but treatment with hydration and bisphosphonates may be required (Section 19).

17.3.3. OTHER

Thyrotoxicosis or excessive administration of thyroid hormone can lead to hypercalcemia by accelerating bone turnover with bone resorption exceeding mineralization *(58)*. Vitamin A intoxication can also stimulate osteoclastic activity and cause hypercalcemia. Enhanced osteoclastic reabsorption has also been reported with type 1 Gaucher's disease, juvenile idiopathic arthritis, and other non-specific inflammatory disorders.

17.4. Renal Induced

Excretion of calcium by the kidneys acts as an essential defense by ridding the body of excess calcium absorbed by the GI tract or released by bone *(46)*. Hypercalciuria is often an early warning of impending hypercalcemia when the calcium entering the extracellular fluid exceeds the ability of the kidney to excrete it. Hypercalcemia can cause a decrease in its own excretion by direct effects on glomerular filtration and by disrupting urinary concentrating ability leading to a dehydration and increased calcium reabsorption. In any acute or chronic renal failure disorder, the loss of normal calcium excretion makes the individual more susceptible to hypercalcemia. Other causes of hypercalcemia described above including PTH and PTHrP activate renal reabsorption of calcium as part of the mechanism by which they increase serum calcium. Thiazide diuretics, which enhance renal tubular reabsorption of calcium, have been associated with hypercalcemia when given to patients on vitamin D or other potential causes of hypercalcemia.

17.5. Diet

Increases in dietary calcium leads to decreased fractional absorption by feedback mechanisms involving PTH and vitamin D. An exception is the once common entity milk–alkali syndrome in which massive amounts of milk was consumed for peptic ulcer disease (59). With the advent of H_2-antagonists and proton pump inhibitors, this syndrome is rarely seen today but still reported with the ingestion of calcium carbonate in amounts of 2–8 g of day. The clinical features are hypercalcemia, alkalosis with hyperphosphatemia, and progressive renal failure. The pathophysiology involves the effect of inhibition of calcium excretion by alkalosis and renal failure. Another dietary cause of hypercalcemia is with total parenteral nutrition, when there are excessive amounts of calcium or vitamin D in the formulation. Aluminum contamination of amino acids in TPN solutions was once a common cause of hypercalcemia but this should be a condition of the past.

17.6. Hypercalcemia in Infants

The causes of hypercalcemia that present in infancy deserves special consideration because many of the conditions are unique to that period because of such factors as maternal influences on the fetus, decreased ability of the immature kidneys to excrete a calcium load and the role of high bone turnover. There are other conditions in which the severity is so great that potentially life-threatening hypercalcemia presents during the first few weeks to months of life (1, 60).

17.6.1. NEONATAL HYPERPARATHYROIDISM

Hyperparathyroidism (HPT) in the neonate is the result of diminished calcium transport across the placenta resulting in stimulation of fetal parathyroid tissue and disorders of the CaSR, especially the homozygous form (51, 60). In addition to the non-specific signs of hypercalcemia that include dehydration, hypertension, lethargy, hypotonia, constipation and respiratory distress, neonates with HPT also present with bone manifestations including decreased mineralization, fractures, and assorted bone deformities. The biochemical features of HPT besides elevated PTH levels include hypercalcemia that can be in the 15–30 mg/dL in neonatal severe primary hyperparathyroidism (NSHPT), mild hypophosphatemia, high alkaline phosphatase, and anemia. In the most severe cases, nephrocalcinosis may be present.

Neonatal HPT can be a secondary adaptive phenomenon as result of inadequate transport of calcium across the placenta. The most common reason for this is maternal hypocalcemia as result of such conditions as poorly controlled maternal hypoparathyroidism, pseudohypoparathyroidism, or renal tubular acidosis. We recently described three cases of neonatal HPT in infants with mucolipidosis II disease where the primary disorder appeared to interfere directly with placental calcium transport (61). Infants with secondary HPT due to maternal hypocalcemia characteristically are not as hypercalcemic as other causes of neonatal HPT but can have severe demineralization. With good supportive care, the secondary hyperparathyroidism usually resolves, as does the bone disease by 6 months of age.

Disorders of the CaSR, which are discussed under FHH (Section 17.1.2), are the most common cause of neonatal HPT *(1, 51)*. Infants are more likely than adults to have symptomatic hypercalcemia and bone disease with the heterozygous form of the CaSR defect, especially if the infant is the offspring to an affected father but normal mother. In this setting the normocalcemic mother cannot transport adequate calcium across the placenta to maintain the fetal calcium concentration at a level that will suppress the fetal parathyroid glands expressing the abnormal CaSR. Infants expressing homozygous CaSR abnormalities have neonatal severe primary hyperparathyroidism that should be considered a life-threatening emergency because of the extreme degree of hypercalcemia coupled with renal and skeletal findings. The diagnosis may be suspected due to family history or prenatal skeletal changes and will develop the most profound symptoms as described above. With a reported mortality rate of 25% in the literature, the treatment of choice has been emergency total parathyroidectomy. However a role for intravenous pamidronate to stabilize the patient has recently been suggested.

17.6.2. SUBCUTANEOUS FAT NECROSIS

Subcutaneous fat necrosis (SFN) is a relatively common disorder observed in full term infants after a traumatic or difficult delivery with resulting areas of indurated subcutaneous nodules typically found on the buttocks, trunk, thighs, cheeks, or extremities *(60)*. Monocytic infiltrates are typically found in the areas of induration and in a minority of infants, hypercalcemia develops over a period of days to weeks. The mechanism, which can be severe, may be due to prostaglandin E_2 or in other instances secondary to 1,25(OH)$_2$D formation as described in Section 17.2.2 in other granulomatous disorders. In addition to hypercalcemia and possibly high 1,25(OH)$_2$D, other biochemical features include low PTH and high phosphate levels. The treatment of these infants until the inflammation resolves includes typical treatments (Section 6) corticosteroids, saline, and furosemide but also low calcium and vitamin D formula (CalciloXD, Ross Laboratories, North Chicago, IL). One must monitor for vitamin D deficiency if this formula is used.

17.6.3. WILLIAMS SYNDROME

Williams syndrome is a chromosomal abnormality of 7q11.23 characterized by infantile presentation of supravalvular aortic stenosis, mental defects, a distinctive "elfin" facies, and in 15% of the cases hypercalcemia *(60)*. The hypercalcemia when present usually resolves in the first year of life but there can also be more persistent hypercalciuria and nephrocalcinosis. Although the affected gene defect appears to be the elastin gene, studies suggesting abnormalities in vitamin D function suggest a possible contiguous gene defect. The diagnosis can usually be made by a fluorescent in situ hybridization (FISH) for the elastin gene. Treatment is usually with dietary restriction of calcium and vitamin D.

17.6.4. IDIOPATHIC INFANTILE HYPERCALCEMIA

First described in the 1950s by Lightwood, idiopathic infantile hypercalcemia (IIH) first appeared to be a disorder causes by excessive maternal vitamin D supplementation *(60)*. This syndrome, which shares features with Williams syndrome but is not associated with a positive FISH test for elastin, has been associated with elevated PTHrP. Hypercalcemia with IIH is usually more persistent that with Williams syndrome and may require treatment with glucocorticoids and a low calcium and vitamin D formula like Calcilo XD.

17.6.5. SKELETAL DYSPLASIAS

Two rare skeletal dysplasias have been associated with hypercalcemia *(60, 62)*. The severe, infantile form of hypophosphatasia in which there is a deficiency of tissue non-specific alkaline phosphatase is associated with a defect in skeletal mineralization, rachitic changes on X-ray and hypercalcemia. The latter is likely the result of poor osteoblast function in the face of continued osteoclastic bone resorption. Besides low serum alkaline phosphatase, the classic biochemical changes are an increase in both urinary phosphoethanolamine and serum pyridoxal-5-phosphate. The second condition is Jansen syndrome associated with hypercalcemia and metaphyseal dysplasia and later development of a characteristic X-ray picture. The etiology appears to be due to constitutively active PTH/PTHrP receptors.

17.6.6. DIETARY AND IATROGENIC CAUSES

Neonates, especially premature infants are particularly susceptible to a variety of imbalances that can lead to hypercalcemia *(60)*. Probably the most common cause of moderate hypercalcemia in premature infants is phosphorus deficiency with insufficient phosphorus to allow normal bone mineralization leading to excess serum and urinary calcium. This is most commonly seen when very low birth weight infants fed unsupplemented human milk or inappropriate term formulas deficient in phosphorus. In addition to very low levels of serum phosphorus, this disorder features osteopenia and elevated alkaline phosphatase and can be treated with appropriate supplementation. Hypercalcemia may occur with excessive calcium during ECMO, exchange transfusion or excessive vitamin D supplementation. Vitamin A if given in excess can stimulate bone turnover and hypercalcemia.

17.6.7. OTHER

There are a number of other conditions that are rare or are common but rarely reported to be associated with hypercalcemia in infants (Table 12) *(6, 51)*.

Table 12
Rare Causes of Neonatal Hypercalcemia

Primary oxalosis
Congenital lactase deficiency
Down's syndrome
Renal tubular acidosis
Thyrotoxicosis
Infantile hypothyroidism
Congenital mesoblastic nephroma
Adrenal insufficiency
Prostaglandin E syndrome

18. DIAGNOSTIC EVALUATION OF HYPERCALCEMIA

Identification of the cause of hypercalcemia requires a detailed history and physical in combination with an appropriate use of the laboratory studies (Table 13). Section 5 describes in more detail the interpretation of studies of divalent ion metabolism. The first step in laboratory evaluation of the child or infant with suspected hypercalcemia is to confirm the diagnosis with total serum calcium, electrolytes, BUN, creatinine, phosphorus, and albumin. We do not recommend the use of "corrected" serum calcium but the albumin and electrolytes may point to the need for ionized calcium measurement. In a patient with hypoalbuminemia, acidosis or severe illness, ionized calcium should be measured to confirm the diagnosis. The severity of the diagnosis is important for treatment but may also point to likely etiologies. In patients with confirmed hypercalcemia, the serum phosphorus may help to identify the cause. In disorders involving PTH or PTHrP, the stimulation of renal phosphorus excretion may lead to a low serum phosphate concentration. Normal to high serum phosphate concentrations is seen with vitamin D mediated states, renal failure, and disorders described above as related to bone. The next step is the measurement of PTH, which will be increased in PTH-mediated conditions but should be suppressed in other causes of hypercalcemia.

Table 13
Laboratory Features of Hypercalcemic Syndromes

Condition	PO$_4$	PTH	1,25(OH)$_2$D	Special test
1° Hyperparathyroidism	⇓	⇑	nl to ⇑	Urine Ca/cr ⇑
Familial hypercalciuric hypercalcemia	nl to ⇓	nl to ⇑	nl to ⇓	Urine Ca/cr ⇓
Vitamin D intoxication	⇑	⇓	nl to ⇑	25(OH)D ⇑
Granulomatous disorders	nl to ⇑	⇓	⇑	1,25(OH)$_2$D ⇑
Humoral hypercalcemia of malignancy	⇓	⇓	nl to ⇓	PTHrP ⇑
Immobilization	nl to ⇑	⇓	⇓	Urine Ca/cr ⇑
Subcutaneous fat necrosis	⇑	⇓	nl to ⇑	

The measurement of 25(OH)D is diagnostic in states of vitamin D intoxication and the more esoteric 1,25(OH)2D and PTHrP are helpful in patients in whom the history and other clinical information point to the possibility of their involvement. The urinary concentrations of calcium and creatinine can be a useful indicator of hypercalciuria as seen in most states or can be used to detect hypocalciuria in FHH patients and family members by measuring the ratio of calcium clearance to creatinine clearance.

19. MANAGEMENT OF HYPERCALCEMIA

The management of hypercalcemia in children will depend on the severity and cause of the hypercalcemia (Table 14). Ideally, the therapy should be directed at treatment of the underlying disorder. Otherwise the management is directed to lower serum calcium non-specifically by increasing renal excretion, reducing calcium absorption, or decreasing the flux out of bone (45, 46, 63). These processes may be affected in differing degrees depending on the etiology of the hypercalcemia. Renal calcium excretion can be increased by hydration, preferably with isotonic saline to first treat any ongoing dehydration and then to establish a saline diuresis with an infusion of isotonic saline at 2–3 times maintenance requirements. These measures with increase calcium filtration by increasing the glomerular filtration rate and decreasing the sodium dependent calcium reabsorption. Calcium reabsorption at the thick ascending limb can be further decreased with the addition of the loop diuretic furosemide but the intravascular volume status must be maintained with careful fluid balance or tubular reabsorption may increase worsening the hypercalcemia. Furosemide can lead to electrolyte disturbances such as hypokalemia if not monitored closely. Maximizing calcium excretion with these maneuvers has the ability to lower serum calcium approximately 1–3 mg/dL, but by itself cannot totally correct severe hypercalcemia. Gastrointestinal calcium absorption can be decreased by limiting the calcium and vitamin D in the diet especially in disorders mediated by 1,25(OH)$_2$D, using glucocorticoids, which block the action of

Table 14
Treatment of Hypercalcemia in Children*

Agent	Dose	Comment
Furosemide	0.5–1 mg/kg/dose IV q6–24 h	Avoid volume depletion
Methylprednisolone	1 mg/kg/day IV	Useful in vitamin D mediated hypercalcemia
Salmon Calcitonin	4–8 IU/kg q 12 h	Give IM or SQ
Pamidronate	0.5–1 mg/kg IV	Give in 10 ml/mg over 4 h minimum
Zoledronic acid	0.025–0.05 mg/kg IV	Give over 15–30 min

*Patient must be made euvolemic before and during therapy with normal saline 150–250 ml/kg/day.

vitamin D. The most severe hypercalcemic states generally involve increase bone resorption, so measures that decrease bone resorption are the most powerful in lowering serum calcium. The bisphosphonates, which inhibit osteoclast function, are the most potent agents in treating hypercalcemia. In children, the greatest experience is with intravenous pamidronate. There is a more potent analogue zoledronic acid, which has been introduced for hypercalcemia of malignancy in adults. Pamidronate has been given safely to children with metabolic bone disease at a dose of 1 mg/kg given intravenously in 10 ml isotonic saline per mg pamidronate to be given over 4 h. There is limited experience with the use of zoledronic acid in children although it has been reported to be safe when given at a dose of 0.025–0.05 mg/kg up to a maximum dose of 4 mg. An advantage of zoledronic acid is that it can be given over a minimum of 15–30 min rather than the 4 h required for pamidronate. Both agents should be avoided in the presence of renal failure and can be associated with transient fever and hypophosphatemia, and possibly an overshoot hypocalcemia. A much older agent to inhibit bone resorption is calcitonin. Calcitonin works to lower calcium in hours but a resistance to its effects develops over 24–48 h. Therefore it is useful when given in combination with one of the bisphosphonates. Several agents given in the past that are no longer recommended are plicamycin, gallium nitrate, and intravenous phosphate. Each of these agents has significant toxicities and has been replaced by the bisphosphonates.

With mild hypercalcemia (total serum calcium < 12 mg/dL, ionized < 1.5 mM), asymptomatic children often do not require treatment other than avoiding dehydration and reducing the calcium in the diet. In patients with moderate hypercalcemia (total serum calcium 12–14 mg/dL), dehydration should be expected and aggressive rehydration with normal saline should be instituted. Hydration is unlikely to normalize the serum calcium and the next step should be directed to treat the primary etiology if known. Bisphosphonates should be used only with caution with moderate hypercalcemia to avoid an over shoot hypocalcemia. In patients with severe hypercalcemia (total serum calcium > 14 mg/dL or who are symptomatic) are at greater risk for morbidity and mortality. In addition to the hydration, the careful addition of furosemide at a dose of 0.25–0.5 mg/kg can be given every 12 h after the patient is adequately hydrated with isotonic saline. Caution to avoid dehydration or hypokalemia must be exercised. Many of these patients will have increased bone resorption as part of their pathophysiology so the use of bisphosphonates, possibly preceded by calcitonin may be considered. There are rare patients with severe hypercalcemia with renal failure in whom peritoneal or hemodialysis using a low calcium dialysate as an emergency measure is indicated.

CASE SCENARIO DISCUSSIONS

Case Scenario 1: Hypercalcemia in a healthy adolescent. This young man is suffering from immobilization hypercalcemia with sudden turn off of his active bone mineralization simultaneous with an increase in bone resorption releasing large amounts of calcium into the blood stream. His lethargy and depression is a direct result as are his GI symptoms. He is hypertensive as result of the effect on the vascular system and his renal manifestations include acute renal failure and a urinary concentrating defect.

The combination of poor intake and renal water wasting has led him to be dehydrated which is exacerbating the direct inhibition of GFR by hypercalcemia. The cause of this patient's hypercalcemia appears to be fairly straightforward but a minimum work-up to look for any surprises in this patient with severe hypercalcemia would be a serum PTH level, which should be suppressed and a spot urine calcium/creatinine which should be elevated.

The definitive treatment would be to get the patient mobilized but that is not likely to be successful anytime soon and intermediate measures such as use of a tilt-table is not effective. The first step would be to correct the dehydration with isotonic saline and to maintain fluid balance by infusing the calcium at 2–3× maintenance. Whereas this is likely to help correct the acute renal failure and decrease the calcium, it is unlikely to lower the total calcium more than about 2 mg/dL. One can add furosemide at a dose of about 0.5–1.0 mg/kg IV every 12 h, the total fluid balance must stay positive or the calcium will start to go back up again. To lower the calcium to the normal range, a bisphosphonate may have to be used. The choices are pamidronate 0.5–1.0 mg/kg IV over 4 h or possibly the newest agent in the class, zoledronic acid 4 IV over 15 min. The patient's calcium, phosphorus, renal function, and electrolytes need to be monitored closely through the treatment phase.

Case Scenario 2: Neonatal hypercalcemia. This infant with the washed-out bones and hypercalcemia either could have a primary abnormality of the skeleton but more likely has neonatal hyperparathyroidism, which is supported by the low phosphorus level. The calcium level is lower than what is generally reported with NSHPT but a CaSR defect cannot be ruled out. Maternal hypocalcemia whether from hypoparathyroidism is an important cause but abnormalities of placental transport of calcium are possible as well. The first step in the diagnosis is to measure an ionized calcium PTH levels on the mother and infant. Urine calcium and creatinine levels may help in the evaluation of a CaSR disorder. In this case, the mother had low calcium and PTH levels because of idiopathic hypoparathyroidism that was not being medically controlled and her infant had an elevated PTH as result. The management of the moderate hypercalcemia was supportive with fluids; initially 150–200 ml/kg/day of normal saline given parenterally followed by oral intake of 2 times the normal maintenance requirements of fluid. With time, the hyperparathyroidism resolved and the skeleton remineralized.

REFERENCES

1. Rubin LP. Disorders of calcium and phosphorus metabolism. In: Taeusch HW, Ballard RA, Gleason CA (eds.) Avery's Diseases of the Newborn, 8th ed., Philadelphia: Saunders, 2005: 1346–1365.
2. Hruska KA, Levi M, Slatopolsky E. Disorders of phosphorus, calcium, magnesium metabolism. In: Schrier RW (ed.) Disorders of the Kidney & Urinary Tract, 8th ed., vol. 3. Philadelphia: Lippincott Williams & Wilkins, 2007:2295–2352.
3. Yu ASL. Renal transport of calcium, magnesium, and phosphate. In: Brenner BM (ed.) Brenner & Rector's the Kidney, 7th ed., vol. 1. Philadelphia: Saunders, 2004:535–571.
4. Vokes, TJ. Blood calcium, phosphate, and magnesium. In: Favus MJ (ed.) Primer on the Metabolic Bone Diseases and Disorders of Mineral Metabolism, 6th ed., Washington DC: American Society of Bone and Mineral Research, 2006:123–127.

5. Favus MJ, Bushinsky DA, Lemann J. Regulation of calcium, magnesium and phosphate metabolism. In: Favus MJ (ed.) Primer on the Metabolic Bone Diseases and Disorders of Mineral Metabolism, 6th ed., Washington DC: American Society of Bone and Mineral Research, 2006:76–83.

6. Rigo J, DE Curtis M. Disorders of calcium, phosphorus, and magnesium metabolism. In: Martin RJ, Fanaroff AA, Walsh MC (eds.) Fanaroff and Martin's Neonatal–Perinatal Medicine, 8th ed., vol. 2. Philadelphia: Mosby, 2006:1491–1520.

7. Marx SJ, Bourdeau JE. In: Narins RG (ed.) Maxwell & Kleeman's Clinical disorders of Fluid and Electrolyte metabolism, 5th ed, New York: McGraw-Hill 1994:XXX.

8. Favus MJ. Intestinal absorption of calcium, magnesium, and phosphorus. In: Coe FL, Favus MJ (eds.), Disorders of Bone and Mineral Metabolism, 2nd ed., Philadelphia: Lippincott Williams & Wilkins, 2002:48–73.

9. McKay CP, Specker BL, Tsang RC, Chesney RW. Mineral metabolism during childhood. In: Coe FL, Favus MJ (eds.) Disorders of Bone and Mineral Metabolism, 2nd ed., Philadelphia: Lippincott Williams & Wilkins, 2002:48–73.

10. Friedman PA. Renal calcium metabolism. In: Alpern RJ, Hebert SC (eds.) Seldin and Giebisch's The Kidney, 4th ed., vol. 2, Boston: Elsevier 2008:1851–1890.

11. Aubin JE, Lian JB, Stein GS. Bone formation: maturation and functional activities of osteoblast lineage cells. In: Favus MJ (ed.) Primer on the Metabolic Bone Diseases and Disorders of Mineral Metabolism, 6th ed., Washington DC: American Society of Bone and Mineral Research, 2006: 20–29.

12. Ross, PF. Osteoclast biology and bone resorption. In: Favus MJ (ed.) Primer on the Metabolic Bone Diseases and Disorders of Mineral Metabolism, 6th ed., Washington DC: American Society of Bone and Mineral Research, 2006:30–35.

13. Kovacs CS. Skeletal physiology: fetus and newborn. In: Favus MJ (ed.) Primer on the Metabolic Bone Diseases and Disorders of Mineral Metabolism, 6th ed., Washington DC: American Society of Bone and Mineral Research, 2006:50–55.

14. Tebben PJ, Kumar R. The hormonal regulation of calcium metabolism. In: Alpern RJ, Hebert SC (eds.) Seldin and Giebisch's The Kidney, 4th ed., vol. 2, Boston: Elsevier 2008: 1891–1909.

15. Hebert SC, Riccardi D, Geibel JP. The calcium-sensing receptor. In: Alpern RJ, Hebert SC (eds.) Seldin and Giebisch's The Kidney, 4th ed., vol. 2, Boston: Elsevier 2008:1785–1802.

16. Holick MF, Garabedian M. Vitamin D: Photobiology, metabolism, mechanism of action and clinical applications. In: Favus MJ (ed.) Primer on the Metabolic Bone Diseases and Disorders of Mineral Metabolism, 6th ed., Washington DC: American Society of Bone and Mineral Research, 2006: 50–55.

17. Deftos LJ. Calcitonin. In: Favus MJ (ed.) Primer on the Metabolic Bone Diseases and Disorders of Mineral Metabolism, 6th ed., Washington DC: American Society of Bone and Mineral Research, 2006:50–55.

18. Portale AA. Blood calcium, phosphate, and magnesium. In: Favus MJ (ed.) Primer on the Metabolic Bone Diseases and Disorders of Mineral Metabolism, 3rd ed., Washington DC: American Society of Bone and Mineral Research, 1996:93–96.

19. Penfield JG, Choudry, Cronin, Knochel JP, Levi M. Disorders of phosphate and magnesium metabolism. In: Coe FL, Favus MJ (eds.), Disorders of Bone and Mineral Metabolism, 2nd ed., Philadelphia: Lippincott Williams & Wilkins, 2002:48–73.

20. Heath H. Laboratory analyses useful in the diagnosis of bone and calcium metabolic disorders. In: Kleerekoper M, Siris ES, McClung M (eds.) The Bone and Mineral Manual, 2nd ed., New York: Elsevier, 2005:11–15.

21. Brown EM, Juppner H. Parathyroid hormone: synthesis, secretion, and action. In: Favus MJ (ed.) Primer on the Metabolic Bone Diseases and Disorders of Mineral Metabolism, 6th ed., Washington DC: American Society of Bone and Mineral Research, 2006:90–99.

22. Mallette LE, Gagel RF. Parathyroid hormone and calcitonin. In: Favus MJ (ed.) Primer on the Metabolic Bone Diseases and Disorders of Mineral Metabolism, 3rd ed., Washington DC: American Society of Bone and Mineral Research, 1996:96–109.

23. Clemens TL, Adams JS. Vitamin D metabolites. In: Favus MJ (ed.) Primer on the Metabolic Bone Diseases and Disorders of Mineral Metabolism, 3rd ed., Washington DC: American Society of Bone and Mineral Research, 1996:109–114.

24. Broadus AE, Nissenson RA. Parathyroid hormone-related protein. In: Favus MJ (ed.) Primer on the Metabolic Bone Diseases and Disorders of Mineral Metabolism, 6th ed., Washington DC: American Society of Bone and Mineral Research, 2006:99–106.

25. Burtis WJ. Parathyroid-hormone-related protein assays. In: Favus MJ (ed.) Primer on the Metabolic Bone Diseases and Disorders of Mineral Metabolism, 3rd ed., Washington DC: American Society of Bone and Mineral Research, 1996:105–109.

26. Marx SJ. Familial hypocalciuric hypercalcemia. In: Favus MJ (ed.) Primer on the Metabolic Bone Diseases and Disorders of Mineral Metabolism, 3rd ed., Washington DC: American Society of Bone and Mineral Research, 1996:190–192.

27. Fitzpatrick LA. The hypocalcemic states. In: Coe FL, Favus MJ (eds.), Disorders of Bone and Mineral Metabolism, 2nd ed., Philadelphia: Lippincott Williams & Wilkins,2002: 568–588.

28. Lebowitz MR, Moses AM. Hypocalcemia. Sem in Nephrol 1992:12:146–158.

29. Heras-Herzig A, Guise TA. Disorders of calcium metabolism. In: Alpern RJ, Hebert SC (eds.) Seldin and Giebisch's The Kidney, 4th ed., vol. 2, Boston: Elsevier 2008:1911–1944.

30. Goltzman D, Cole DEC. Hypoparathyroidism. In: Favus MJ (ed.) Primer on the Metabolic Bone Diseases and Disorders of Mineral Metabolism, 6th ed., Washington DC: American Society of Bone and Mineral Research, 2006:216–219.

31. Downs RW. Hypoparathyroidism in the differential diagnosis of hypocalcemia. In: Bilezekian JP (ed.) The Parathyroids, 2nd ed., San Diego: Academic Press 2001:755–761.

32. Thakker RV. The molecular genetics of hypoparathyroidism. In: Bilezekian JP (ed.) The Parathyroids. 2nd ed., San Diego: Academic Press 2001:779–789.

33. Umpaichitra V, Bastian W, Castells S. Hypocalcemia in children: pathogenesis and management. Clin Pediatr 2001;40:305–312.

34. Pollack MR, Yu ASL. Clinical disturbances of calcium, magnesium, and phosphate metabolism. In: Brenner BM (ed.) Brenner & Rector's The Kidney, 7th ed., vol. 1, Philadelphia: Saunders, 2004: 1041–1076.

35. Whyte MP. Autoimmune hypoparathyroidism. In: Bilezekian JP (ed.) The Parathyroids. 2nd ed., San Diego: Academic Press 2001:791–805.

36. Jan De Beur SM, Levine MA. Pseudohypoparathyroidism. In: Bilezekian JP (ed.) The Parathyroids, 2nd ed., San Diego: Academic Press 2001:807–825.

37. Carpenter TO, Insogna KL. The hypocalcemic disorders: differential diagnosis and therapeutic use of vitamin D. In: Feldman D (ed.) Vitamin D, 2nd ed., vol. 2, Boston: Elsevier 2005: 1049–1063.

38. Downs RW. Miscellaneous causes of hypocalcemia. In: Favus MJ (ed.) Primer on the Metabolic Bone Diseases and Disorders of Mineral Metabolism, 6th ed., Washington DC: American Society of Bone and Mineral Research, 2006:227–229.

39. Benabe JE, Martines-Maldonado M. Disorders of calcium metabolism. In: Narins RG (ed.) Maxwell & Kleeman's Clinical Disorders of Fluid and Electrolyte Metabolism, 5th ed., New York: McGraw-Hill 1994:1009–1044.

40. Carpenter TO. Neonatal hypocalcemia. In: Favus MJ (ed.) Primer on the Metabolic Bone Diseases and Disorders of Mineral Metabolism, 6th ed., Washington DC: American Society of Bone and Mineral Research, 2006:227–229.

41. Rubin LP. Disorders of calcium and phosphorus metabolism. In: Taeusch HW, Ballard RA, Gleason CA (eds.) Avery's Diseases of the Newborn, 8th ed., Philadelphia: Saunders, 2005: 1346–1365.

42. Koo W. Hypocalcemia and hypercalcemia in neonates. In: Kleerekoper M, Siris ES, McClung M (eds.) The Bone and Mineral Manual, 2nd ed., New York: Elsevier, 2005:11–15.

43. Drezner MK. Treatment of hypoparathyroidism. In: Bilezekian JP (ed.) The Parathyroids, 2nd ed., San Diego: Academic Press 2001:827–833.

44. Thakker RV. Hypocalcemia: pathogenesis, differential diagnosis, and management. In: Favus MJ (ed.) Primer on the Metabolic Bone Diseases and Disorders of Mineral Metabolism, 6th ed., Washington DC: American Society of Bone and Mineral Research, 2006:213–215.

45. Shane E, Irani D. Hypercalcemia: pathogenesis, clinical manifestations, differential diagnosis, and management. In: Favus MJ, (ed.) Primer on the Metabolic Bone Diseases and Disorders of Mineral Metabolism, 6th ed., Washington DC: American Society of Bone and Mineral Research, 2006: 176–180.

46. Bilezekian JP, Mulder JE, Silverberg SJ. Hypercalcemic states: differential diagnosis and acute management. In: Coe FL, Favus MJ (eds.), Disorders of Bone and Mineral Metabolism, 2nd ed., Philadelphia: Lippincott Williams & Wilkins, 2002:489–515.

47. Heller HJ, Pak CYC. Primary hyperparathyroidism. In: Coe FL, Favus MJ (eds.) Disorders of Bone and Mineral Metabolism, 2nd ed., Philadelphia: Lippincott Williams & Wilkins, 2002: 516–534.

48. Germain-Lee EL, Levine MA. Primary hyperparathyroidism and other causes of hypercalcemia in children and adolescents. In: Bilezekian JP (ed.) The Parathyroids, 2nd ed., San Diego: Academic Press 2001:743–753.

49. Kollars J, Zarroug AE, van Heerden J, Lteif A, Stavlo P, Suarez L, Moir C, Ishitani M, Rodeberg D. Primary hyperparathyroidism in pediatric patients. Pediatrics 2005;115:974–980.

50. Arnold A. Familial hyperparathyroid syndromes. In: Favus MJ (ed.) Primer on the Metabolic Bone Diseases and Disorders of Mineral Metabolism, 6th ed., Washington DC: American Society of Bone and Mineral Research, 2006:185–188.

51. Marx SJ. Familial hypocalciuric hypercalcemia. In: Favus MJ (ed.) Primer on the Metabolic Bone Diseases and Disorders of Mineral Metabolism, 6th ed., Washington DC: American Society of Bone and Mineral Research, 2006:188–190.

52. Rubin MR, Thys-Jacobs S, Chan FK, Koberle LMC, Bilezikiann JP. Hypercalcemia due to vitamin D toxicity. In: Feldman D (ed.) Vitamin D, 2nd ed., vol. 2, Boston: Elsevier 2005:1355–1377.

53. Bell NH. Hypercalcemia and abnormal vitamin D metabolism. In: Coe FL, Favus MJ (eds.) Disorders of Bone and Mineral Metabolism, 2nd ed., Philadelphia: Lippincott Williams & Wilkins, 2002:48–73.

54. Hathcock JN, Shao A, Vieth R, Heaney R. Risk assessment for vitamin D. Am J Clin Nutr 2007;85: 6–18.

55. Adams JS, Hewison M. Hypercalcemia caused by granuloma-forming diseases. In: Favus MJ (ed.) Primer on the Metabolic Bone Diseases and Disorders of Mineral Metabolism, 6th ed., Washington DC: American Society of Bone and Mineral Research, 2006:200–202.

56. Horwitz MJ, Orloff JJ, Stewart AF. Disorders of serum minerals caused by cancer. In: Coe FL, Favus MJ (eds.) Disorders of Bone and Mineral Metabolism, 2nd ed., Philadelphia: Lippincott Williams & Wilkins, 2002:535–556.

57. McKay CP, Furman WL: Hypercalcemia complicating childhood malignancies. Cancer 1993;72: 256–260.

58. Wysolmerski JJ. Miscellaneous causes of hypercalcemia. In: Favus MJ (ed.) Primer on the Metabolic Bone Diseases and Disorders of Mineral Metabolism, 6th ed., Washington DC: American Society of Bone and Mineral Research, 2006:203–208.

59. Benabe JE, Martines-Maldonado M. Disorders of calcium metabolism. In: Narins RG (ed.) Maxwell & Kleeman's Clinical disorders of Fluid and Electrolyte metabolism, 5th ed., New York: McGraw-Hill 1994:1009–1044.

60. Langman CB. Hypercalcemic syndromes in infants and children. In: Favus MJ (ed.) Primer on the Metabolic Bone Diseases and Disorders of Mineral Metabolism, 6th ed., Washington DC: American Society of Bone and Mineral Research, 2006:209–212.

61. Unger S, Paul DA, Nino M, McKay C, Miller S, Sochett E, Braverman N, Clarke JTR, Cole DEC. Mucolipidosis II presenting as severe neonatal hyperparathyroidism. European J Pediatr 2005;164:236–243.

62. Jacobs TP, Bilezekian JP. Rare causes of hypercalcemia. J Clin Endocrinol Metab 2005;90:6316–6322.

63. Ziegler R. Hypercalcemic crisis. J Am Soc Nephrol 2001;12:S3–S9.

5 Disorders of Magnesium Metabolism

Charles P. McKay

Key Points

1. Serum magnesium concentrations may not reflect the state of whole body magnesium stores.
2. In magnesium depletion states, urinary fractional excretion of magnesium should be less than 2% if renal conservation is normal.
3. Hypomagnesemia is a common electrolyte disturbance that is usually mild but can be associated with refractory hypocalcemia and severe neuromuscular and cardiac disturbances.
4. Recently described genetic abnormalities of intestinal and renal magnesium transport are important causes of hypomagnesemia.

Key Words: Magnesium; hypomagnesemia; hypermagnesemia; hypocalcemia; Bartter syndrome

1. INTRODUCTION

Magnesium is the 4th most abundant cation in the body with an average adult having about 25 g of magnesium and the 2nd most abundant cation in the cell. It shares many characteristics with calcium but does not appear to be regulated by a control system like calcium, which is regulated by PTH and vitamin D. The homeostasis of magnesium is largely controlled by the kidney whereas the level of serum calcium is the result of the net flux from bone, intestine, and kidney. Magnesium is a divalent cation with an atomic weight of 24 and serves in the body as an important cofactor for numerous enzymes, especially those involving ATP. It is therefore very important in the regulation of membrane stability, hormone secretion, neuromuscular, and cardiovascular function. Disorders of magnesium metabolism are characterized by abnormalities in these systems.

2. DISTRIBUTION OF MAGNESIUM IN THE BODY

Sixty six percent of all total body magnesium is in the skeleton as compared to 99% for calcium. Another 33% of total body magnesium is intracellular, with the majority being in muscle and liver and only 1% is extracellular (1).

From: *Nutrition and Health: Fluid and Electrolytes in Pediatrics*
Edited by: L. G. Feld, F. J. Kaskel, DOI 10.1007/978-1-60327-225-4_5,
© Humana Press, a part of Springer Science+Business Media, LLC 2010

2.1. Serum Magnesium

The normal serum level of magnesium is kept in a fairly constant range of 1.6–2.4 mg/dL (1.4–2 mEq/L or 0.7–1.0 mmol/L) (2). Similar to calcium, it is the ionized portion of magnesium, which is physiologically important and that represents 55–70% of serum magnesium with protein-bound and complexed fractions making up about 20–30 and 10–20%, respectively. Because the relative amount of protein-bound magnesium is about half of that of calcium, the effect of low albumin states on the relation between total and the ionized fraction is not as dramatic with magnesium. Total serum magnesium levels correlate well with symptoms of hyper- and hypomagnesemia but do not correlate well with muscle and other tissue stores but there is better correlation with bone stores.

2.2. Tissue Magnesium

The majority of magnesium is in bone where it resides on the surface of the hydroxyapatite crystals and is freely exchangeable (3). The remaining 2/3 of total body magnesium is intracellular where it lies predominantly in organelles, especially the mitochondria. The cytosolic magnesium has a concentration of about 0.5 mM but is largely complexed to proteins and organophosphates with a small component being ionized. The concentration of intracellular magnesium does not vary greatly in the presence of hypomagnesemia or hypermagnesemia. The control of intracellular magnesium is still poorly described but is linked to cellular potassium homeostasis. Magnesium depletion appears to reduce muscle tissue stores of potassium and vice versa with a fall of muscle magnesium of 0.5 mmol for every 10 mmol fall in muscle potassium.

3. MAGNESIUM HOMEOSTASIS

Normal magnesium balance in adults is the result of ingestion of about 300 mg in the diet with secretion of about 30 mg with digestive juices (4). There is net absorption of 30% or 100 mg, which is usually excreted in the urine. Net magnesium absorption is linear with magnesium intake. Magnesium is plentiful in most foods so dietary deficiency is unusual. The daily requirements for magnesium range from 50 mg in the first 6 months of life to 150–250 mg in young children under 10 years of age to 400 mg in adolescent males. Magnesium absorption is not regulated so magnesium balance is generally the result of renal excretion.

3.1. Systemic Transport of Magnesium

3.1.1. INTESTINAL TRANSPORT

The majority of magnesium absorption occurs in the ileum with lesser amounts in the duodenum, jejunum, and colon (5). There appears to be both by saturable transcellular and nonsaturable paracellular transport but the saturable component normally contributes a small portion of total absorption. Nonsaturable paracellular absorption is by passive ionic diffusion and "solvent drag" with water absorption and is most prominent at higher intestinal concentrations of magnesium. At lower magnesium concentrations, there is evidence for active magnesium absorption that appears to involve the cation channel TRMP6. Abnormalities of this transporter appear to be responsible for the condition hypomagnesemia with secondary hypocalcemia (HSH). Unlike calcium absorption, the role for $1,25(OH)_2$ vitamin D regulation of magnesium absorption is controversial. Magnesium does not compete with calcium for absorption but its absorption can be decreased in the presence of substances that bind it like phosphorus.

3.1.2. RENAL HANDLING OF MAGNESIUM

Urinary excretion of magnesium is the product of filtration and renal tubular reabsorption with little evidence for secretion *(4, 6, 7)*. Magnesium balance is maintained by changes in tubular reabsorption, which is remarkable being that there is no system regulation as with PTH for calcium. About 80% of total serum magnesium is ultrafilterable which in adults means that about 2000 mg of magnesium are filtered and about 100 mg or 1–3% of the filtered load is excreted in the urine daily. The amount of excreted magnesium can vary from less than 0.5% with magnesium deficiency to up to 80% of the filtered load during magnesium infusion in renal failure.

The proximal renal tubule only reabsorbs 10–15% of the filtered load in adults but 70% in neonates suggesting a change in the permeability to magnesium during development. This increased permeability in neonates may be a passive paracellular pathway not present in adults. Thus the reabsorption of magnesium is very different in mature subjects from calcium in which 60–70% is reabsorbed proximally. In contrast to the proximal tubule, the descending loop of Henle can reabsorb significant amounts of magnesium. The thick ascending limb (TAL) though is responsible for about 70% of magnesium reabsorption with the cortical TAL reabsorbing the major portion. Magnesium reabsorption is driven by the lumen positive transepithelial voltage generated by potassium recycling in this segment. This recycling requires the entry of Na, K, and chloride into the cell by the Na–K–2Cl transporter, exit of K back in to the lumen by ROMK and basolateral exit of Na by Na–K-ATPase and Cl by the chloride channels ClC-K$_a$ and ClC-K$_b$, both of which require a β-subunit called barttin. The permeability of the paracellular pathway for magnesium and calcium reabsorption has been shown to be controlled by the protein paracellin-1 that is the product of the gene *CLDN16*. There is some evidence for active transcellular reabsorption in the TAL but it is controversial. In the TAL and the distal tubule is found the calcium sensing receptor CaSR, which is responsible for control of magnesium reabsorption (Section 3.2).

The distal tubule is the last segment of the renal tubule demonstrated to reabsorb magnesium and it is responsible for about 10% of the magnesium reabsorption, which is predominantly transcellular and active. Magnesium, driven by the transmembrane negative electrical potential, enters the cell through the divalent ion channel TRPM6. TRPM6 is also found in the intestine and mutations of TRPM6 result in low magnesium GI absorption and renal reabsorption in the condition HSH.

3.2. Regulation of Magnesium Metabolism

Control of magnesium metabolism is predominantly by modulation of renal tubular reabsorption since the intestinal absorption is proportional to intake *(7, 8)*. Multiple

Table 1
Regulation of Magnesium in Renal Tubule

Agent or condition	Thick ascending limb	Distal tubule
Parathyroid hormone	Increase	Increase
Calcitonin	Increase	Increase
Vasopressin	Increase	Increase
1,25(OH)$_2$vitamin D	Unknown	Increase
Aldosterone	Increase	Increase
Insulin	Increase	Increase
Hypomagnesemia	Increase	Increase
Hypermagnesemia	Decrease	Decrease
Hypercalcemia	Decrease	Decrease
Volume expansion	Decrease	Decrease
Potassium depletion	Decrease	Decrease
Hypophosphatemia	Decrease	Decrease
Metabolic acidosis	Decrease	Decrease
Metabolic alkalosis	Increase	Increase
Loop diuretics	Decrease	No effect
Thiazide diuretics	No effect	Increase
Amiloride	No effect	Increase

hormones, metabolic conditions and diuretics influence magnesium reabsorption in the TAL and distal tubule (Table 1) but in contrast to calcium, there is no one system dedicated to the regulation of serum magnesium. In the TAL limb, magnesium reabsorption is modulated by changes in the transepithelial voltage, Na–K–2Cl transporter, potassium recycling and paracellin-1 regulation of the paracellular permeability and the agents and conditions that modify magnesium work through these mechanisms. One of the most important regulators of magnesium and calcium reabsorption in both the TAL and distal tubule is the divalent sensing receptor CaSR that is present in many tissues but most importantly the parathyroid and renal tubule. The CaSR responds to changes in plasma magnesium and calcium with a decrease in the paracellular transport of these two divalent cations possibly by affecting paracellin-1. This may be the predominant mechanism by which hypomagnesemia stimulates its renal conservation.

The distal tubule is responsible for determining the final amount of magnesium excreted. It increases magnesium reabsorption not only in response to PTH, calcitonin, and vasopressin but also in response to 1,25(OH)$_2$vitamin D. The systemic effect of 1,25(OH)$_2$vitamin D administration though may be increased magnesium excretion because of the effect of 1,25(OH)$_2$vitamin D on GI absorption and serum calcium and magnesium levels through which CaSR decreases magnesium reabsorption. Other metabolic conditions such as acidosis and intravascular volume status also affect magnesium excretion. Finally, certain diuretics have an important effect on renal tubular magnesium handling. Loop diuretics, which inhibit Na–K–2Cl transporter, acutely decrease magnesium reabsorption in the TAL but its chronic effects are lessened due to enhanced reabsorption in other parts of the nephron, especially the distal tubule. Thiazide diuretics, which inhibit the $Na^+–Cl^-$ cotransporter, increase magnesium excretion but this may be in part due to associated hypokalemia when given on a chronic basis. In contrast, the potassium sparing diuretic amiloride is also magnesium sparing.

4. NEONATAL MAGNESIUM METABOLISM

Magnesium is transported across the placenta to the fetus with daily accumulation of approximately 5 mg/day (9). Unlike calcium in which the transport appears greatest in the third trimester, placental magnesium transport appears greatest in the first trimester. The transport mechanism is distinct from the one that transports calcium and maintains a fetal magnesium concentration that is greater than the maternal concentration. The magnesium transport is affected by maternal stores so that infants born to mothers who are magnesium depleted will be born with abnormally low stores as well. After birth, intestinal magnesium absorption appears to be greater than that demonstrated later in childhood. There also appears to be greater tubular reabsorption of magnesium by the kidney which in part may be due to increased permeability in the proximal tubule as described in Section 3.1.2. Fractional excretion of magnesium ($FE_{mg} = (U_{mg} \div S_{mg})/U_{cr} \div S_{cr})$ $\times$ 100) less than 1% has been described as compared to excretion in older children and adults of 1–3%. These processes likely contribute to the higher serum magnesium concentrations described in premature infants, especially those less than 35 weeks gestation. The suggested intake for magnesium is 4–15 mg/100 kcal in term infants and 7–17 mg/dL in preterm infants.

5. MEASUREMENT OF MAGNESIUM

Evaluation of magnesium metabolism for the most part is concerned with the determination of the status of magnesium stores to evaluate for evidence of depletion or excess. Since no hormone system is responsible for control of magnesium as is true for calcium with parathyroid hormone and vitamin D, study of such a system is unnecessary.

5.1. Serum Magnesium

Serum magnesium shares several features with serum calcium; first, total magnesium is comprised of three fractions ionized, protein-bound and complexed, secondly, the ionized fraction is physiologically and clinically the most important, and finally, protein binding by magnesium is mostly to albumin and is pH dependent (10). In contrast to calcium, total serum magnesium is not as dependent on the levels of serum albumin since only 20–30% of total magnesium is protein-bound. Therefore, direct measurement of ionized magnesium is usually not available in the clinical setting even though magnesium-specific electrodes have been developed and normal ionized magnesium levels in the serum are 0.44–0.59 mmol/L. The total serum magnesium may be "corrected" for the level of magnesium with the formula: ($Mg_c = Mg_T + (4 - Salb)$) where Mg_c is the "corrected" magnesium, Mg_T is the total magnesium in mmol/L, and Salb is the albumin concentration in g/dL, but generally in clinical practice such "correction" is not performed.

Total serum magnesium is measured by a spectrophotometric method using calmagite as the indicator. Total magnesium is usually measured in serum but heparinized plasma can be used if caution is exercised to avoid certain heparins such as lithium heparin known to artifactually increase plasma magnesium. Citrate and EDTA that can complex magnesium and lower measured levels should never be used. Serum and plasma must be quickly separated from RBCs while avoiding hemolysis to avoid leakage of magnesium out of the cells. For the most part, the serum magnesium status is evaluated by total magnesium with the normal range being 1.6–2.4 mg/dL (1.4–2 mEq/L or 0.7–1.0 mmol/L).

5.2. Evaluation of Body Tissue Stores

Clinical investigators for years have studied methods to evaluate the state of magnesium stores by measuring magnesium levels in bone, erythrocytes, and other tissues (1, 3). Erythrocyte magnesium correlates poorly with whole body magnesium and is not clinically useful. For the most part serum magnesium is used to estimate bone and total body magnesium but there are times where hypomagnesemia may be present without magnesium depletion. To further investigate the possibility of magnesium depletion, the so-called Magnesium Tolerance Test (MTT) has been described for adults (11). It is based on the principle that in the presence of magnesium depletion, an administered magnesium load will be taken up by bone and other tissue and not be excreted in the urine. The protocol is described in Table 2. The test has not been standardized in children but there is no reason to think that the results would be significantly different in older children than adults. The one caveat is that with abnormal renal magnesium wasting, the test cannot be used.

Table 2
Magnesium Tolerance Test Protocol

---

1.   Collect 24 h urine for baseline magnesium/creatinine ratio.
2.   Infuse 0.2 mEq (2.4 mg) elemental magnesium per kilogram lean body
        weight in 50 ml D5W over 4 h.
3.   Collect 24 h urine for magnesium/creatinine starting with the
        beginning of the infusion,
4.   Calculate percentage magnesium retained with the formula: %Mg
        retained = 1 – [Postinfusion 24 h urine Mg – Preinfusion urine
        Mg/creatinine × postinfusion creatinine – total elemental Mg infused
        × 100]
5.   Definition of magnesium deficiency:
        >50% retention at 24 h = definite deficiency
        >25% retention at 24 h = probable deficiency

---

6. CLINICAL EVALUATION MAGNESIUM RENAL HANDLING

Magnesium balance is maintained by either intestinal absorption or renal excretion. Renal excretion of magnesium usually matches the intestinal absorption and in the presence of magnesium depletion the renal excretion of magnesium should be quite low

(2, 4). In adults it has been shown to be 12 mg/day or less with severe depletion. To test whether there is appropriate renal conservation of magnesium or if the kidney is contributing to the condition by inappropriate magnesium loss into the urine, fractional excretion of magnesium (Fe$_{Mg}$) can be measured in a spot urine using the formula:

$$FEMg = UMg \times PCr/0.7 \times PMg \times UCr \times 100$$

in which Cr = creatinine, P = plasma, and U = urine.

In non-renal disorders causing hypomagnesemia, the FEMg should be <2% but in renal wasting of magnesium it is typically >5% and is often 15% or greater.

7. GENETIC TESTING OF MAGNESIUM DISORDERS

The genetic cause of many of the hypomagnesemic disorders (Table 5) have been identified and can be measured clinically. At the time of the writing of this chapter, there are CLIA approved laboratories for a number of the described genetic defects. Information for the laboratories can be accessed through GeneTests©, University of Washington, Seattle, WA; www.geneclinics.org, which is funded by the National Library of Medicine, NIH and the National Human Genome Research Institute, NIH. This site provides current information about the different disorders, labs providing testing, what tests are offered, methods used, CLIA status, and contact information.

8. HYPOMAGNESEMIA – INTRODUCTION

Magnesium depletion is a very common and important condition whose severity is often underestimated by the level of serum magnesium. It is almost always the result of decreased gastrointestinal absorption or increased renal loss. Hypomagnesemia can be from rare inherited disorders or be associated with many common GI disorders and medications. Nutritional deficiency of magnesium is also an important contributing factor. The signs and symptoms of hypomagnesemia are usually the result of neuromuscular hyperexcitability or cardiac disturbances. Hypomagnesemia is also an important cause of refractory electrolyte disturbances of calcium and potassium homeostasis.

HYPOMAGNESEMIA CASE SCENARIOS

Case Scenario #1: Multiple electrolyte abnormalities in 12-year-old. You are called to see 12-year-old male who was admitted 2 days prior with diarrhea and weakness. Labs show Na-132 mEq/L, K-2.8 mEq/L, Cl-98 mEq/L, HCO$_3$-18 mEq/L, calcium-6.8 mg/dL, and albumin 2.8 g/dL. He has been on IV fluids with 40 mEq/L potassium and oral calcium supplements but his labs have not improved. He has a PMH of prematurity with necrotizing enterocolitis, short-gut syndrome, and chronic diarrhea. You perform a physical and he has short stature, and has a positive Trousseau's and Chvostek's signs. You ask the lab to add a magnesium level to the morning labs and the result comes back 0.85 mg/dL.

What is the likely cause of the hypomagnesemia? How does it relate to the other electrolyte disturbances? How would you treat this patient?

Case Scenario #2: Two-day-old neonate with seizures. Full term AGA infant who is a product of a term pregnancy and born by a spontaneous vaginal delivery without complications develops poor feedings followed by a generalized seizure at 48 h of age. Stat labs show normal electrolytes and total serum calcium 5.8 mg/dL and an IV dose of calcium is given without correction of the hypocalcemia. Review of the record shows that the mother has diabetes.

What is the most likely cause and how would you make the diagnosis? What are the emergency steps in the treatment?

9. DEFINITION OF HYPOMAGNESEMIA AND MAGNESIUM DEPLETION

Hypomagnesemia may be defined as serum magnesium levels less than 1.6 mg/dL (1.4 mEq/L or 0.7 mmol/L) *(10)*. Due to lesser protein binding, "pseudohypomagnesemia" due to hypoalbuminemia is not the problem that "pseudohypocalcemia" is with low serum albumin. Whereas hypomagnesemia is relatively easy to define, the characterization of whole body magnesium stores is much more difficult and is discussed in Section 5.2. The evaluation of urinary excretion of a magnesium load with the so-called Magnesium Tolerance Test has been accepted in adults as the best measurement of tissue stores but it has not been well studied in children.

10. CLINICAL FEATURES OF HYPOMAGNESEMIA

The clinical manifestations of hypomagnesemia can be separated into its neuromuscular and cardiac effects and disturbances on calcium and potassium homeostasis (Table 3) *(2, 12)*. The exact role of magnesium depletion on the heart and nervous system is often difficult to separate from concomitant hypocalcemia, hypokalemia, or associated clinical conditions. Conversely, magnesium deficiency must be considered in patients with hypocalcemia, hypokalemia, and any of the signs and symptoms outlined below.

10.1. Neuromuscular Effects

The earliest sign of hypomagnesemia may be neuromuscular irritability, which can be manifested by a positive Trousseau's and Chvostek's signs as described with hypocalcemia *(13)*. Trousseau's sign is elicited by pumping a sphygmomanometer cuff 20 mmHg above the systolic BP for 5 min to produce ischemia of the ulnar nerve. A positive sign is when the metacarpophalangeal joints flex, interphalangeal joints extend, and the thumb adducts. Chvostek's sign is elicited by tapping with three fingers over the facial nerve anterior to the ear. A positive sign can be arranged from twitching of the lip at the angle of the mouth to twitching of nasolabial fold, lateral angle of the eye or finally all of the facial muscles on that side. Although isolated magnesium depletion has been shown to cause neuromuscular irritability, many or most children with positive Trousseau's and Chvostek's signs will have concurrent hypocalcemia.

Table 3
Clinical Manifestations of Hypomagnesemia

Neuromuscular
    Positive Trousseau's and Chvostek's signs
    Muscle tremor
    Muscle weakness
    Vertical nystagmus
    Seizures
Cardiac
    EKG changes
        Prolonged PR and QT intervals
    Arrhythmias
        Supraventricular
        Ventricular
    Sudden death
    Enhancement of digoxin toxicity
    Hypertension
Electrolyte
    Hypokalemia
    Hypocalcemia

Central nervous systems symptoms include seizures that may be tonic–clonic, multifocal motor or generalized. Other symptoms described with hypomagnesemia include vertigo, ataxia, choreo-athetoid movements, and psychiatric changes. A rare but fairly specific sign for hypomagnesemia is vertical nystagmus that may not resolve immediately after correction of hypomagnesemia.

10.2. Cardiac Effects

The cardiac manifestations involve mainly conduction disturbances but in adults there is great interest in the role of magnesium in myocardial infarction (2). The pathophysiology of the abnormality involves the role of magnesium, calcium and potassium on depolarization and repolarization of the myocardium. Electrocardiogram disturbances include prolongation of the PR and QT intervals and widening of the QRS complex. Abnormal T and U waves may develop as well as the electrolyte disturbances become more severe. Mild hypomagnesemia is not associated with arrhythmias but adults with severe hypomagnesemia have developed atrial and most importantly ventricular arrhythmias. Digoxin toxicity is an important condition that can be exacerbated in the presence of hypomagnesemia and hypokalemia.

10.3. Electrolyte Disturbances

Patients with hypomagnesemia often also present with hypocalcemia and hypokalemia (3). Several features of these two disturbances with hypomagnesemia are refractory to treatment unless the underlying magnesium deficiency is corrected. Hypocalcemia and hypokalemia likely play a large role in the symptoms associated with hypomagnesemia and there are numerous inherited and acquired causes of hypo-magnesemia, which also cause wasting of potassium and calcium.

Hypokalemia and potassium depletion has long been recognized as a feature of mag-nesium depletion. The cause and effect or "chicken and egg" question of which comes first is difficult to discern with hypokalemia and hypomagnesemia. There is both loss of intracellular potassium and renal wasting of potassium in the presence of hypomagne-semia. The pathophysiology may relate to effects of magnesium on intracellular mecha-nisms involving ATP as well as the functioning of potassium channels. Nevertheless, in patients with refractory hypokalemia, concomitant hypomagnesemia should be sought and treated.

Severe refractory hypocalcemia has long been recognized in pediatrics to be associ-ated with hypomagnesemia. This is not seen with mild hypomagnesemia when magne-sium stimulates the CaSR on parathyroid cells similar to calcium but typically is seen with severe hypomagnesemia when the serum magnesium is less than 1.1 mg/dL *(4)*. The mechanism may be due to inhibition of PTH secretion secondary to interference in the generation of second messengers by adenylate cyclase and phospholipase C in part by enhancing the inhibitory action of the CaSR on PTH secretion. There is also a resistance to the action of PTH with magnesium depletion at the level of bone and the kidney so even in the presence of PTH; there is a subnormal tissue effect. The result is refractory hypocalcemia resistant to even IV calcium and 1,25-$(OH)_2$ vitamin D unless magnesium is administered concurrently. In patients with severe hypocalcemia and hypomagnesemia who are given magnesium, the PTH secretory response and rise in calcium can occur in minutes but the peripheral response to PTH may take days to fully correct.

11. CAUSES OF HYPOMAGNESEMIA

11.1. Decreased Intake

Hypomagnesemia can be seen with a variety of illnesses associated with decreased intake (Table 4). In these states the renal excretion will decrease to less than 12 mg per day but continued unregulated stool losses from GI secretions result in net negative balance *(1, 14)*. This can result from starvation or unusual diets or with protein-calorie malnutrition. Children with protein-calorie malnutrition may have diarrhea and other factors that contribute to the hypomagnesemia. Also hospitalized patients, especially those in ICU settings on prolonged parenteral therapy are at high risk for magnesium depletion.

11.2. Decreased GI Absorption

A large number of GI illnesses that are associated with chronic diarrhea even without malabsorption can have hypomagnesemia due to the high concentration of magnesium in diarrheal fluid *(11, 14)*. Intestinal malabsorption in conditions such as celiac disease can develop magnesium depletion as result of magnesium binding to free fatty acids to form soaps. The hypomagnesemia can be correlated with the rate of excretion of fecal fat and can be lessened with the institution of a low fat diet. Hypomagnesemia with

Table 4

Causes of Hypomagnesesemia

Decreased dietary intake
    Starvation
    Protein–calorie malnutrition
    Total parenteral nutrition
Decreased intestinal absorption
    Chronic diarrhea
    Malabsorption syndromes – celiac, short gut
    Steatorrhea
    Hypomagnesemia with secondary hypocalcemia
Increased renal tubular disorders
    Gitelman and some Bartter syndrome
    Autosomal dominant hypoparathyroidism, Bartter-like phenotype
    Familial hypomagnesemia with hypercalciuria and nephrocalcinosis
    Isolated dominant and recessive hypomagnesemia
    Mitochondrial hypomagnesemia
Secondary renal magnesium wasting
    Diabetes, DKA
    Post-obstructive and post-ATN diuresis
    Volume expansion, hyperaldosteronism
    Medications
        Diuretics, except potassium sparing diuretics
        Cisplatin
        Amphotericin
        Cyclosporin, Tacrolimus
        Amphotericin
Other
    Pancreatitis
    Hyperthyroidism
    Burns

secondary hypocalcemia is a rare genetic disorder of the TRPM6 gene on chromosome 9q22 resulting severe hypomagnesemia presenting in infancy with refractory seizures *(15)*. Hypocalcemia unresponsive to calcium replacement results from suppression of PTH secretion (Section 10.3) but which can respond to parenteral or sometimes high-dose enteral magnesium.

11.3. Renal Magnesium Wasting

11.3.1. FUNCTIONAL MAGNESIUM WASTING

There are a variety of disorders in which there is renal wasting of magnesium due to the inhibition of tubular reabsorption of magnesium as described in Section 3.1.2 *(8)*. The first group of disorders are associated with polyuria and can be associated with an osmotic diuresis as is seen with diabetic ketoacidosis or when there is abnormal salt and water reabsorption as seen in the recovery phase of acute tubular necrosis or during the diuretic phase after relief of urinary obstruction. Renal magnesium wasting is also seen when salt and water reabsorption are inhibited after volume expansion with saline or as a result of hyperaldosteronism. Finally there can be magnesium losses in the urine with tubular dysfunction from interstitial nephritis or after renal transplantation.

11.3.2. MEDICATIONS

A number of medications cause hypomagnesemia including the loop diuretics and the thiazides, which inhibit salt and water reabsorption and hence the forces driving magnesium reabsorption in the thick ascending limb (TAL) and distal convoluted tubule (DCT), respectively *(8)*. Osmotic diuretics induced by mannitol or with hyperglycemia and glucosuria can also cause magnesuria. Another important cause of renal magnesium wasting is due to tubular toxicity seen with cisplatin, amphotericin B, aminoglycosides, and cyclosporin A. The mechanism and clinical course of each is unique. The magnesium wasting with cisplatin is associated with hypocalciuria suggesting involvement of the DCT and can last for months after the discontinuation of the drug. Amphotericin B induced magnesuria is related to the total cumulative dose and is also associated with hypocalciuria but has the other classic features of renal potassium wasting and distal renal tubular acidosis. Aminoglycosides renal toxicity can present with hypomagnesemia, hypokalemia, hypocalcemia, and tetany and has been associated with high doses. More commonly, mild hypomagnesemia is seen during therapy but reverses shortly after its discontinuation. Finally, the hypomagnesemia of cyclosporine A is common with its use in transplant patients but does not correlate with serum cyclosporine levels or other signs of renal toxicity.

11.3.3. INHERITED RENAL MAGNESIUM WASTING DISORDERS

Recent developments in molecular biology have allowed the identification of several inherited disorders of renal wasting and better understanding of the mechanisms of normal and abnormal renal magnesium transport (Table 5) *(8, 15)*. Disorders of salt and water transport in the TAL and DCT are primarily responsible for renal magnesium wasting. Hypomagnesemia has been long recognized as a feature in many patients with Bartter syndrome. We have a much better understanding of the biologic nature of this group of illnesses, which we now subdivide based on the molecular defect and specific features. Whereas most patients who present with the so-called antenatal Bartter syndrome (aBS), which is a disorder of the NKCC2 cotransporter or the ROMK potassium channel do not have significant hypomagnesemia, those with antenatal Bartter syndrome and sensorineural deafness (BSND) can have magnesium levels of 1.2 mg/dL or less. The defective gene product has been creatively named "barttin" and is the B subunit activating the renal chloride channels CLC-Ka and CLC-Kb. This abnormality, which inhibits salt and water reabsorption in both the TAL and DCT, explains the magnesium wasting. These patients can be distinguished from those with aBS by the absence of hypercalciuria and nephrocalcinosis as well as the presence of the deafness. They often require parenteral fluid replacement and can advance to end-stage renal disease.

Table 5

Inherited Causes of Hypomagnesemia with OMIM Numbers

Disease	OMIM®	Gene	Protein
Hypomagnesemia with secondary hypocalcemia	602014	TRPM6	TRPM6
Familial hypomagnesemia with hypercalciuria and nephrocalcinosis	603959	CLDN16	Paracellin-1
Familial hypomagnesemia with hypercalciuria and nephrocalcinosis with ocular	610036	CLD19	Claudin 19
Autosomal dominant hypomagnesemia with hypocalciuria	154020	FXYD2	γ Subunit Na^+–K^+–ATPase
Activating mutations of divalent ion sensing receptor	601199	CASR	Ca^{2+}/Mg^{2+}-sensing receptor
Gitelman syndrome	263800	SLC12A3	NCCT
Antenatal Bartter syndrome type I	601678	SLC12A1	NKCC2
Antenatal Bartter syndrome type II	241200	KCNJ1	ROMK
Classic Bartter syndrome type III	607364	CLCNKB	CLCKB
Bartter syndrome with sensorineural deafness type IV	602522	BSND or CLCNKA +CLCNKB	Barttin or CLCKA and CLCKB

Adapted from Naderi et al. *(10)*. OMIM is the Online Mendelian Inheritance in Man® (Johns Hopkins University, Baltimore, MD; www.ncbi.nih.gov/sites/entrez?db=OMIM)

Mutations in the *CLCNKB* gene coding for CLC-Kb chloride channel are the cause for classic Bartter syndrome, which is only associated with hypomagnesemia in some of the affected patients. The features of this syndrome are hypokalemic metabolic alkalosis with variable hypercalciuria.

Gitelman syndrome, which is caused by mutations of *SLC12A3*, which codes for the thiazide-sensitive sodium–chloride cotransporter NCCT, is a defect of the DCT and is characterized by hypokalemia, hypomagnesemia, metabolic alkalosis, and hypocalciuria. The cause of magnesium wasting with this defect is not well understood with hypotheses ranging from the abnormal sodium entry into the DCT cells to apoptosis of the early DCT cells, which are responsible for magnesium transport.

Disorders of the divalent ion receptor CaSR, which is expressed in the TAL, cells as well as the parathyroid glands, are also associated with abnormalities in magnesium handling. Autosomal dominant hypoparathyroidism is due to activating mutation of CaSR and patients with this disorder typically have hypomagnesemia in the 1.2–1.4 mg/dL range in addition to hypocalcemia. Treatment with calcium and vitamin D can lead to worsening of the hypercalciuria and hypomagnesemia and should be reserved only for symptomatic hypocalcemia. There is another group of patients with complete activation of CaSR, who have hypomagnesemia due to more severe magnesium wasting and a "Bartter syndrome like" phenotype.

There are several recently described genetic abnormalities of renal magnesium wasting and varying degrees of hypomagnesemia. Familial hypomagnesemia with hypercalciuria and nephrocalcinosis (FHHNC) is a defect of the *CLDN16* gene, which codes for the protein called either claudin-16 or paracellin. Paracellin is essential for the paracellular reabsorption of magnesium in the TAL. These patients present during childhood with the triad of hypomagnesemia, hypercalciuria, and nephrocalcinosis as well as with polyuria, failure to thrive, urinary tract infections, and ocular manifestations including myopia, chorioretinitis, and nystagmus. The hypomagnesemia tends to be severe and so seizures and tetany are common in these patients. Treatment has included magnesium and thiazides to help prevent nephrocalcinosis but the long-term prognosis has been poor with progression to chronic renal failure in early adolescence.

Hypomagnesemia with secondary hypocalcemia (HSH) is a disorder of the *TRPM6* gene that codes for the TRPM6 cation channel. Presenting in the neonatal period, these children can have some of the most severe degrees of hypomagnesemia to the 0.5 mg/dL range resulting in hypoparathyroidism, hypocalcemia, seizures, and tetany. Treatment is with magnesium infusions followed by high-dose oral magnesium with or without parenteral magnesium therapy. Other rare causes of hypomagnesemia are isolated hypomagnesemia of dominant and recessive inheritance. Whereas in the former the gene defect is the *FXYD2* gene, in the latter is not known. Isolated dominant hypomagnesemia is associated with low calcium excretion where as the recessive form usually has normal calcium excretion. Finally, hypomagnesemia has been found to be due to a defect in mitochondrial DNA in a kindred with hypomagnesemia, hypercholesterolemia, and hypertension.

11.4. Hypomagnesemia in Neonates

Hypomagnesemia can present in the neonatal period (Table 6) with hypocalcemia, tremors, and seizures *(16)*. It can often present as a medical emergency with refractory hypocalcemia and seizures that require correction of the hypomagnesemia before other clinical manifestations will respond to treatment. Neonatal hypomagnesemia results from one of the following mechanisms: lack of fetal accumulation due to inadequate placental transport, usually as result of maternal depletion, abnormal gastrointestinal absorption, or renal wasting. The most common etiology presenting within a few days after birth is with infants of diabetic mothers (IDM) where it correlates to the lack of diabetic control and magnesium depletion in the mother but it can also be seen in infants whose mothers have gestational diabetes only. Fetal magnesium depletion can also result from other causes of maternal magnesium depletion and intrauterine growth retardation.

Neonates, especially sick premature infants can suffer from a variety of gastrointestinal disorders resulting in a variety of nutritional deficiencies including hypomagnesemia. Infants with surgery after necrotizing enterocolitis and short gut are at increased risk. In addition to the acquired disorders, hypomagnesemia with secondary hypocalcemia usually presents in infancy (described under Section 11.3.3). Magnesium loss in the urine is a common etiology of mild to severe hypomagnesemia in neonates. Generalized tubular dysfunction is important cause as in older children but the sick neonate

Table 6
Causes of Neonatal Hypomagnesemia

Inadequate placental transport
    Maternal insulin dependent diabetes mellitus
    Maternal gestational diabetes
    Maternal magnesium depletion
    Intrauterine growth retardation (IUGR)
Decreased GI absorption
    Severe diarrhea or malabsorption
    Liver disease
    Hypomagnesemia with secondary hypocalcemia
Renal loss
    Volume expansion, diuresis
    Diuretics – loop diuretics, thiazides
    Aminoglycosides
    Inherited tubular disorders
        Familial hypomagnesemia with hypercalciuria and nephrocalcinosis
        Isolated dominant or recessive hypomagnesemia
        Hypomagnesemia with secondary hyperparathyroidism
Other
    Exchange transfusion with citrated blood
    Maternal hyperparathyroidism

who is on loop diuretics for lung disease and who have treated with aminoglycosides for infection is a real set-up for clinically significant hypomagnesemia. There are several rare inherited tubular disorders described above in Section 11.3.3 that typically present in infancy.

12. DIAGNOSTIC EVALUATION OF HYPOMAGNESEMIA

The first step in the diagnosis of hypomagnesemia is recognition that a disorder of magnesium may be present in a patient with the signs and symptoms outlined in Table 3 because serum magnesium is not included in any of the popular laboratory "panels." As previously noted, ionized magnesium or "corrected" magnesium values are not needed as with calcium due to the fact that only about 20% of magnesium is protein-bound. A chemistry panel including potassium and calcium should also be measured because of the commonly associated deficiency states of these ions as well as looking for evidence of renal disease or diabetes mellitus. If hypomagnesemia is present, one should review the history and physical for evidence of any of the conditions or treatments listed in Table 4 as a possible cause *(11)*. Renal handling of magnesium should be with the measurement of the fractional excretion of magnesium (Fe_{Mg}) in a spot urine using the formula:

$$FEMg = UMg \times PCr/0.7 \times PMg \times UCr \times 100$$

in which Cr = creatinine; P = plasma; and U = urine. The FEMg should be <2% in the presence of hypomagnesemia and if the FE_{Mg} > 5% then renal wasting should be considered *(2)*. If the renal excretion is very low then nutritional or malabsorptive disorders should sought. Due to the possibility that an important cardiac rhythm disturbance may be present, all patients with moderate to severe hypomagnesemia probably should have an electrocardiogram performed.

13. MANAGEMENT OF HYPOMAGNESEMIA

There are several important principals in the treatment of hypomagnesemia. First, severe hypomagnesemia may be life threatening with hypocalcemia, seizures, and tetany and the serum must be brought up to greater than 1 mg/dL with intravenous replacement over a 5–10 min period *(2, 11, 16)*. Secondly, the total body magnesium deficit may not be reflected by the serum magnesium level, especially after treatment and may need prolonged therapy for complete replacement. Thirdly, as serum magnesium rises with intravenous therapy there is significant ongoing renal loss that requires additional therapy. In contrast, if there is renal insufficiency present, magnesium replacement must proceed with caution. Finally, simultaneous deficits of potassium may be present and should be replaced as well. During intravenous therapy monitoring of the deep tendon reflexes may allow detection of hypermagnesemia with levels greater than 2.5 mg/dL.

For severe hypomagnesemia the following doses have been recommended:

1. Neonates. Give 0.1–0.2 ml/kg per dose of 50% magnesium sulfate (0.4–0.8 mEq/kg or 50–100 mg/kg) IV slowly under constant cardiac monitoring, can repeat every 12–24 h.
2. Older children. Give 0.12 ml/kg per dose of 50% magnesium sulfate (0.5 mEq/kg or 60 mg/kg) IV over 1–4 h, can repeat every 12 h.
3. Large adolescents and adults. Give 16–24 ml of 50% magnesium sulfate (64–96 mEq) in 500 ml D5 over 6–8 h, can repeat every 12 h. Use 1/2 dose with renal failure.

For mild hypomagnesemia without significant ongoing loss, avoidance of factors leading to magnesium wasting such as certain diuretics and the addition of magnesium containing foods such as meat, seafood, dairy products, and green vegetables may be sufficient. For moderate hypomagnesemia, oral replacement of magnesium is probably adequate. The dose of elemental magnesium (Table 7) is 10–20 mg/kg/dose up to a maximum of 250–500 mg/dose given 3–4 times per day to avoid the development of diarrhea.

HYPOMAGNESEMIA CASE SCENARIO DISCUSSIONS

Case Scenario #1: This patient has hypocalcemia, hypokalemia, mild hyperchloremic acidosis, and hypomagnesemia. He likely has chronic malabsorption and diarrhea which can contribute to all of the abnormalities but the persistence of the hypocalcemia and hypokalemia suggests that magnesium depletion may be playing a role in the etiology of these disturbances by blocking PTH secretion and action and affecting intracellular K and renal K handling. One could perform a Magnesium Tolerance Test as described

Table 7
Common Oral Formulations of Magnesium

Magnesium salt	Common brand names (OTC)	Elemental Mg
Magnesium oxide	Mag-Ox® 400 Tablet	242 mg
Magnesium hydroxide	Phillips'® Milk of Magnesia	165 mg/5 ml
Magnesium gluconate	Magonate®	54 mg/5 ml
	Magonate® Tablet	27 mg
Magnesium L-aspartate HCl	Maginex™ Granules	122 mg
	Maginex™ Tablet	61 mg
Magnesium chloride	Slow-Mag® Tablet	64 mg

in Section 5.2 to assess whole body magnesium stores but measurement of fractional excretion of magnesium in this hypomagnesemic child will at least give a measure of whether renal conservation is occurring or if the kidney is contributing to the magnesium depletion. The FE_{Mg} described in Section 6 was performed and was 1.8%, which is appropriate in the presence of hypomagnesemia. Other studies to be considered include an ionized calcium to better assess the hypocalcemia as well as a PTH and 25(OH)D levels, which may be causing the low serum calcium. Correction of the hypomagnesemia is likely necessary to allow correction of the hypokalemia and hypocalcemia and you order two doses of 0.12 ml/kg per dose of 50% magnesium sulfate (0.5 mEq/kg or 60 mg/kg) IV each given over 2 h and 12 h apart. The next, the serum potassium is up to 3.8 mEq/L and the calcium is now 9.2 mg/dL with ionized calcium normal at 1.1 mM demonstration the causative nature of the hypomagnesemia on the associated electrolyte disorders. Long-term correction of the total body magnesium depletion with oral magnesium supplements will be required.

Case Scenario #2: Two-day-old neonate with seizures. This infant presents with early neonatal hypocalcemia. There is no history of asphyxia but the infant is an IDM, which is one of the common causes of early neonatal hypocalcemia. Hypomagnesemia is common in IDM due to renal magnesium wasting in the mothers, even with gestational diabetes. It is important to recognize and treat the hypomagnesemia because the hypocalcemia will prove refractory to treatment until the serum magnesium is corrected. You send off blood for serum magnesium and it comes back 0.85 mg/dL. With serum magnesium levels less than 1.0–1.1 mg/dL, there is both inhibition of PTH secretion and its effects on peripheral tissues. With restoration of the serum magnesium levels to above 1.1 mg/dL, this can be rapidly corrected. You give 0.1–0.2 ml/kg per dose of 50% magnesium sulfate (0.4–0.8 mEq/kg or 50–100 mg/kg) IV over 15 min with constant cardiac monitoring or by IM injection. After administration of magnesium the level of calcium and magnesium is monitored and further correction given as needed. There is often a need to repeat the IV magnesium dose after 12–24 h. There may be an underlying abnormality in magnesium metabolism (Sections 11.2 and 11.3, above) but these usually present later than Day 2 of life and will require more long-term and aggressive magnesium therapy.

14. HYPERMAGNESEMIA – INTRODUCTION

Due to the ability of the kidney to excrete a load of magnesium as serum magnesium exceeds the normal range, clinically significant hypermagnesemia is an uncommon disorder in the presence of normal renal function. Hypermagnesemia is almost always the result of either decreased renal function or an increased enteral or parenteral magnesium load. Newborns whose mothers have received parenteral magnesium for preeclampsia are susceptible for hypermagnesemia in part due to their developmentally low glomerular filtration rate.

HYPERMAGNESMIA CASE SCENARIOS

Case Scenario #1: Lethargy in a child in long-term care facility. Five-year-old child with multiple congenital abnormalities is admitted from a long-term care facility with lethargy and hypotension. He has a long history of constipation, which had been treated with resultant diarrhea. His low blood pressure is thought to be due to dehydration as a result of the diarrhea. Fleets enemas were being avoided because of his known chronic renal insufficiency from hypoplastic kidneys as part of an unknown syndrome.

What studies do you want to order? What is the most likely treatment?

Case Scenario #2: Newborn with suspected sepsis. One-day-old term infant noted to be lethargic in the delivery suite develops worsening respiratory depression after treatment with ampicillin and gentamicin are initiated for suspected sepsis. There were no premature rupture of membranes or other risk factors for sepsis.

What other information do you need to assess the cause of the respiratory depression? What lab studies are needed? What is the prognosis?

15. DEFINITION

Serum magnesium levels in the excess of 2.4 mg/dL or (2.0 mEq/L or 1 mmol/L) is considered elevated *(10)* but hypermagnesemia in neonates has been defined as levels in excess of 2.8 mg/dL (2.3 mEq/L or 1.15 mmol/L) *(16)*. Mild elevations of serum magnesium are relatively common in hospitalized patients but have little clinical significance. Unlike serum calcium, where the ionized portion is commonly measured in the clinical setting, measurement of ionized magnesium is not generally available. Also in contrast to hypomagnesemia, where serum levels and total body stores may not correlate with depletion, with magnesium intoxication the level of serum magnesium is sufficient to evaluate the severity of the condition.

16. CLINICAL FEATURES

The clinical features of hypermagnesemia are directly related to the level of serum magnesium and typically are not seen until the level exceeds 3–5 mEq/L *(11, 14)*. The signs and symptoms of hypermagnesemia arise predominantly from its effects on the cardiovascular and nervous symptoms and generally progress from mild to life threatening severity as the level of magnesium rises but the exact levels at which symptoms occur can vary from patient to patient (Table 8) *(12)*. Magnesium causes flushing and

Table 8
Clinical Manifestations of Hypermagnesemia
by Severity

Serum magnesium 3–5 mEq/L
  Mild reduction in BP
  Drowsiness, lethargy
  Flusing
  Nausea, vomiting
Serum magnesium 5–10 mEq/L
  EKG changes
  Hypotension
  Decreased deep tendon reflexes
  Suppressed ventilation
Serum magnesium >10 mEq/L
  Coma
  Muscle paralysis
  Respiratory paralysis
  Refractory hypotension
  Complete heart block
  Cardiac arrest

---

hypotension through vasodilatation of the vasculature by blocking calcium channels and induction of prostacyclin as well as by inhibition of norepinephrine release. The effects on the heart progress from prolongation of the PR, QRS, and QT intervals to worsening heart block and ultimately asystole in the most severe cases. The effects on the nervous system are the result of inhibition of acetylcholine release. As serum magnesium increases the effects on the musculature can result in weakness and hyporeflexia to complete paralysis and respiratory failure. Nausea and vomiting are likely the result of smooth muscle inhibition. The central nervous system is also affected and can result in drowsiness to coma as the level of magnesium rises.

17. CAUSES OF HYPERMAGNESEMIA

Hypermagnesemia is usually the result of decreased glomerular filtration rate or increased load. Newborns whose mothers are treated with magnesium for preeclampsia are also at high risk and should be evaluated for hypermagnesemia. Other unusual causes of mild hypermagnesemia are listed in Table 9. Patients with familial hypocalciuric hypercalcemia who have inactivating defects of the CaSR often have mild hypermagnesemia which is usually not clinically significant.

17.1. Renal Failure

Due to the ability of the kidney to increase the fraction excretion of magnesium to virtually 100% of the filtered load, hypermagnesemia does not appear in acute or chronic

Table 9
Causes of Hypermagnesemia

Renal failure
   Acute renal failure
   Chronic renal insufficiency
   End-stage renal disease
Magnesium load
   Magnesium containing antacids
   Magnesium cathartics
   Magnesium enemas
   Magnesium infusion
Miscellaneous
   Familial hypocalciuria hypercalcemia
   Hypothyroidism
   GH deficiency
   Addison's disease
Neonatal hypermagnesemia
Unknown

---

renal failure until the GFR falls below 20–30% of normal *(2)*. Significant hypermagnesemia is usually the result of a magnesium load in the setting of renal insufficiency. Therefore, patients known to have renal insufficiency or failure should avoid or limit magnesium containing antacids, cathartics, and enemas. Magnesium containing phosphate binders should be used with caution. An unusual cause of hypermagnesemia in hemodialysis patients is the result improperly treated water for dialysate.

17.2. Excess Magnesium Load

In the presence of normal renal function, severe hypermagnesemia is rare with ingestion of magnesium but mild elevations in serum magnesium are common with the use of magnesium for bowel clean out *(1)*. Patients with inflammatory bowel disease, obstruction or with bowel perforation are at greater risk for clinically significant hypermagnesemia. When magnesium is given parenterally, there is an even greater risk for severe hypermagnesemia. Hypermagnesemia has been induced during pregnancy as a standard treatment for preeclampsia and premature labor for many years.

17.3. Neonatal Hypermagnesemia

Hypermagnesemia in neonates is usually the result of magnesium crossing the placenta after magnesium sulfate administration to the mother for treatment of preeclampsia and premature labor *(16)*. Severe hypermagnesemia is unusual and typically resolves in a few days. Other causes of hypermagnesemia in neonates are the administration of magnesium with total parenteral nutrition and with intravenous magnesium sulfate for the treatment of persistent pulmonary hypertension. Studies have shown that total serum magnesium levels are greater in very premature infants as compared to term infants but that the more physiologically important ultrafilterable fraction of magnesium is not significantly different. The presentation of hypermagnesemia in neonates is that of a depressed infant with hypotonia but in the worst cases it can be severe and lead to respiratory failure due to a curare-like effect. Hypocalcemia may be present as well as result of inhibition of PTH secretion by the high magnesium.

18. DIAGNOSIS OF HYPERMAGNESEMIA

One should suspect the diagnosis of hypermagnesemia when the cardiac and neuromuscular symptoms as outlined in Table 8 are seen in a patient with renal insufficiency or after administration of magnesium with enterally or parenterally. A careful history is important to look for potential causes (Table 9), in particular, the maternal record needs to be reviewed in the management of a depressed newborn. In addition to the measurement of total serum magnesium, renal function, electrolytes, and serum calcium should be measured in the initial lab evaluation. An electrocardiogram should be performed to look for any cardiac electrical disturbances.

19. MANAGEMENT OF HYPERMAGNESEMIA

In the presence of normal renal function the management is largely supportive as one waits for the kidneys to excrete the excess magnesium (3, 14). Hydration and loop diuretics may augment the renal excretion. In severe hypermagnesemia, some of the manifestations can be acutely reversed by the administration of intravenous calcium. In older children, the dose is 100–200 mg of elemental calcium IV over 5–10 min and in neonates it is calcium gluconate, 100 mg/kg (9 mg/kg elemental calcium) over 20 min. The calcium can be repeated but the levels of total and ionized calcium should be monitored. In the most severe cases or in the setting of renal failure, peritoneal or hemodialysis with a low magnesium bath is able to rapidly correct the hypermagnesemia. In neonates, exchange transfusion with citrated blood has been used in life threatening cases to more effectively lower serum magnesium.

CASE SCENARIO DISCUSSIONS

Case Scenario #1: Lethargy in a child in a long-term care facility. This child with lethargy and hypotension could have many reasons for his signs and symptoms including sepsis. A careful review of events finds that he has been given an excessive amount of magnesium citrate, which resulted in diarrhea and dehydration. A serum magnesium level is added to a chemistry panel and comes back at 7.2 mg/dL and his serum creatinine is 4.2 mg/dL as compared to his baseline of 2.8 mg/dL. The dehydration from the cathartic caused an acute deterioration of his renal function that then contributed to his inability to handle the magnesium load. The treatment is support of his blood pressure with normal saline and the careful use of loop diuretics after rehydration to aide renal excretion of magnesium but not to exacerbate the dehydration is indicated. A bolus of intravenous calcium at a dose of 100 mg of elemental calcium over 10 min may reverse some of the effects of the hypermagnesemia. If the renal function and hypermagnesemia are severe enough, dialysis may be necessary.

Case Scenario #2: Newborn with suspected sepsis. This infant presents with lethargy and respiratory distress like so many infants but the history revealed that this case differs in that the mother had preeclampsia and had been treated with magnesium. Unfortunately for her and her infant, the dose was excessive and both developed hypermagnesemia. The serum magnesium in the fetus was 6.4 mg/dL, total calcium 8.9 mg/dL, and ionized calcium 0.95 mM. The mild hypocalcemia is the likely result of suppression of PTH secretion by high levels of magnesium. In this case the therapy is supportive with IV calcium gluconate at a dose of 100 mg/kg (9 mg/kg elemental calcium) over 20 min to help reverse the respiratory depression, hydration to help assist urinary excretion and possibly the use of a loop diuretic like furosemide to enhance renal excretion. The electrolyte disturbance should resolve in 48 h with good supportive care.

REFERENCES

1. Agus ZS, Massry SG. Hypomagnesemia and hypermagnesemia. In: Narins RG, ed., Maxwell & Kleeman's Clinical Disorders of Fluid and Electrolyte Metabolism, 5th ed., New York: McGraw-Hill, 1994:1099–1119.
2. Reikes S, Gonzalez EA, Martin KJ. Abnormal calcium and magnesium metabolism. In: DuBose TD, Hamm LL, ed., Acid–Base and Electrolyte Disorders. Philadelphia: Saunders, 2002: 453–487.
3. Alfrey AC. Disorders of magnesium metabolism. In: Seldin DW, Giebisch G, eds., The Kidney: Physiology and Pathophysiology, 2nd ed., New York: Raven Press, 1992:2357–2373.
4. Hruska KA, Levi M, Slatopolsky E. Disorders of phosphorus, calcium, magnesium metabolism. In: Schrier RW, ed., Disorders of the Kidney & Urinary Tract, 8th ed., Vol. 3. Philadelphia: Lippincott Williams & Wilkins, 2007:2295–2352.
5. Favus MJ. Intestinal absorption of calcium, magnesium and phosphorus. In: Coe FL, Favus MJ, eds., Disorders of Bone and Mineral Metabolism, 2nd ed., Philadelphia: Lippincott Williams & Wilkins, 2002:34–47.
6. Yu ASL. Renal transport of calcium, magnesium, and phosphate. In: Brenner BM, ed., Brenner & Rector's The Kidney, 7th ed., Vol. 1. Philadelphia: Saunders, 2004:535–571.
7. Quamme GA, Cole DEC. Physiology and pathophysiology of renal magnesium handling. In: Coe FL, Favus MJ, eds., Disorders of Bone and Mineral Metabolism, 2nd ed., Philadelphia: Lippincott Williams & Wilkins, 2002:34–47.
8. Quamme GA, Schlingmann KP, Konrad M. Mechanisms and disorders of magnesium metabolism. In: Alpern RJ, Hebert SC, eds., Seldin and Giebisch's The Kidney, 4th ed., Vol. 2. Boston: Elsevier, 2008:1747–1767.
9. Rigo J, De Curtis M. Disorders of calcium, phosphorus, and magnesium metabolism. In: Martin RJ, Fanaroff AA, Walsh MC, eds., Fanaroff and Martin's Neonatal–Perinatal Medicine, 8th ed., Vol. 2. Philadelphia: Mosby, 2006:1491–1520
10. Vokes TJ. Blood calcium, phosphate, and magnesium. In: Favus MJ, ed., Primer on the Metabolic Bone Diseases and Disorders of Mineral Metabolism, 6th ed., Washington DC: American Society of Bone and Mineral Research, 2006:123–127
11. Rude RK. Magnesium depletion and hypermagnesemia. In: Favus MJ, ed., Primer on the Metabolic Bone Diseases and Disorders of Mineral Metabolism, 6th ed., Washington DC: American Society of Bone and Mineral Research, 2006:123–127.
12. Penfield JG, Choudhury D, Cronin RE, Knochel JP, Levi M.. Disorders of Phosphate and Magnesium Metabolism. In: Coe FL, Favus MJ, eds., Disorders of Bone and Mineral Metabolism, 2nd ed., Philadelphia: Lippincott Williams & Wilkins, 2002:589–615.

13. Fitzpatrick LA. The hypocalcemic states. In: Coe FL, Favus MJ, eds., Disorders of Bone and Mineral Metabolism, 2nd ed., Philadelphia: Lippincott Williams & Wilkins, 2002:568–588.

14. Pollack MR, Yu ASL. Clinical disturbances of calcium, magnesium, and phosphate metabolism. In: Brenner BM, ed., Brenner & Rector's The Kidney, 7th ed., Vol. 1. Philadelphia: Saunders, 2004: 535–571.

15. Naderi ASA, Reilly RF. Hereditary etiologies of hypomagnesemia. Nature Clinical Practice Nephrology 2008;4:80–89.

16. Rigo J, De Curtis M. Disorders of calcium, phosphorus, and magnesium metabolism. In: Martin RJ, Fanaroff AA, Walsh MC, eds., Fanaroff and Martin's Neonatal–Perinatal Medicine, 8th ed., Vol. 2. Philadelphia: Mosby, 2006:1491–1520.

6 Disorders of Phosphorus Homeostasis

Valerie L. Johnson

Key Points

1. Relationship between ADHR, XLH, and ARHP.
2. Clinical assessment of phosphate excretion and TmPi/GFR.
3. FGF-23 and CKD.
4. Acute management of hypophosphatemia.
5. How phosphate needs are met in the growing child.

   Key Words: FGF-23; hypophosphatemia; hyperphosphatemia; rickets; 25-hydroxy vitamin D; 1,25-dihydroxy vitamin D

1. PHOSPHORUS BALANCE

Phosphate is fundamental to cellular metabolism and skeletal mineralization. It is of critical importance when it comes to growth – as a constituent of bone mineral. The body content of phosphorus increases from 0.6% body weight in the newborn to 1% or 600–700 g in the adult reflecting the increasing proportion of mineralized bone and soft tissue per unit of body mass *(1)*. In the growing individual phosphorus balance must be positive to meet the needs of growth. Balance studies indicate that a 1- to 3-month-old infant fed a standard formula retains 32 ± 25 (SD) mg/kg body weight of phosphate *(2, 3)*, while the adult retains zero.

The terms *phosphate concentration* and *phosphorus concentration* are often used interchangeably. The plasma phosphate concentration is usually measured in units of mg/dL or mmol/L. The following calculations may be used to convert between these units:

- 1 mmol of phosphate = 31 mg of elemental phosphorus
- 1 mmol/L of phosphate = 3.1 mg/dL (or 31 mg/L) or phosphorus
- 1 mg of phosphorus = 0.032 mmol of phosphate
- 1 mg/dL of phosphorus = 0.32 mmol/L of phosphate

The content of phosphate in plasma, urine, tissue, or foodstuffs is measured and expressed in terms of the amount of elemental phosphorus contained in the specimen or

From: *Nutrition and Health: Fluid and Electrolytes in Pediatrics*
Edited by: L. G. Feld, F. J. Kaskel, DOI 10.1007/978-1-60327-225-4_6,
© Humana Press, a part of Springer Science+Business Media, LLC 2010

phosphorus concentration. Phosphorus in the form of phosphate ion circulates in blood as an organic form consisting principally of phospholipids and phosphate esters and an inorganic form (Pi). From a clinical standpoint only the inorganic form of phosphate is measured. Ninety percent of plasma Pi is filtered at the glomerulus as phosphate ions, the ratio of HPO_4^{2-} to $H2PO_4^{-}$ depending on pH, or as phosphate complexed with sodium, calcium, or magnesium. The other 10% of the remaining plasma phosphate is as noted protein-bound and not filterable. Correcting the volume occupied by plasma proteins (7%) raises the ultrafiltrate Pi concentration by an additional 7.5%, negating the effect of the reduction in plasma protein-bound Pi. Both in vivo and in vitro measurements show that the ratio of ultrafilterable Pi to total plasma Pi is close to 1 *(4)*.

The serum phosphorus concentration exhibits a circadian rhythm characterized by a rapid decrease in early morning to a nadir shortly before noon, a subsequent increase to a plateau in late afternoon and a small further increase to a peak shortly after midnight *(5, 6)*. Restriction or supplementation of dietary phosphorus induces a substantial decrease or increase, respectively, in serum concentrations of phosphorus during the late morning, afternoon, and evening, but induces less or no change in the morning phosphorus concentration *(6)*. Morning fasting bloods are therefore least affected by dietary changes on the serum phosphorus concentration.

There are substantial differences in serum phosphorus concentrations depending on age. Phosphorus levels are highest in infants, ranging from 4.8 to 7.4 mg/dL in the first 3 months of life and decreasing to 4.5–5.8 mg/dL by 1–2 years of age. In mid-childhood values range from 3.5 to 5.5 mg/dL and decrease to adult values by late adolescence *(7–9)*. In adult males, serum phosphorus levels decrease with age from approximately 3.5 mg/dL at age 20 years to 3.0 mg/dL at age 70 *(10)*. In females values are similar to those of males until after menopause, when they increase slightly from approximately 3.4 mg/dL at age 50 years to 3.7 mg/dL at 70 years of age *(10)*.

1.1. Renal Phosphate Transport

1.1.1. CELLULAR ASPECTS

The kidney is the major regulator of Pi homeostasis and can increase or decrease its Pi reabsorptive capacity in response to need. Under normal physiologic conditions, 80–97% of the filtered load of phosphate is reabsorbed by the renal tubule. The rate limiting step in renal Pi reabsorption involves the transport of Pi from the tubular lumen across the apical BBM. Pi then moves across the cell and effluxes at the basolateral membrane. Pi transport across the BBM is saturable, Na-dependent and driven by a Na-gradient (outside > inside) that is maintained by the basolateral membrane-associated Na,K-ATPase. Na/Pi co-transport across the BBM is electrogenic, sensitive to pH, with 10- to 20-fold increases documented when the pH is increased from 6 to 8.5, and the target for physiologic/pathophysiologic regulation. The mechanism of phosphate efflux at the basolateral membrane has not been elucidated. Current data suggest that phosphate can exit the cell down its electrochemical gradient via a low capacity Na/Pi co-transport system that couples flux of one sodium with that of one divalent phosphate ion or a high-capacity phosphate anion exchange mechanism *(11)*.

Approximately 70% of the filtered load of phosphate is reabsorbed by the proximal tubule, with three times as much occurring in the proximal straight tubules as in proximal convoluted tubules *(12–14)*. Due to axial heterogeneity most of the phosphate reabsorption by the proximal tubule occurs within the first 25% of the proximal tubule length. Little or no phosphate transport has been shown to occur in the Loop of Henle. Phosphate reabsorption in the distal nephrons is controversial. Results from micropuncture studies suggest that up to 10% of the filtered phosphate load is reabsorbed by the distal convoluted tubules *(15)*. Other studies have failed to uncover evidence of distal Pi transport *(16)*. Terminal nephrons segments may reabsorb an additional 3–7% of the filtered phosphate load based on the fact that a higher fraction of filtered phosphate remains in the late distal tubules than appears in the final urine *(15–17)*. Although some studies have failed to demonstrate phosphate reabsorption in isolated perfused cortical collecting tubules *(18)*, others have shown a small but significant net efflux of phosphate from this nephron segment *(19, 20)*.

1.1.2. MOLECULAR CHARACTERIZATION

Three classes of Na/Pi co-transporters have been identified in mammalian kidney *(21–23)*. The type I Na/Pi co-transporter (Npt1) is expressed predominantly in the BBM of the proximal tubular cells *(24, 25)* and mediates fluxes of chloride and organic anions as well as Pi. Dietary phosphorus or PTH does not seem to alter type I Na/Pi co-transporter protein or mRNA expression. Thus, the type I co-transporter is not thought to be a major determinant of proximal tubule phosphate handling.

The type II family of Na/Pi co-transporters exhibit 25% homology with Npt1. The type II co-transporter is largely responsible for renal phosphate reabsorption as indicated by knockout experiments. Targeted inactivation of type II (Npt2) in mice leads to severe phosphate wasting (85% reduction in phosphate reabsorption), hypercalciuria, and skeletal abnormalities. There are three highly homologous isoforms; type IIa *(Npt2a)* and type IIc *(Npt2c)* are expressed almost exclusively in the BBM of the renal proximal tubule *(26, 27)*. The type IIb is not expressed in the kidney *(28)*. The type IIb is expressed in the BBM of the small intestine and plays a role in the physiologic regulation of intestinal reabsorption of phosphate *(29–31)*

1.1.3. ROLE OF DIETARY PHOSPHORUS

The dietary intake of phosphorus is one of the most important physiologic regulators of Na/Pi co-transport. An increase in dietary phosphorus is associated with an increased total and fractional urinary excretion of phosphorus. This may occur even in the absence of detectable changes in the serum level and filtered load of phosphorus. PTH plays an important role in this phosphaturic response to a phosphorus load. However, the phosphaturic response may be observed in hypoparathyroid patients as well. In the presence of dietary phosphate restriction or hypophosphatemia, phosphate homeostasis is preserved by short-term intrinsic renal and intestinal adaptations in transport processes, and by more long-term hormonal mechanisms, which regulate the efficiency of phosphate transport in the kidney and intestine. The net effect of these adaptations is virtual abolition of phosphate excretion in the urine, and an increase in the plasma phosphate concentration toward normal. This response is achieved with only a slight increment in the plasma Ca^{2+} concentration.

The renal tubule can adapt quickly to changes in dietary intake or plasma concentrations of phosphorus. During Pi deprivation the abundance of the apically localized Na/Pi co-transporters, Na/Pi type IIa in the kidney BBM, and Na/Pi type IIb in the intestinal BBM increase with a concomitant increase in Pi reabsorption. These alterations in Na/Pi co-transport take place within hours and are independent of changes in PTH, 1,25 $(OH)_2D_3$ or serum calcium levels. This adaptation, in addition, has been shown not to be inhibited by cycloheximide or actinomycin D (inhibitors of protein synthesis), which suggests that new protein synthesis is not required *(32)*.

Adaptation induced after long-term (4 days) phosphorus restriction, on the other hand, has been shown to be inhibited by cycloheximide and actinomycin D, which suggests that new protein synthesis is required for the long-term response. Again there is an adaptive increase in the abundance of the type II Na/Pi co-transporter protein, but also mRNA.

It is important to remember that the renal reabsorption of Pi is very rapidly altered by a number of factors, e.g., $paCO_2$, HCO_3, sodium delivery, adrenergic agents, dopamine, etc (see Table 1). These effects may be totally independent of hormones and secreted factors. The well-described hormones involved in the adaptation to high or low Pi diets in both animal models and humans include PTH and 1,25 $(OH)_2D_3$.

1.1.4. ROLE OF PARATHYROID HORMONE

PTH is the major hormonal regulator of renal phosphate reabsorption (see above). Type II Na/Pi transporters represent the major pathway of renal phosphate reabsorption and are the major target with respect to inhibition of proximal tubular reabsorption by PTH. PTH produces a greater inhibition of Pi transport in the proximal straight tubules than proximal convoluted tubules *(33)*.

It also has been demonstrated that the N-amino-terminal fragment PTH sequence 1–34 reproduces all physiologic effects of the PTH sequence 1–84. It has been demonstrated that the amino acid sequences 10–15 and 24–34 of PTH are necessary for binding to the receptor. With regard to the biologic effects of PTH, it has been shown that the first two N-terminal amino acids 1 and 2 are required for activation of the adenylate cyclase–protein kinase A pathway, whereas the amino acid sequences 28–34 are required for the activation of the phospholipase C–protein kinase C pathway. Recent work demonstrated that the addition of PTH 1–34 (which signals through both the protein kinase A and protein kinase C pathways) to either the apical or the basolateral surface of isolated perfused proximal tubules caused internalization of the type II Na/Pi transport protein. On the other hand, PTH 3–34, which signals only through the protein kinase C pathway, has an effect apically but not basolaterally. It can be concluded from these studies that type-II Na/Pi protein transporter activity and internalization are regulated by c-AMP-dependent and independent mechanisms, and that functional PTH receptors are located on both the apical and basolateral membranes of the proximal tubule.

Table 1
Factors Affecting Renal Reabsorption of Phosphorus

Factor	Proximal tubular reabsorption
Volume expansion	Decreased
Phosphate loading	Decreased
Phosphorus restriction	Increased
Hypercalcemia	
Acute	Increased
Chronic	Decreased
Metabolic acidosis	
Acute	No change
Chronic	Decreased
Metabolic alkalosis	
Acute	Decreased
Chronic	Increased
Respiratory acidosis	Decreased
Respiratory alkalosis	Increased
Hormones	
Parathyroid hormone	Decreased
Vitamin D (chronic)	Decreased
Growth hormone	Increased
Calcitonin	Decreased
Thyroid hormone	Increased
Insulin	Increased
FGF-23	Decreased
Dopamine	Decreased
Diuretics (mannitol, loop diuretics, thiazides, acetazolamide)	Decreased
Glucose	Decreased (osmotic diuresis)
Glucocorticoids	Decreased

1.1.5. ROLE OF VITAMIN D

The main source of vitamin D in humans is endogenous vitamin D_3 (also known as cholecalciferol), which is produced by the ultraviolet irradiation of 7-dehydrocholesterol in the skin. Cholecalciferol is metabolized by the liver into 25-hydroxy cholecalciferol (25-hydroxyvitamin D_3 [25(OH)D_3]). After enterohepatic circulation 25(OH)D_3 is further metabolized in the kidney to 1,25-dihydroxycholecalciferol (calcitriol [1,25(OH)$_2$D$_3$]), which is the most active known metabolite of vitamin D. It has recently been shown that 25(OH)D_3 in complex with its carrier protein, the vitamin D binding protein, is filtered through the glomerulus and reabsorbed in the proximal tubules by the endocytic receptor megalin. Endocytosis is required to preserve 25(OH)D_3 and deliver it to the cells as the precursor for generation of 1,25(OH)$_2$D$_3$. PTH seems to act as a trophic hormone in stimulating the production of $1,25(OH)_2D_3$. Thus, with intact parathyroid glands, changes in serum calcium indirectly regulate renal production of $1,25(OH)_2D_3$ by altering the secretion of PTH. In addition there is evidence that calcium acts directly to alter the synthesis of calcitriol. Low serum phosphorus stimulates and high serum phosphorus suppresses the renal formation of $1,25(OH)_2D_3$ independent of PTH. Growth hormone by virtue of increased synthesis of insulin-like growth factor 1 stimulates the activity of $25(OH)D$ 1α-hydroxylase. Chronic metabolic acidosis also increases serum levels of calcitriol. This latter effect could be mediated by acidosis-induced urinary losses of phosphate leading to cellular phosphate depletion.

The effect of vitamin D on the renal handling of phosphorus has been the subject of numerous investigations. One of the difficulties in interpreting the changes in urinary excretion of phosphorus has been related to the calcemic actions of vitamin D, which by suppressing PTH secretion, indirectly alter the renal handling of phosphorus. $1,25(OH)_2D_3$ may have a phosphaturic or phosphate sparing effect based on the state of phosphate balance. When hypophosphatemic due either to vitamin D deficiency or phosphate deprivation or when baseline phosphate excretion is high (e.g., volume expansion, administration of PTH or calcitonin) $1,25(OH)_2D_3$ is antiphosphaturic. On the other hand, $1,25(OH)_2D_3$ is phosphaturic with hyperphosphatemia or in phosphate replete states. The duration of $1,25(OH)_2D_3$ therapy also affects phosphate transport. Chronic administration of $1,25(OH)_2D_3$ is associated with a decrease in renal phosphate reabsorption. This response is thought to be a consequence of an increase in intestinal phosphate and positive phosphate balance, which, in turn, induces an adaptive decrease in phosphate reabsorption by the proximal tubule. Acute $1,25(OH)_2D_3$ administration is associated with a change in the lipid composition of the membrane and increases renal phosphate reabsorption – but also depends on the experimental conditions of the study such as prior administration of vitamin D, PTH, and phosphorus balance of the organism.

Type IIa co-transport protein has been thought to be the target of $1,25(OH)_2D_3$ regulation. In vitamin D deficient, but not parathyroidectomized rats, $1,25(OH)_2D_3$ increased renal type II-mediated co-transport, mRNA, and protein levels (34).

1.1.6. ROLE OF GROWTH HORMONE

Growth hormone (GH) has been shown to be a factor that increases the renal reabsorption of phosphate. When GH is elevated or administered on a chronic basis to adult humans or adult animals there is a reduction in the urinary Pi excretion and elevation in plasma Pi levels. The removal of GH in the adult rat (through hypophysectomy) causes a significant decline in the maximum capacity to reabsorb Pi (TmPi) by the whole kidney and results in increased phosphaturia. However, this effect cannot be attributed solely to GH because all pituitary hormones were removed. In addition, Hammerman et al. (35) reported that the effects of pharmacologic doses of GH results in a selective stimulation of proximal tubular BBM Na/Pi transport systems.

Mulroney et al. (36) using a peptidic antagonist to GH-releasing factor to suppress the pulsatile release of GH from the anterior pituitary over a 2-day period showed a doubling of the urinary excretion of Pi and attenuation of somatic body growth. These effects were attributed to a decrease in the TmPi. On the other hand, short-term use of the GH-releasing factor antagonist had no effect of lowering the TmPi and increasing urinary Pi excretion. Woda et al. *(37)* have demonstrated that using the GH-releasing factor antagonist for 48 h is associated with a 30% reduction in Vmax of Pi transport in proximal tubule BBM prepared from weaning rats, implicating GH in proximal tubule Pi uptake. Furthermore, these authors have shown that the mechanism for the enhanced Na/Pi co-transport activity in the juvenile rat appears to be through the action of GH on the expression of proximal tubular BBM type IIa Na/Pi co-transporter protein.

1.1.7. OTHER FACTORS

A number of other hormones also target the type II co-transporter in the regulation of renal Pi handing. Amongst these are thyroid hormone, dexamethasone, epidermal growth factor, insulin, etc. Please see Table 1 for additional factors affecting the renal transport of Pi.

1.1.8. THE ROLE OF PHOSPHATONINS IN PHOSPHATE HOMEOSTASIS

In the last several years a new class of regulators have surfaced called phosphatonins that control systemic phosphate homeostasis linking bone metabolism and mainly the renal handling of phosphate. A number of different molecules have been identified such as FGF-23 (fibroblast growth factor 23) mainly expressed in regions of active bone formation and remodeling (particularly in osteocytes and lining cells), FGF-7 (fibroblast growth factor 7), MEPE (matrix extracellular phosphoglycoprotein) expressed in odontoblasts and osteocytes embedded in mineralized matrix, and more specifically its carboxy-terminal MEPE/acidic serine–aspartate-rich MEPE associated motif (ASARM peptide), and sFRP4 (secreted frizzled related protein-4). These phosphatonins, and especially FGF-23, decrease serum phosphate via two simultaneous actions in the proximal convoluted tubules: they decrease the expression of the Na/Pi co-transporters, thus increasing phosphate excretion and they reduce the production of $1,25(OH)_2D_3$, thus decreasing the ability of the intestine to absorb phosphate (Fig. 1).

Phosphatonins were first identified in patients with tumor-induced osteomalacia (TIO). Patients with TIO typically exhibit low serum Pi concentrations, normal or slightly low serum calcium concentrations, normal PTH concentrations, inappropriately low $1,25(OH)_2D_3$ concentrations, renal Pi wasting, and rickets and osteomalacia. It was demonstrated that conditioned medium from a tumor associated with TIO produced a factor or factors that inhibited Na^+–Pi-dependent transport in cultured OK cells *(38)*. Several laboratories subsequently showed that FGF-23, sFRP-4, FGF-7, and MEPE are present in these tumors and contribute to the phosphaturia associated with this syndrome *(39–47)*.

FGF23 has been studied most extensively and clearly has been established as a potent regulator of systemic phosphate transport and balance at the level of bone, intestine, and kidney (Figs. 2 and 3). FGF-23 inhibits Na^+–Pi uptake in cultured renal epithelial cells and also inhibits Pi reabsorption when infused into rodents in vivo *(39, 43, 48, 49)*. Similar findings are reported for sFRP-4, MEPE *(42)*, and FGF-7 *(43)*.

INTESTINE

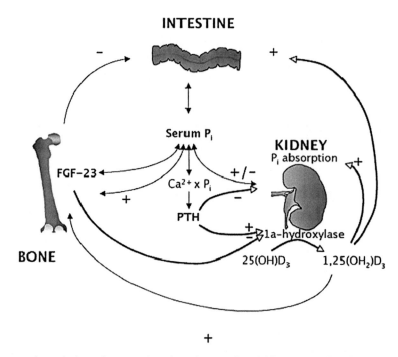

Fig. 1. Hormonal regulation of serum phosphate by parathyroid hormone, vitamin D_3, and FGF-23. *Serum* phosphate levels are influenced by dietary intake and intestinal absorption, the rate of renal excretion of reabsorption, respectively, and skeletal deposition and release from bone. Changes in serum phosphate concentration alter the calcium × phosphate product and a fall in free calcium triggers release of parathyroid hormone (PTH). PTH inhibits renal phosphate reabsorption and at the same time stimulates 1α-hydroxylase expression and activation of $1,25(OH)_2D_3$ from its inactive precursor $25(OH)D_3$. The active vitamin D_3 stimulates in turn renal and intestinal phosphate absorption as well as deposition of phosphate in bone. An increase in serum phosphate concentrations also directly increases FGF-23 synthesis and release from bone independent from the PTH axis. FGF-23 lowers phosphate concentrations by inhibiting renal and intestinal phosphate transport as well as preventing activation of $1,25(OH)_2D_3$, which in turn controls levels of bone synthesis of FGF-23 (from Wagner *(134)* (Fig. 1)).

In addition to inhibiting Pi reabsorption in the kidney FGF-23 alters vitamin D metabolism such that serum $1,25(OH)_2D_3$ concentrations are reduced or fail to increase despite the presence of hypophosphatemia *(43, 49)*. The reduction in serum concentrations of $1,25(OH)_2D_3$ reduces Pi absorption in the intestine and possibly in the kidney as well, suggesting an inhibitory effect of these proteins on 25-hydroxyvitamin D 1α-hydroxylase activity *(43, 49)*. As might be expected, in FGF-23 knockout mice, 25-hydroxyvitamin D 1α-hydroxylase expression is increased and elevated serum levels of $1,25(OH)_2D_3$ cause significant hypercalcemia and hypophosphatemia. MEPE, on the other hand, increases circulating $1,25(OH)_2D_3$ concentrations.

The intake of dietary phosphorus and serum Pi concentrations might be expected to play a role in the regulation of phosphatonin concentrations. In humans, however, short-term alterations in dietary intake do not appear to influence concentrations of FGF-23. In rodents, on the other hand, following changes in dietary Pi, the data suggest that FGF-23, PTH, and $1,25(OH)_2D_3$ are all involved in the adaptation to dietary Pi *(50)*.

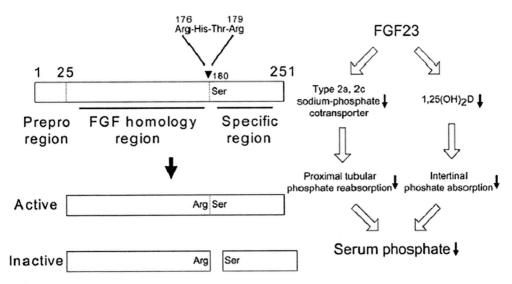

Fig. 2. Structure and function of FGF-23. FGF-23 is a protein with 251 amino acids. There is a signal peptide with 24 amino acids in the N-terminal portion of the FGF-23 protein. A part of FGF-23 is cleaved between Arg[179] and Ser[180] by furin recognizing Arg[176]-X-X-Arg[179] motif. FGF-23 has an FGF homology region in the N-terminal portion of this processing site. FGF-23 reduces serum phosphate by suppressing proximal tubular phosphate reabsorption and intestinal phosphate absorption (from Fukumoto *(135)* (Fig. 2)).

$1,25(OH)_2D_3$ in turn has been shown to regulate FGF-23 in rats. Saito et al. *(51)* showed that serum FGF-23 levels increased following the administration of $1,25(OH)_2D_3$ to intact rats in a dose-dependent manner. There, in addition, was a direct correlation between the serum phosphorus concentrations and serum FGF-23 concentrations. In thyroparathyroidectomized rats, $1,25(OH)_2D_3$ also increased serum FGF-23 concentrations. In the thyroparathyroidectomized rats, serum FGF-23 levels were at the low end of normal despite elevated serum phosphorus concentrations. In contrast in hypoparathyroid humans, serum FGF-23 levels are elevated.

FGF-23 interacts with FGF receptors that belong to type 1 transmembrane phosphotyrosine kinase receptors to elicit its biological response *(52)*. Recent studies indicate that FGF-23 requires Klotho, as a co-factor for receptor activation *(52, 53)*. The Klotho/Klotho gene encodes a single-pass membrane protein, which has homologies to β-glucosidases *(54–57)*. Two transcripts formed through alternative RNA splicing are transcribed from the gene and encode a membrane or secreted klotho protein *(54)*. Klotho is expressed in several tissues including the kidney, reproductive tissues, and brain *(56)*. The role of Klotho as an FGF-23 receptor is supported by the fact that Klotho-deficient mice have a phenotype similar to FGF-23 null mice *(55)*.

In summary, FGF-23, sFRP-4, MEPE, and FGF-7 have been shown to inhibit Pi reabsorption. FGF-23 and sFRP-4 also modulate the synthesis of $1,25(OH)_2D_3$. FGF-23 synthesis, in turn, is regulated by $1,25(OH)_2D_3$ as $1,25(OH)_2D_3$ action is required for maintaining normal FGF-23 production in osteoblasts. It also seems that FGF-23 acts on the parathyroid gland to inhibit both PTH biosynthesis and secretion. By inhibiting the circulating level of PTH, FGF-23 thus appears to counteract its inhibition of tubular

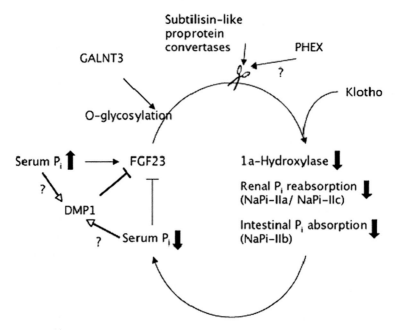

Fig. 3. Regulation and function of FGF-23. FGF-23 is released from bone upon elevated serum phosphate levels. To be biologically active, FGF-23 requires O-glycosylation by GALNT3 (UDP-*N*-acetyl-α-D-galactosamine: polypeptide *N*-acetylgalactosaminyltransferase 3). FGF-23 lowers serum phosphate levels by decreasing the expression of renal (Na/Pi-IIa and Na/Pi-IIc) and intestinal (Na/Pi-IIb) phosphate transporters thereby reducing phosphate uptake from diet and increasing renal excretion of phosphate. Furthermore, FGF-23 inhibits 1α-hydroxylase expression in kidney reducing the final step in vitamin D_3 activation and thereby prevents a compensatory increase in intestinal and renal phosphate transport. High vitamin D_3 levels itself may also directly stimulate FGF-23 synthesis providing for a regulatory circuit and feedback mechanism. FGF-23 is cleaved and inactivated by subtilisin-like proprotein convertases requiring a recognition motif consisting of Arg[176]-X-X-Arg[179] at position 176. PHEX is not directly involved in FGF-23 degradation but may indirectly contribute to cleavage (from Wagner, CA *(134)* (Fig. 2)).

phosphate reabsorption and enhance its suppression of $1,25(OH)_2D_3$ biosynthesis. Data in rodents show that FGF-23 and sFRP-4 concentrations may be regulated by the intake of dietary Pi. The data in human subjects are much less clear with respect to the effects of dietary Pi on the concentrations of these peptides. Thus, FGF-23 is in the position to keep serum phosphate levels low and to act as a bone phosphate sensor controlling intestinal and renal phosphate handling.

1.2. Renal Phosphate Transport – Changes as a Function of Age

The kidneys of infants and children reabsorb a high fraction of filtered Pi appropriate to the needs of the growing child. Spitzer and Barac-Nieto *(58)* recently reviewed the body of literature pertaining to the role of the newborn kidney in Pi balance. Early experiments in dogs *(59)* and rats *(60)* had suggested that this high reabsorptive capacity is intrinsic to the kidneys. That this is indeed the case was demonstrated by Johnson and Spitzer *(61)* in isolated kidneys containing phosphate concentrations varying between

3 and 15 mg/dL. The slopes of the regression lines describing the relationship between the filtered load of Pi and the amount reabsorbed per unit of kidney weight (Fig. 4) illustrate that at any filtered load of Pi the kidney of the newborn reabsorbed almost four times as much Pi than that of the adult. Micropuncture experiments by Kaskel et al. *(62)* confirmed the avid nature of Pi reabsorption by the newborn. Studies at comparable locations along the proximal tubule revealed that the fraction of filtered Pi reabsorbed was significantly higher in immature than in mature guinea pigs (Fig. 5). Eighty-five percent of the age-related difference in the renal reabsorption of Pi could be explained by the higher rates of Pi reabsorption in the proximal segments of the nephron and the remaining 15% by differences in reabsorption at more distal nephron sites. Woda et al. *(63)* also examined the renal tubular sites of increased phosphate transport as well as Na/Pi expression in the juvenile rat. Renal micropuncture experiments were performed

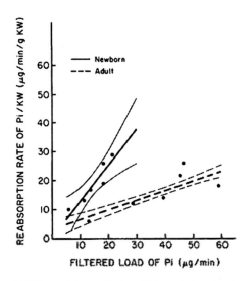

Fig. 4. Regression lines and 95% confidence limits of the relationship between the reabsorption of phosphate (Pi) and the filtered load of Pi by the isolated perfused kidneys of newborn ($y = 1.25x + 0.09$) and mature ($y = 0.34x + 3.1$) guinea pigs (used with permission from Johnson and Spitzer *(61)*).

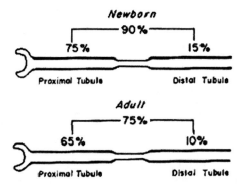

Fig. 5. Schematic representation of the changes in fractional reabsorption of Pi along the renal tubule during maturation (based on data from Kaskel et al. *(62)*) (from Spitzer and Barac-Nieto *(58)* (Fig. 2)).

in acutely thyroparathyroidectomized adult (>14 weeks old) and juvenile (4 weeks old) male rats fed a normal phosphate or low phosphate diet. Phosphate reabsorption was greater in the proximal convoluted and straight tubules of the juvenile compared to the adult fed a normal phosphate diet.

Neiberger and Barac-Nieto *(64)* further studied the mechanism underlying the high renal reabsorption of Pi during growth looking at the Na^+–Pi co-transport system in luminal brush-border membrane vesicles (BBMV) obtained from the kidneys of newborn and adult animals (Fig. 6). At both ages, most transport of Pi into vesicles was found to be Na^+ gradient dependent. The uptake was concentrative, i.e., the intravesical Pi concentration exceeded the equilibrium concentration as long as an inwardly directed Na^+ gradient subsisted across the brush-border membrane. As the gradient dissipated, the vesicular Pi content diminished to reach equilibrium. The initial rate of Na^+-dependent Pi uptake was linear with time and was much higher from vesicles obtained from newborn than from adult animals. Kinetic analysis of the initial transport rates revealed that the Vmax of the Na^+–Pi was substantially higher in BBMV from

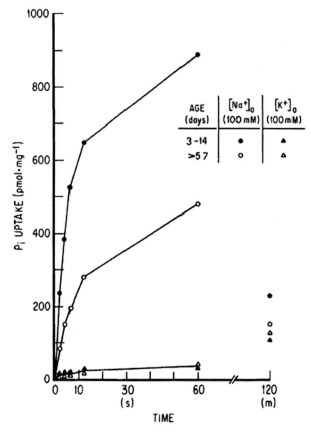

Fig. 6. Time course of Pi (0.1 mM) uptake in brush-border membrane vesicles (BBMV) of 3- to 14-day-old and >57-day-old guinea pigs; *Circles,* uptake in the presence of 100 mM Na^+ gradient. *Triangles,* uptake in the presence of 100 mM inwardly directed KCl gradient (used with permission from Neiberger et al. *(64)*).

newborns (650 pmol/s per mg protein) than those of adults (144 pmol/s per mg protein). The K_m, a measure of the apparent affinity of the co-transporter for Pi did not differ with age. The capacity for Na^+–Pi co-transport across the luminal brush-border membrane of the renal proximal tubular cells was reported to be four-fold higher in the newborn than the adult. Dietary modifications in which the diet was supplemented with Pi for 3 days decreased by about 50% the V_{max} for Na^+–Pi co-transport in renal BBMV from adult animals but only about 25% in the newborn. On the other hand, low dietary Pi resulted in a doubling of the Na^+–Pi co-transport capacity in renal BBMV of the adult (from 144 to 318 pmol/mg per s), but no significant change in the V_{max} of the Na^+–Pi co-transport system of the newborn. Based on these studies Spitzer and Barac-Nieto (58) conclude that the newborn Na^+–Pi co-transport system is characterized by a high transport capacity and low adaptability to changes in dietary Pi. Woda et al. (63) similarly showed greater Pi uptake in BBMV from both superficial and outer juxtamedullary cortices of juvenile rats. Western blot analysis revealed a 2- and 1.8-fold higher amount of Na/Pi-2 protein in the superficial and outer juxtamedullary cortices, respectively, in juvenile rats. Immunofluorescence microscopy also indicated that Na/Pi-2 expression was present in the proximal tubule BBM to a greater extent in juvenile rats. These features of the co-transport system may explain, in part, the hyperphosphatemia observed in newborns fed a diet of cow's milk, which is rich in Pi (75).

The high capacity of the developing kidney for Pi reabsorption appears to persist independent of extracellular factors known to modulate renal Pi transport in vivo. As Bojour and Fleish (65) present evidence that renal phosphate reabsorption may be affected by total body stores of Pi, Barac-Nieto et al. (66) set out to determine if the high Pi demand associated with growth may, similar to a reduction in Pi supply, result in a low level of intracellular Pi, and that this low level is responsible for initiating and maintaining a high renal Pi co-transport capacity. Nuclear Magnetic Resonance (NMR) spectroscopy and chemical methods were used to determine the effect of age and Pi intake on intracellular Pi in the perfused kidney. The findings from these studies indicate that changes in intracellular Pi related to age or diet are not a consequence of changes in abundance or maximum mobility of Na^+–Pi co-transporters and are consistent with earlier observations. In animals fed a normal phosphate diet intracellular Pi was twice as high (1.85 ± 0.23 vs. 0.90 ± 0.02 mM) while the fractional reabsorption of Pi was lower (0.70 vs. 0.90) in >4-week-old than in <1-week-old animals. Diet induced changes in intracellular Pi were associated with changes in V_{max} of similar magnitude in mature and immature animals, but in opposing directions. However, as seen in Fig. 7, at any given intracellular Pi concentration, V_{max} was substantially higher in microvilli prepared from kidneys of newborn than of older animals.

Woda et al. (63) also showed that dietary phosphate restriction in juvenile rats resulted in a significant increase in Na/Pi expression in the proximal tubule BBM as well as the expression of intracellular NaPi-2 protein. Dietary phosphate restriction in the juvenile rat upregulated BBM Na/Pi-2 expression, which was associated with the further increase in proximal tubular Pi reabsorption. As a result of this study and others (67, 68) a specific type IIa-related Na/Pi co-transporter protein was postulated to account for the high Pi transport rate in weanling animals. Evidence for this was obtained by antisense experiments and transport expression in *Xenopus oocytes*. When mRNA isolated from

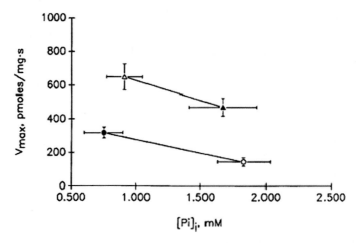

Fig. 7. Relationship between intracellular Pi (*[Pi]*) in kidney and Vmax in renal microvilli of newborn guinea pigs fed standard (*open triangle*) or high (*solid triangle*) Pi diets and mature guinea pigs fed standard (*open circles*) or low (*solid circle*) Pi diets (used with permission from Barac-Nieto et al. *(66)*).

kidney cortices of rapidly growing rats was treated with type IIa transporter antisense oligonucleotides or was depleted of type IIa-specific mRNA by a subtraction hybridization procedure, Na$^+$-dependent Pi uptake was still detected in injected oocytes *(67)*. The type IIa transporter-depleted mRNA contained an mRNA species that showed some sequence homology to the type IIa transporter encoding message. This is compatible with the fact that young type IIa knock-out mice lacking type IIa mRNA and protein retain the capacity to reabsorb phosphate at a rate that cannot be explained by the presence of type I and III Na/Pi transporter *(69)*. Segawa et al. *(67)* isolated a cDNA from the human and rat kidney that encodes a growth-related Na$^+$-dependent Pi co-transporter, type IIc. The transport activity was dependent on extracellular pH. In electrophysiological studies, type IIc Na/Pi was electroneutral, while type IIa was highly electrogenic (see above). In Northern blotting analysis, the type IIc protein was shown to be localized at the apical membrane of the proximal tubular cells in superficial and corticomedullary nephrons of the weanling rat kidney. Hybrid depletion experiments showed that type IIc could function as a Na/Pi co-transporter in weanling animals, with its role reduced in adults. Segawa's studies *(67, 68)* suggest that the type IIc is a growth-related renal Na/Pi co-transporter, which has a high affinity for Pi and is electroneutral.

Parathyroid hormone in the adult decreases the excretion of Pi by inhibiting BBM Na/Pi co-transport. The response to PTH is different during early post-natal life. Linarelli *(70)* showed that infusion of PTH into newborn babies resulted in minimal depression of the tubular reabsorption of Pi. In the isolated kidney of the newborn guinea pig addition of PTH to the perfusion fluid caused a marked increase in tubular calcium (Ca^{2+}) reabsorption and in urinary excretion of c-AMP, but had little effect on the excretion of Pi.

Growth hormone equally plays an important role in renal reabsorption of Pi during development. Woda et al. *(71)* studied the regulation of renal Na/Pi-2 expression and tubular phosphate reabsorption in the juvenile rat and have demonstrated that GH is responsible independently of PTH, for the enhanced Pi uptake in both the proximal convoluted tubule and straight tubule of juvenile rats on a normal Pi diet. In addition, the authors found that GH contributes significantly to the blunted phosphaturic response to PTH in the juvenile rat. The proposed mechanism for the enhanced Na/Pi co-transport activity appears to be through the action of GH on the expression of proximal tubular BBM type IIa Na/Pi transporter protein. Overall phosphate handling by the immature kidney is regulated so that phosphate retention is promoted to meet the phosphorus needs of the growing organism.

2. CLINICAL ASSESSMENT OF RENAL PHOSPHORUS EXCRETION

Under normal physiologic conditions 80–97% of the filtered load of phosphate is reabsorbed by the renal tubules *(72)*. For those solutes not undergoing tubular secretion, the difference, $100 - FE_{Pi}$, where FE_{Pi} represents the fractional excretion of phosphate, is the percentage of phosphate that is reabsorbed or the fractional tubular reabsorption of Pi (TRPi). If renal function is normal and dietary intake average, calculation of the TRPi gives a rough guide as to whether or not tubular Pi reabsorption is normal or not. The TRPi may be calculated on random urine samples without the need for a timed urine collection. Calculation of the TRPi requires drawing a blood sample at the time of the urine collection. The TRPi is calculated as follows: TRPi (%) = $(1 - U_{pi} \times P_{cr}/U_{cr} \times P_{pi}) \times 100$, where U_{pi} and P_{pi} represent the plasma and urinary concentrations of Pi and P_{cr} and U_{cr} represent the plasma and urinary concentrations of creatinine, respectively.

The TRPi is markedly influenced by changes in GFR as well as dietary phosphate intake, and a more reliable means of assessing phosphate reabsorption is to measure the TmPi/GFR. Clearance studies in humans and experimental animals show that as the filtered load of phosphate is progressively increased, phosphate reabsorption rises until a maximum tubular reabsorptive rate for phosphate (Pi), or TMPi, is reached, after which phosphate excretion increases in proportion to its filtered load *(73)*. The TmPi/GFR or the maximum tubular reabsorption of phosphate per unit volume of GFR therefore is thought to be the most reliable measure of overall tubular reabsorptive capacity. Ideally, the TmPi should be calculated by performing a phosphate titration study. However, the TmPi may be calculated using a more practical method. Walton and Bijvoet *(74)* have shown that TmPi/GFR can be derived from the TRPi and plasma Pi and have produced a nomogram to simplify the calculation. The validity of the Walton–Bijvoet nomogram was questioned in children who are known to have higher concentrations of P_{Pi} and lower GFRs *(7, 8, 75, 76)*. Brodehl et al. *(77)* have shown that the Walton–Bijvoet nomogram, while derived from studies in normal adults, gives good agreement with directly measured TmPi/GFR in infants and children at high rates of filtered Pi load. Brodehl et al. *(14)* also showed that as predicted on theoretical grounds TmPi/GFR could be calculated from the formula TmPi/GFR = $P_{Pi} - (U_{Pi} \times P_{Cr}/U_{Cr})$. For clinical evaluation this equation may be used regardless of the phosphate load. Stark et al. *(78)* showed that there were no differences between morning fasting and non-fasting serum phosphate values. Furthermore, timed urinary collections are not necessary.

3. HYPOPHOSPHATEMIC DISORDERS

The causes of hypophosphatemia may be classified into one of three groups: increased urinary phosphate excretion, decreased GI absorption of phosphate, and shifts of phosphorus from the extracellular compartment (Table 2). Mild hypophosphatemia does not usually result in symptoms. Serum phosphate levels generally have to be below 1 mg/dL for patients to become symptomatic. A number of the clinical manifestations of severe hypophosphatemia may be seen in Table 3. The focus of this chapter is on a number of the disorders that result in increased urinary phosphate excretion and treatment of these conditions. *Treatment*: For the other causes listed in Table 2 the clinical circumstances will generally suggest whether severe underlying phosphate deficiency is present, as serum levels may not always be a good reflection of body stores. In some patients who may be hypophosphatemic from antacid or diuretic use correction of the underlying cause may be all that is necessary. In mild to moderate hypophosphatemia (~2 mg/dL) oral repletion with skim milk (0.9 mg phosphorus per mL) or Neutra-phos, Neutra-phos K, or Fleet phosphorus soda preparations may be useful. Intravenous phosphorus repletion is reserved for severe (~1 mg/dL) hypophosphatemia. The most frequently recommended regime is to administer 2.5 mg/kg body weight (0.08 mmol/kg body weight) of elemental phosphorus over a 6-h period for

Table 2

Causes of Hypophosphatemia

Increased urinary phosphate excretion
    Volume expansion
    Fanconi syndrome
    Hyperparathyroidism
    Acetazolamide and other diuretics acting on the proximal tubule
    Acute renal failure and recovery from acute tubular necrosis
    Corticosteroids
    Tumor-induced osteomalacia*
    Inherited defects*
    Vitamin D deficiency (or resistance)*
    Post-renal transplant*
Decreased GI absorption of phosphate
    Inadequate phosphate intake
    Chronic diarrhea
    Phosphate-binding antacids
    Chronic alcoholism
Altered distribution of phosphate
    Acute respiratory alkalosis
    Post-parathyroidectomy "hungry bone syndrome"
    Diabetic ketoacidosis
    Refeeding in chronically malnourished individuals and in chronic alcoholism
    Leukemia during the acute phase and in the leukemic phase of lymphomas

*Topics discussed in detail in this chapter.

Table 3
Clinical Manifestations of Hypophosphatemia

Hematologic
    Predisposition to hemolysis
    Decrease in erythrocyte 2,3-diphosphoglycerate levels, which increases
        hemoglobin-oxygen affinity
    Diminished white cell phagocytosis
Musculoskeletal
    Impaired muscle function with overt cardiac and respiratory failure
    Proximal myopathies
    Rhabdomyolysis
    Increased bone resorption with development of rickets and osteomalacia
Kidney
    Decreased proximal tubule reabsorptive function
    Decreased renal conservation of calcium with possible frank hypercalciuria

---

severe asymptomatic hypophosphatemia and 5 mg/kg body weight (0.16 mmol/kg body weight) of elemental phosphorus over a 6-h period for severe symptomatic hypophosphatemia. Parenteral administration should be discontinued when the serum phosphorus concentration is greater than 2 mg/dL.

3.1. Hereditary Hypophosphatemic Rickets with Hypercalciuria

Hereditary hypophosphatemic rickets with hypercalciuria (HHRH) is an autosomal recessive disorder characterized by hypophosphatemia secondary to renal Pi wasting, an appropriate increase in the serum concentration of $1,25(OH)_2D_3$ with associated intestinal calcium hyperabsorption and hypercalciuria, and rickets and osteomalacia (Table 4). The most probable mechanism for the hypercalciuria in this disorder is increased intestinal calcium absorption. The increased renal phosphate clearance (TmP/GFR) is usually 2–4 standard deviations below the age-related normal range.

Initial clinical studies suggested that HHRH was a primary renal Pi wasting disorder since all abnormalities, with the exception of decreased renal Pi reabsorption, are completely corrected by dietary Pi supplementation. The Npt2a gene and a fragment of the Npt2a promoter gene, though, were not found to have mutations in affected individuals. The disease locus was mapped to human chromosome region 9q34, which contains Slc34A3, the gene encoding the type IIc Na/Pi co-transporter. The mutation is predicted to truncate the type IIc protein in the first transmembrane domain and to result in complete loss of function in individuals homozygous for the deletion. Compound heterozygotes are similarly affected supporting the conclusion that this disease is caused by Slc34A3 mutations affecting both alleles. The phosphaturic factor FGF-23 is at normal or low-normal serum levels in patients with HHRH, further supporting a primary renal defect as the cause of the disease.

It is not entirely clear why loss of function of the less abundant type IIc Na/Pi co-transporter causes rickets and osteomalacia in humans where as mutations in the more abundant type IIa Na/Pi co-transporter elicits a mild skeletal phenotype that lacks the typical features of rickets and osteomalacia in mice *(79)*. Possibly the type IIc co-transporter may be a more important regulator of Pi homeostasis in humans than mice. Differences in developmental expression patterns of type IIa and type IIc Na/Pi co-transporters in relation to skeletal maturation, which is critically dependent on Pi supply may also be at issue. Extrarenal expression of type IIa and type IIc Na/Pi co-transporters in addition may have an impact on skeletal phenotype.

Treatment: Patients with HHRH frequently develop renal stones as a result of increased urinary excretion of both calcium and phosphate. Long-term phosphate supplementation as the sole therapy leads, with the exception of the persistently decreased TmP/GFR, to reversal of the clinical and biochemical abnormalities. Elemental phosphorus (as Neutra-Phos or Neutra-Phos K) is administered several times daily. The addition of $1,25(OH)_2D_3$ runs the risk of development of nephrocalcinosis and nephrolithiasis. The goal of therapy is to improve mineralization of osteoid, and to decrease circulating levels of $1,25(OH)_2D_3$, thereby reducing the intestinal absorption of calcium.

3.2. Tumor-Induced Osteomalacia (TIO)

TIO is a rare paraneoplastic syndrome with symptoms including chronic muscle and bone pain, weakness, and fatigue in association with a high risk of fragility fractures due to osteomalacia. The pathogenesis of TIO results from the production and secretion of the phosphaturic tumor factors (phosphatonins), which as noted above specifically inhibit Na/Pi co-transport. FGF-23, sFRP-4, FGF-7, and MEPE all have been identified in relation to this condition. FGF-23, the first to be identified in TIO by Shimada et al. *(80)*, is normally produced in bone and is markedly elevated in the tumors and serum of patients with TIO. As a consequence of the elevated FGF-23 the renal expression of Npt2a and Npt2c is decreased and there is reduced renal reabsorption of Pi (with resultant decrease in serum Pi; Table 4). FGF-23 downregulates the conversion of $25(OH)D_3$ to $1,25(OH)_2D_3$ (with ensuing rickets and osteomalacia) *(80)*. Cure of the disease phenotype and decreases in FGF-23 serum concentrations after tumor removal in patients with TIO support the role of FGF-23 in the pathogenesis of this condition.

Treatment: Location of the tumor in TIO is often difficult and may require extensive and repeated surveys with conventional imaging techniques. Magnetic resonance skeletal survey may be improved by using magnetic resonance gradient recall echo imaging. Alternatively, sst-based molecular imaging scintigraphies have been developed, based on the possibility that these tumors are somatostatin receptor positive (sst1–sst5). Finally, the anatomical localization of the tumor may be more precise when combining PET and CT using a using a radiopharmaceutical compound coupling octreotide, a DOTA chelator, and [68]gallium *(81)*. Unless the location of the tumor has been found and its size enables surgical removal treatment usually consists of chronic oral treatment with phosphate and calcitriol. There are preliminary reports that Cinacalcet may also be of benefit to individuals with this condition *(82)*.

3.3. Autosomal Dominant Hypophosphatemic Rickets (ADHR), X-Linked Hypophosphatemic Rickets (XLH), and Autosomal Recessive Hypophosphatemic Rickets (ARHP)

ADHR, XLH, and ARHP are characterized by hypophosphatemia, decreased renal Pi reabsorption and rickets, and osteomalacia. These disorders are inherited, and are easily distinguished from HHRH by the absence of appropriate increases in the serum concentration of 1,25(OH)$_2$D$_3$ in the setting of hypophosphatemia, and the absence of associated intestinal calcium reabsorption and hypercalciuria (Table 4).

ADHR is characterized by hypophosphatemia due to isolated renal phosphate wasting. Children with ADHR present with skeletal defects including severe bowing of long bones and widening of metaphyseal regions of the bones that is most prominent at costochondral joints. Interestingly, study of a large family cohort with ADHR has revealed evidence of incomplete penetrance, variable onset (pre-pubertal vs. post-pubertal, and spontaneous recovery of renal phosphate reabsorption) *(83–85)*.

ADHR is caused by heterozygous mutations in the gene encoding FGF-23 *(86, 87)*. Mutations identified in ADHR are missense mutations and in each case, the mutation alters an arginine residue at either position 176 or 179. The mutations, which involve a proprotein convertase (furin) cleavage site, prevent the proteolytic processing of FGF-23 to its inactive N- and C-terminal peptides. Mutant FGF-23 proteins exhibit increased stability, and are more active than wild-type FGF-23 in vivo *(88)*, and are likely present at elevated concentrations in ADHR patients *(89)*. In these patients FGF-23 acts by not only suppressing the reabsorption of phosphate in the proximal tubule, but also the biosynthesis of 1,25(OH)$_2$D$_3$. The latter is consistent with the inappropriately low or normal levels of 1,25(OH)$_2$D$_3$ observed in patients with ADHR.

Table 4
Biochemical Features of ARHR, XLH, ADHR, HHRH and TIO

	XLH	ADHR	TIO	HHRH	ARHR
Mutated gene	Phosphate-regulating gene with homologies to endopeptidases on the X chromosome (PHEX)	Fibroblast growth factor 23 (FGF-23)	-	Type IIc Na/Pi transporter-SLC34A3	Dentin matrix protein 1 (DMP1)
Serum Pi	low	low	low	Low	low
Serum Ca	normal	normal	normal	normal/high	normal
25(OH)D$_3$		normal	normal	normal	normal
1,25(OH)$_2$D$_3$	normal	normal/low	normal/low	normal/high	normal
PTH	normal/high	normal	normal	low	normal
Urine Ca	decreased	decreased	decreased	increased	decreased
FGF-23	normal/high	normal/high	high	low	high

XLH (vitamin D resistant rickets) is the most common inherited phosphate wasting disorder with a prevalence of 1/20,000. The defective gene is on the X-chromosome, but female carriers are affected so that it is an X-linked dominant disorder. It frequently becomes manifest during late infancy when the child begins walking. The patient develops skeletal deformities that primarily include bowing of the long bones and widening of the metaphyseal region. The latter is most common at costochondral junctions (rachitic rosary). These deformities are associated with diminished growth velocity, often resulting in short stature. Later in life patients show osteomalacia, enthesopathy (calcified ligaments and teno-osseous junctions), degenerative joint disease, and continued dental disease in particular tooth decay and dental abscesses.

Early parabiosis and kidney cross-transplantation experiments showed that there was a circulating hypophosphatemic factor present in the serum of *Hyp* mice (the mouse homolog of human XLH) *(90–92)*. In *Hyp* mice, the defect in renal phosphate reabsorption is a consequence of a decrease in BBM abundance of Npt2a and Npt2c cotransporter proteins *(93)*. In addition, Pi regulation of the renal enzymes involved in the synthesis and catabolism of $1,25(OH)_2D_3$ is abnormal in the mouse mutants. These findings are consistent with the action of phosphatonins.

Genetic linkage analysis has revealed inactivating mutations in *PHEX*, a gene located on Xp22. PHEX (**PH**osphate regulating gene with homology to **E**ndopeptidases on the **X** chromosome) protein is expressed in various tissues, including the kidney, but is most abundant in mature osteoblasts and odontoblasts. There is significant sequence homology between PHEX and members of the M13 family of zinc metallopeptidases, which are integral membrane glycoproteins that show proteolytic activity immediately outside the cell. Since it does not appear to circulate it has been suggested that PHEX mediates inactivation by proteolytic cleavage of FGF-23. Serum FGF-23 concentrations are, in fact, elevated in about two-thirds of patients with XLH *(94, 95)* and in all *Hyp* mice. The *Hyp* phenotype is dependent on FGF-23 *(96)*. The phenotype of FGF-23-null mice is indistinguishable from the phenotype of animals that are null for both PHEX and FGF-23 further supporting the fact that FGF-23 is required for the development of hypophosphatemia and is downstream from PHEX *(97, 98)*. *Hyp* mice, which have been injected with inactivating antibodies to FGF-23, normalized their blood phosphorus concentrations and, furthermore, healed their rachitic changes, also supporting the conclusion that PHEX is directly or indirectly involved in the metabolism of FGF-23 *(99)*. PHEX-dependent cleavage of FGF-23, however, has not been yet demonstrated in vivo and there is limited data in vitro supporting this possibility *(48, 100)*. Alternatively, there is data to suggest that accelerated FGF-23 synthesis rather than decreased FGF-23 degradation may characterize this disorder *(97)*.

ARHP: Study of the clinical and biochemical abnormalities of affected individuals with ARHP indicates a great deal of similarity to ADHR and XLH. Clinical features include rickets, skeletal deformities, dental defects, and affected individuals develop osteosclerotic bone lesions and enthesopathies later in life. Hypophosphatemia resulting from renal phosphate wasting is accompanied by normal or low $1,25(OH)_2D_3$ levels and high alkaline phosphatase levels. PTH is normal and urinary calcium excretion is normal. FGF-23 levels appear to be either elevated or normal in ARHP, which is inappropriate to the low serum phosphorus levels. The families of these patients showed no mutations in FGF-23 (causing its resistance to degradation) or the PHEX gene that is linked to the degradative pathway of FGF-23. Subsequently, mutations in the dentin matrix protein 1 (DMP-1) were identified *(101, 102)*. DMP-1 is widely expressed but particularly abundant in bone where it is synthesized by osteoblasts. It is involved in the regulation of transcription in undifferentiated osteoblasts. DMP-1 belongs to the SIB-LING protein family, which includes osteopontin, matrix extracellular phosphoglyco-protein (MEPE), bone sialoprotein II, and dentin sialoprotein, and whose genes are clus-tered on chromosome 4q21. DMP-1 undergoes phosphorylation during the early phase of osteoblasts maturation and is subsequently exported into the extracellular matrix where it regulates the nucleation of hydroxyapatite.

Of the several DMP1 mutations identified, one mutation alters the translation ini-tiation codon (MIV), two mutations are located in different intron–exon boundaries, and three are frameshift mutations within exon 6. These mutations all appear to be inactivating.

Studies using a DMP-1 knock-out mouse model showed highly elevated levels of FGF-23 in bone and serum. Moreover, DMP-1 deficient mice showed abnormal matura-tion of osteoblasts to osteocytes and an altered structure of bone, dentine, and cartilage, as well as hypophosphatemia and osteomalacia *(102)*. Thus DMP1 may play a dual role in phosphate homeostasis. It may act as a negative regulator of FGF-23. In addition, as DMP-1 has a well established importance in osteoblast function, loss of DMP-1 function in osteoblasts, and extracellular matrix may also contribute to the bone abnormalities typical of ARHP.

Treatment Strategies for XLH, ADHR, ARHP: Treatment for the above hypophos-phatemic conditions depends on the underlying genetic defect. Those disorders caused by genetic mutations associated with low or inappropriately normal $1,25(OH)_2D_3$ levels (as a consequence of elevated FGF-23 that suppresses the renal 25-hydroxyvitamin D 1α-hydroxylase activity) are generally treated with oral phosphate and oral $1,25(OH)_2D_3$. This includes XLH, ADHR, and ARHP. Elemental phosphorus (as Neutra-phos or Neutra-phos K) is administered several times daily. Since the oral phos-phate leads to the development of secondary hyperparathyroidism, $1,25(OH)_2D_3$ (avail-able as calcitriol in capsular form or liquid) is also given. Therapy with $1,25(OH)_2D_3$ is adjusted to avoid the development of hypercalcemia and hypercalciuria, yet to maxi-mize the suppression of PTH synthesis and secretion. The therapeutic goal is to maintain serum calcium and PTH levels within the normal range, to improve alkaline phosphatase activity, and to prevent the development of increased calcium excretion. Phosphate ther-apy in some cases is limited by the development of diarrhea and abdominal discomfort. A renal ultrasound should be performed before treatment and subsequently at 1–2 year intervals. Radiographs of the knees and over the hand/wrist should be performed before treatment and subsequently at yearly intervals.

3.4. Other Genetic Disorders of Hypophosphatemia

Phosphaturia, hypophosphatemia, and rickets/osteomalacia have been reported in *fibrous dysplasia (FD)*. The disorder is characterized by fibrous skeletal lesions and associated localized mineralization defects. FD can result in pain, fracture, and deformity in affected areas. FD is a classic feature of *McCune Albright Syndrome* (MAS; triad of precocious puberty, café-au-lait lesions and polyostotic bone dysplasia). FD and MAS are caused by activating mutations of GNAS1, the gene encoding the alpha-subunit of the stimulatory G protein. While somatic activating mutations in GNAS1 gene are responsible for this disease it is unclear whether or not increased cyclic AMP level causes enhanced expression of FGF-23. Recent studies confirm that FD by itself may also be associated with increased FGF-23 levels, in turn, inversely correlated with serum phosphorus, and $1,25(OH)_2D_3$ levels. *Treatment*: Treatment with bisphosphonates has been shown to reduce serum FGF-23 levels, which result in a reduction of renal phosphate wasting. The mechanisms underlying the reduction of FGF-23 by bisphosphonates are unclear.

Borzani et al. *(103)* a number of years ago reported a patient with a condition called *Hypophosphatemic Bone Disease (HBD)*. This disorder of phosphate metabolism previously has been described by Scriver et al. *(104, 105)* in a kindred with autosomal dominant inheritance. Frymoyer and Hodgkin *(106)* describe a similar kindred with X-linked disease. Although the condition is in some ways analogous to XLH, there are important differences between the two diseases. For example, there is selective impairment in the tubular reabsorption of phosphate in HBD but the defect is less severe and it is clearly different from that described in XLH. Clinical manifestations of HBD appear in infancy, but the dwarfism and the bone changes are less severe than in XLH at comparable concentrations of serum phosphorus in the two diseases. While in both conditions there is osteomalacia of endostal trabecular bone, only in XLH is florid rickets present, affecting the epiphyses and compromising linear growth. The phosphaturic response to PTH infusion is abnormal in qualitative aspects, but it is present in HBD, and this differs from that described in XLH. *Treatment*: The treatment with oral phosphates and $1,25(OH)_2D_3$ in patients with HBD is accompanied by increases in serum phosphorus, with improved tubular reabsorption of phosphate and bone healing; this combination of responses is not present in XLH.

Linear nevus sebaceous syndrome (LNSS)/epidermal nevus syndrome (ENS) or Schimmelpenning–Feuerstein–Mims syndrome is another rare condition with hypophosphatemia that may lead to the development of rickets. Two recent case reports have described elevated FGF-23 levels in two patients. While the skin lesions appeared to be the source of the FGF-23 in one patient *(107)*, the bone lesions were thought to secrete FGF-23 in the other patient *(108)*.

3.5. Other Causes of Hypophosphatemic Rickets

As discussed above ADHR, ARHR, XLH, TIO, and hypophosphatemic rickets osteomalacia associated with MAS/FD are characterized by hypophosphatemia and low $1,25(OH)_2D_3$ levels. FGF-23 levels are basically high in patients with these hypophosphatemic diseases. However, the mechanisms of excess actions of FGF-23 in these disorders are variable. *Adolescent hypophosphatemic osteomalacia* is similar to XLH except for the fact that with this condition patients develop the hypophosphatemic rickets at an advanced age, compared with the classic X-linked disturbance. Increased levels of biologically active FGF-23 has been observed in this group of patients *(109)*. This is a diagnosis of exclusion and careful follow-up of the patients is required as TIO is a much more common condition and the responsible tumor is often small and difficult to locate on initial careful clinical examination. The mechanism for the elevated FGF-23 level in this condition is unclear. *Treatment*: Drug therapy is based on phosphate supplements together with a large dose of $1,25(OH)_2D_3$.

3.5.1. VITAMIN D-DEPENDENT RICKETS, TYPE I

25-Hydroxy vitamin D_3-1α hydroxylase deficiency, also known as vitamin D-dependent rickets, type 1 (VDDR-1) is inherited as an autosomal recessive disorder. It is characterized by the early onset of rickets with hypocalcemia and is caused by mutations of the 25-hydroxy vitamin D_3-1α hydroxylase gene. The human gene encoding the 1α-hydroxylase is located on chromosome 12q14, and comprises nine exons, and eight introns. The enzyme is specifically expressed in the proximal tubule. It results from inactivating mutations. Vitamin D is metabolized by sequential hydroxylations in the liver (25-hydroxylation) and the kidney (1α-hydroxylation). Hydroxylation of 25-hydroxyvitamin D3 is mediated by 25-hydroxy vitamin D_3-1α hydroxylase in the kidney (Fig. 8). Patients usually appear normal at birth and develop muscle weakness, tetany, convulsions, and rickets starting at 2 months of age. Serum phosphorus and calcium levels are low, and PTH levels are high with low to undetectable levels of $1,25(OH)_2D_3$. Patients with this disorder have elevated levels of $25(OH)D_3$ as opposed to children with deprivational rickets where $25(OH)D_3$ levels are reduced or absent. *Treatment*: Treatment with physiologic doses of $1,25(OH)_2D_3$ results in healing of the rickets with restoration of the plasma phosphate, calcium, and PTH levels.

3.5.2. HEREDITARY $1,25(OH)_2D_3$-RESISTANT RICKETS (VITAMIN D-DEPENDENT RICKETS, TYPE II)

This rare autosomal recessive disorder is similar to selective deficiency of $1,25(OH)_2D_3$. It usually presents with rachitic changes not responsive to vitamin D treatment (with either $1,25(OH)_2D_3$ or $1(OH)D_3$) with elevated circulating levels of $1,25(OH)_2D_3$, thus differentiating it from vitamin D-dependent rickets, type 1 (Fig. 8). Alopecia of the scalp or the body is seen in approximately 50% of families with this condition. In a subset of affected families the disease has been found to be due to mutations in the vitamin D-receptor gene. In one family a nonsense mutation coding for a premature stop codon in exon 7 of the gene encoding the vitamin D receptor was identified, resulting in the absence of the ligand-binding domain *(110)*. In other families the genetic abnormality has been a point mutation within the steroid-binding domain of the vitamin D-receptor gene *(111)*. In another patient with type II vitamin D-resistant rickets with normal receptor function, failure of $1,25(OH)_2D_3$ to stimulate the enzyme $25(OH)_2D_3$-24-hydroxylase was demonstrated *(112–114)*. The latter may represent a step in the physiological action of $1,25(OH)_2D_3$ that is lacking in some patients with type II vitamin D-dependent rickets.

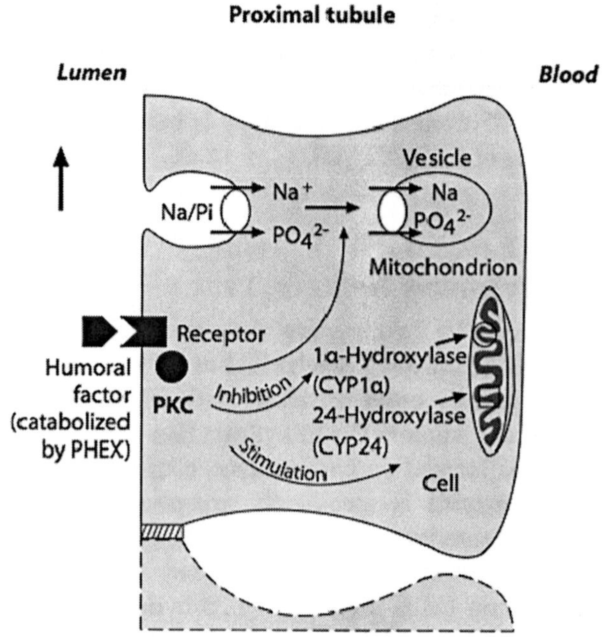

Proximal tubule

Fig. 8. Schematic representation of the molecular genetic basis of three inherited forms of rickets. Vitamin D-dependent rickets type 1 (VDDR-1) is secondary to mutations in the 1α-hydroxylase gene. This gene is responsible for the 1α-hydroxylation of 25-hydroxyvitamin D_3 ($25(OH)D_3$) that occurs in the proximal renal tubule. This 1α-hydroxylation is catalyzed by 25-hydroxyvitamin D_3-1α-hydroxylase (1α-hydroxylase), a mitochondrial cytochrome P450 enzyme that is subject to complex regulation by parathyroid hormone, calcium, phosphorus, and 1,25-hydroxyvitamin D_3 ($1,25(OH)_2D_3$) itself. Vitamin D-dependent rickets type 2 or hereditary $1,25(OH)_2D_3$-resistant rickets is thought to be due in many cases to a mutation in the gene for the vitamin D receptor. In contrast X-linked hypophosphatemic (XLH) rickets results from loss-of-function mutations in the PHEX gene (from Bonnardeaux and Bichet *(136)* (Fig. 40.5)).

Treatment: In contrast to patients with vitamin D-dependent rickets, type I, in type II serum $1,25(OH)_2D_3$ is elevated and the patients either respond to pharmacologic doses of $1,25(OH)_2D_3$ or do not respond at all. Prolonged periods of therapy are usually required. Parenteral therapy with $1,25(OH)_2D_3$ with the administration of oral or parenteral calcium is often necessary. The response to therapy likely is dependent on the exact defect.

3.6. Osteoglophonic Dysplasia (OGD)

OGD is an autosomal dominant disorder characterized by skeletal abnormalities including craniosynostosis, prominent supraorbital ridges and mild facial hypoplasia, rhizomelic dwarfism, and non-ossifying bone lesions. Affected individuals have hypophosphatemia due to renal phosphate wasting associated with inappropriately normal $1,25(OH)_2D_3$ levels *(115, 116)*. White et al. *(117)* recently identified several heterozygous missense mutations in fibroblast growth factor receptor 1 (FGFR1) that are located within or close to the receptor's membrane spanning domain. These mutations all affect amino acid residues that are highly conserved across species and seem to lead to constitutive receptor activation *(117, 118)*. It is thought that the skeletal lesions develop because the constitutive activation of the FGFR1 leads to an up-regulation of FGF-23 secretion in the metaphyseal growth plate. The elevated FGF-23 results in the renal phosphate wasting seen in this condition. Patients with a worse radiographic picture seem to have the most profound hypophosphatemia. *Treatment*: Prosthetic dental replacement has been difficult because of distorted jaw relationship and large alveolar ridges *(119)*. Craniofacial reconstruction may be compromised by obstruction of the nasal airways, difficulty in intubation, and postoperative respiratory problems.

3.7. Post-renal Transplant Hypophosphatemia

Persistent hypophosphatemia has been noted in some patients with chronic kidney disease following renal transplantation, despite relatively modest increases in PTH levels. In these patients FGF-23 levels have been noted to be elevated, and it is possible that FGF-23 plays a role in the hypophosphatemia seen in this situation. *Treatment*: Generally elemental Phosphorus (as Neutra-phos or Neutra-phos K) is administered several times daily. Phosphorus supplementation may aggravate mild hyperparathyroidism, if present; if hyperparathyroidism is absent, phosphate supplementation is the recommended therapy.

4. HYPERPHOSPHATEMIC DISORDERS

The causes of hyperphosphatemia may be classified into three groups: decreased urinary phosphate excretion, redistribution of phosphate, and exogenous administration of phosphate (Table 5). Clinical manifestations of hyperphosphatemia are seen in Table 6. Pseudohyperphosphatemia may be seen in states of paraproteinemia. Hyperlipidemia, hyperbilirubinemia, and sample dilution are much more rare causes of pseudohyperphosphatemia. *Treatment*: Dietary phosphate restriction and oral phosphate binders are generally used for treatment of chronic hyperphosphatemia. Chronic hyperphosphatemia is most commonly seen in chronic kidney disease (see below). Chronic hyperphosphatemia may also be seen in association with tumoral calcinosis/hyperostosis hyperphosphatemia syndrome (see below) and is treated similarly. Acute hyperphosphatemia in association with hypocalcemia requires immediate attention. Severe hyperphosphatemia as seen in patients with acutely reduced renal function, particularly in those with tumor lysis syndrome, may require hemodialysis or a continuous form of renal replacement therapy. Volume expansion also may increase urinary phosphate excretion as can the administration of diuretics such as acetazolamide. Redistribution of phosphorus from the intracellular to the extracellular space can sometimes be rapidly corrected by the administration of glucose and insulin.

4.1. Familial Tumoral Calcinosis (FTC)

Another condition for which the basis of disease has become clearer is tumoral calcinosis. Patients with this condition manifest hyperphosphatemia, mild hypercalcemia, reduced renal phosphate excretion, and elevated $1,25(OH)_2D_3$ concentrations *(120, 121)*. The physical chemical product of calcium × phosphorus is greater than 70 and soft tissue calcifications are present. Extraskeletal calcifications including periarticular,

Table 5
Causes of Hyperphosphatemia

Decreased urinary phosphate excretion
　　Hypoparathyroidism, pseudohypoparathyroidism
　　Abnormal circulating parathyroid hormone
　　Acromegaly (related to growth hormone excess)
　　Bisphosphonates
　　Chronic kidney disease*
　　Familial tumoral calcinosis*
　　Hyperostosis hyperphosphatemia syndrome*
Redistribution of phosphate
　　Tumor lysis syndrome
　　Respiratory acidosis
　　Increased catabolism
　　Severe trauma/traumatic rhabdomyolysis
Exogenous administration of phosphate
　　Administration of phosphate containing enemas (in chronic kidney disease
　　　or following oral sodium phosphate administration for bowel preps)
　　Intravenous phosphate
　　Pharmacologic administration of vitamin D metabolites
Pseudohyperphosphatemia
　　Multiple myeloma
　　Waldenstrom macroglobulinemia

*Topics discussed in detail in this chapter

Table 6
Clinical Manifestations of Hyperphosphatemia

Secondary hyperparathyroidism
Secondary hypocalcemia
　　From calcium precipitation
　　Decreased production of $1,25(OH)_2D_3$
　　Decreased intestinal calcium reabsorption
Ectopic calcifications (of skin, vasculature, cornea, and joints); of
　　significant risk when the physical chemical product of serum calcium
　　and serum phosphorus (in mg/dL) exceeds 70

vascular, and other soft tissue calcium deposits are present in patients with this syndrome. Affected individuals report recurrent painful subcutaneous masses often resulting in ulceration leading to sinus tracts and infection. Masses as much as 1 kg in weight are reported. Three different types of mutations have been reported with this condition. The first type occurs in the gene encoding UDP-N-acetyl-α-D-galactosamine: polypeptide N-acetylgalactosaminyltransferase 3 (GalNAc transferase 3; GALNT3; mapped to 2q24-q31). GalNAc transferase 3 is a Golgi-associated biosynthetic enzyme, which initiates mucin-type O-glycosylation of proteins. O-glycosylation of FGF-23 by

GalNAc transferase 3 is essential for the secretion of intact FGF-23 because O-glycosylation at a subtilisin-like proprotein convertase recognition sequence motif prevents cleavage of FGF-23 *(120)*. Some patients with this syndrome have low concentrations of FGF-23, but high concentrations of FGF-23 fragments. It has been thought that the fragments lack biological activity, but in vivo studies have shown that carboxyl-terminal fragments maintain their biological activity *(122)*. This has caused uncertainty as to precisely how GalNAc transferase 3 mutations cause the syndrome.

A second gene for FTC, encoding FGF-23, has also been found. A missense mutation in the FGF-23 gene abrogates FGF-23 function by absent or extremely reduced secretion of intact FGF-23 *(123, 124)*. A third group of mutations resulting in FTC occurs in the gene for Klotho, which encodes the co-receptor for FGF-23 *(125)*. This results in a diminished ability of FGF-23 to signal via its cognate FGF receptors.

Treatment: Treatment of FTC has not been very successful. Apart from surgery, no modality has been shown to be efficient in managing the calcium deposition of this condition. Low phosphate diet, phosphate-binding antacids, and radiation therapy have been tried. A recent report has suggested that the phosphate-binding agent sevelamer in combination with the carbonic anhydrase inhibitor acetazolamide may be of benefit *(126)*.

4.2. Hyperostosis Hyperphosphatemia Syndrome (HHS)

HHS is a rare metabolic disorder characterized by hyperphosphatemia, inappropriately normal or elevated $1,25(OH)_2D_3$ and cortical hyperostosis. Pain in the long bones is associated with erythema and warmth of the overlying skin. Typical radiographic features of affected bones include cortical hyperostosis, diaphysitis, and periosteal apposition. Prior to gene identification HHS and FTC were thought to share a common pathologic mechanism based on the fact that cortical hyperostosis and ectopic calcifications co-existed in some patients *(127–129)*. HHS is caused by mutations in the GalNAc transferase 3 (GALNT3), which encodes UDP-*N*-acetyl-α-D-galactosamine: polypeptide *N*-acetylgalactosaminyltransferase 3. These inactivating mutations and the low FGF-23 levels found in HHS are the same as that seen in FTC, providing evidence that HHS and FTC are two different phenotypic manifestations of the same disorder. The different phenotypic manifestations in these disorders are thought to result from GALNT3 mutations expressed in different environments or genetic backgrounds.

4.3. Chronic Kidney Disease

The ability of the kidneys to control Pi becomes impaired at glomerular filtration rates of approximately 50–60 mL/min. As the glomerular filtration continues to fall a number of changes occur that affect phosphorus balance, the most important being a decrease in calcitriol level due to deficient 1α-hydroxylation with consequent lower intestinal calcium absorption, hypocalcemia, and stimulation of PTH production. There is also a decrease in the filtered amount of phosphorus with resultant hyperphosphatemia, hypocalcemia, and again stimulation of PTH production. The maintenance of normal levels of Pi when the GRF is between 50 and 30 mL/min has been thought to occur at the expense of continued increase in PTH secretion. FGF-23 production, though, is increased as well. Moreover, the increase in FGF-23 levels correlate with the decline in glomerular filtration rate *(130–132)*. The elevated PTH levels will enhance urinary clearance of phosphorus by lowering proximal tubular reabsorption, thus returning plasma levels to normal, but at the expense of the development of secondary hyperparathyroidism (the classical trade-off hypothesis) and also the higher FGF-23 level, which in itself inhibits the 1α-hydroxylation of $25(OH)D_3$, resulting in further lowering of calcitriol levels and more stimulation of PTH production. Whether the elevated serum FGF-23 levels found in chronic kidney disease are sufficient to correct the hyperphosphatemia of early and advanced chronic kidney disease is not clear. The normal regulatory mechanisms are unable to compensate for phosphorus retention once the glomerular filtration rate falls below approximately 50–30 mL/min. At this point there is a subtle rise in serum phosphorus. Frank hyperphosphatemia becomes manifest once the patient's chronic kidney disease reaches the need for dialysis where the lack of significant kidney function combined with the inefficiency of the dialysis therapy in facilitating phosphorus clearance results in positive phosphate balance unless the amount of absorbed phosphorus is diminished through diet as well as the use of phosphate binders. The secondary hyperparathyroidism causes the development of osteitis fibrosa cystica, which presents radiographically as subperiosteal bone resorption. These lesions most commonly are seen in the middle phalanges of the hands, distal ends of the clavicles, and proximal ends of the tibia. The role of FGF-23 in osteitis fibrosa cystica has not been established. As renal failure advances hyperphosphatemia assumes a major role in the aggravation of secondary hyperparathyroidism. The serum levels of $1,25(OH)_2D_3$ decrease and the intestinal absorption of calcium is low. In many of these patients with advanced renal failure, the hyperplastic parathyroid glands begin not to respond to physiologic regulation and become refractory to treatment. The parathyroid glands may become "autonomous," which may require surgical removal of excessive parathyroid tissue.

Treatment: Strategies to lower plasma phosphorus in chronic kidney disease include dietary phosphate (dietary protein) restriction and the use of medications (phosphate binders) that inhibit intestinal absorption of phosphorus. These agents form poorly soluble complexes with phosphorus in the intestinal lumen. They are most effective when administered concomitantly with meals. Medications that inhibit the absorption of phosphorus include calcium, magnesium, iron and lanthanum salts, and sevelamer hydrochloride. Long-term use of aluminum-based binders have been associated with dementia, refractory anemia, and osteomalacia. If they are used, the duration of therapy should be limited to 2–3 months. The concomitant use of citrate compounds should be avoided as citrate enhances the intestinal absorption of aluminum. Soft tissue and vascular calcification has been found to be associated with a higher serum calcium level and higher calcium intake. The concurrent administration of vitamin D sterols further increases this risk. This has limited the use of calcium-containing binders to 1500–2000 mg/day from both dietary and medication sources *(133)*.

4.4. Case Scenario 1

A 14-month-old male infant presents to his primary care physician's office with failure to thrive. The mother was noted to have short stature. On physical exam of the infant bowing of the lower extremities was noted. Length was 68 cm (<5th percentile for age). Weight was 9.0 kg (12th percentile for age). Initially, a chemistry panel was obtained which was significant for a serum potassium of 4.0 mmol/L, total CO_2 of 24 mmol/L, serum calcium of 9.5 mg/dL, serum phosphorus of 2.6 mg/dL, and alkaline phosphatase of 806 IU/L. Because of the low serum phosphorus and elevated alkaline phosphatase his PCP was prompted to send additional laboratory studies including a PTH, spot urine for phosphate, spot urine for calcium, 25-hydroxyvitamin D, and 1,25-dihydroxyvitamin D. The PTH level was 80 pg/mL (normal range 12–88 pg/mL), 1,25-dihydroxyvitamin D 60 pg/mL (normal range 27–71 pg/mL), and 25-hydroxyvitamin D 26 ng/mL (normal range 13–67 ng/mL). The total reabsorption of phosphate was 45.5% (normal ~80–97%) and the urine calcium creatinine ratio 0.5 (normal range for age <0.6). An x-ray of the long bones confirmed rachitic changes

Autosomal recessive hypophosphatemic rickets (ARHR), X-linked hypophosphatemic rickets (XLH), autosomal dominant hypophosphatemic rickets (ADHR), hereditary hypophosphatemic rickets with hypercalciuria (HHRH), and tumor-induced osteomalacia (TIO) share many of the biochemical features noted in Table 4. In this patient the normal PTH level and absence of hypercalciuria excludes a diagnosis of HHRH. The family history excludes ARHR as this condition is autosomal recessive. The laboratory findings, though, do not distinguish between XLH, ADHR, and TIO. FGF-23 is the circulating phosphaturic factor in XLH, ADHR, and TIO. In XLH the circulating level of FGF-23 is thought to be determined by the rate of its proteolytic cleavage by PHEX protease, while in ADHR there appears to be a gain in function mutation in FGF-23 and in TIO an overproduction of FGF-23. As TIO is an acquired form of hypophosphatemic rickets caused by a variety of benign mesenchymal tumors that secrete FGF-23, this diagnosis seems quite unlikely in this scenario. FGF-23 levels do not help in distinguishing between XLH and ADHR even if they were available. Further family history will help distinguish between the two. As it stands there is insufficient history above, as XLH is an X-linked dominant condition. Sequence analysis for the entire coding region for both of these conditions, though, is available since mutations in these conditions have been identified and will differentiate between the two when the family history is not sufficient to do so.

The treatment for both involves a combination of oral phosphorus and $1,25(OH)_2D_3$. The daily need for phosphorus supplementation is 1–3 g of elemental phosphorus divided into four to five doses. Frequent dosing helps maintain the serum phosphorus level throughout the day, but also decreases the incidence of diarrhea. Calcitriol is administered at a dose of 30–70 ng/kg/day divided into two doses. Complications of treatment occur when there is not an adequate balance between phosphorus supplementation and calcitriol. Phosphorus excess, by decreasing enteral calcium absorption, may lead to secondary hyperparathyroidism and a worsening of the bone disease. Excess calcitriol leads to hypercalciuria and nephrocalcinosis and may even result in hypercalcemia. Laboratory monitoring as well as periodic renal ultrasounds to check for nephrocalcinosis of treatment is essential. Normalization of alkaline phosphatase is a more useful way to monitor therapeutic response than serum phosphorus. For children with significant short stature, growth hormone is an effective treatment option.

4.5. Case Scenario 2

A 17-7/12-year-old young lady presents with blurry vision. She was taken to an ophthalmologist and retina specialist who found her to have cotton wool exudates and ischemia of the retina. Her physical examination otherwise was unremarkable with the exception of her blood pressure, which was 177/121 mmHg. She was admitted to the hospital for management of the blood pressure and further evaluation. Blood pressure was brought under control with Procardia and Atenolol.

Her laboratory evaluation revealed the following: serum Na 139 mmol/L, K 3.8 mmol/L, chloride 109 mmol/L, CO_2 19 mmol/L, glucose 102 mg/dL, BUN 61 mg/dL, creatinine 4.9 mg/dL, total protein 6.2 g/dL, albumin 3.7 g/dL, calcium 8.4 mg/dL, and phosphorus 5.7 mg/dL. Spot urine: protein 53, creatinine 27. UAs were 30–100 mg/dL for protein. Based on her serum creatinine the estimated creatinine clearance was 18 mL/min/1.73 m^2. By renal US the kidneys were small (<5th percentile for age). A PTH was subsequently obtained that was 275 pg/mL (normal range 12–88 pg/mL).

The fact that the kidneys are small for age indicates that this patient has chronic kidney disease. Her kidney disease appears to be far advanced in view of the low creatinine clearance. As would be anticipated normal renal regulatory mechanisms are unable to compensate, and she has started to develop phosphorus retention. Phosphorus retention and hyperphosphatemia develop in virtually all patients with advanced chronic kidney disease. In this aged patient current recommendations are that the phosphorus be kept between 3.5 and 5.5 mg/dL. Hyperphosphatemia leads to secondary hypocalcemia as seen here by causing calcium precipitation, by decreasing the production of $1,25(OH)_2D_3$, and by decreasing intestinal calcium absorption. The hypocalcemia has resulted in the development of secondary hyperparathyroidism. The calcium phosphorus product in this patient is 48, fortunately, making the risk for ectopic calcifications low.

Treatment of the hyperphosphatemia in this case involves a reduction in dietary protein and introduction of phosphate binders. Calcium carbonate and calcium acetate are both used widely for this purpose. Sevelamer is a synthetic polymer that binds phosphorus within the lumen of the gastrointestinal tract and reduces its absorption as well. Small doses of calcitriol are useful for enhancing intestinal calcium absorption with correction of the hypocalcemia. Calcitriol therapy lowers plasma PTH levels in patients who already have biochemical evidence of secondary hyperparathyroidism. Calcium concentrations need to be measured regularly to avoid the complication of hypercalcemia.

REFERENCES

1. Forbes GB (1987) Body Composition. Springer, Berlin, Heidelberg, New York, pp. 170–182.
2. Hohenhauer L, Rosenberg TS, Oh W (1970) Calcium and phosphorus homeostasis on the first day of life. Biol Neonate, 15:49–56.
3. Nordin BCE (1976) Calcium, phosphate and magnesium metabolism. Churchill Livingstone, New York, p. 78.
4. Harris CA, Baer PG, Chirito E, Dirks JH (1974) Composition of mammalian glomerular filtrate. Am J Physiol, 227:972–976.
5. Markowitz M, Rotkin L, Rosen JF (1981) Circadian rhythms of blood minerals in humans. Science, 213:672–674.

6. Portale AA, Hallorhan BP, Morris RC Jr. (1987) Dietary intake of phosphorus modulates the circadian rhythm in serum concentrations of phosphorus: implications for the renal production of 1,25-dihydroxyvitamin D. 80:1147–1154.

7. Brodehl J, Gellissen K, Weber HP (1982) Postnatal development of tubular phosphate reabsorption. Clin Nephrol, 17:163–171.

8. Arnaud SB, Goldsmith RS, Stickler GB, et al. (1973) Serum parathyroid hormone and blood minerals; interrelationships in normal children. Pediatr Res, 7:485–493.

9. Greenberg BG, Winters RW, Graham JB (1960) The normal range of serum inorganic phosphorus and its utility as discriminant in the diagnosis of congenital hypophosphatemia. J Clin Endocrinol, 20:364–379.

10. Keating FR Jr, Jones JD, Elveback LR, et al. (1969) The relation of age and sex to distribution of values in healthy adults of serum calcium, inorganic phosphorus, magnesium, alkaline phosphatase, total proteins, albumin and blood urea. J Lab Clin Med, 73:825–834.

11. Mount DB, Yu ASL (2008) Transport of inorganic solutes: sodium, chloride, potassium, magnesium, calcium and phosphate. In: Brenner BM Levine SA (eds.) Brenner and Rector's The Kidney. Philadelphia. Saunders Elsevier, pp. 156–213.

12. Straum BB, Hamburger RJ, Goldberg M (1972) Tracer microinjection study of renal tubular phosphate reabsorption in the rat. J Clin Invest, 51:2271–2276.

13. Strickler JC, Thompson DD, Klose RM, Giebisch G (1964) Micropuncture study of inorganic phosphate excretion in the rat. J Clin Invest, 43:1596–1607.

14. Dennis VW, Woodhall PB, Robinson RR (1976) Characteristics of phosphate transport in isolated proximal tubule. Am J Physiol, 231:979–985.

15. Pastoriza-Munoz E, Colindres RE, Lassiter WE, Lechene C (1978) Effect of parathyroid hormone on phosphate reabsorption in rat distal convolution. Am J Physiol, 235:F321–F330.

16. Lang F, Greger R, Marchand GR, Knox FG (1977) Stationary microperfusion study of phosphate reabsorption in proximal and distal nephrons segments. Pflugers Arch, 368:45–48.

17. De Rouffignac C, Morel F, Moss N, Roinel N (1973) Micropuncture study of water and electrolyte movements along the loop of Henle in psammomys with special reference to magnesium, calcium and phosphorus. Pflugers Arch, 344:309–326.

18. Dennis VW, Bello-Reuss E, Robinson RR (1977) Response of phosphate transport to parathyroid hormone in segments of rabbit nephrons. Am J Physiol, 233:F29–F38.

19. Shareghi GA, Agus ZS (1982) Phosphate transport in the light segment of the rabbit cortical collecting duct. Am J Physiol, 242:F379–F384.

20. Peraino RA, Suki WN (1980) Phosphate transport by isolated rabbit cortical collecting tubule. Am J Physiol, 238:F358–F362.

21. Murer H, Hernando N, Biber J (2000) Proximal tubular phosphate reabsorption: molecular mechanisms. Physiol Rev, 80: 1373–1409.

22. Murer H, Forster I, Biber J (2004) The sodium-phosphate cotransporters family SLC34. Pflugers Arch, 447:763–767.

23. Collins JF, Bai I, Ghishan FK (2004) The SLC20 family of proteins: dual functions as sodium phosphate cotransporters and viral receptors. Pfleugers Arch, 447:647–652.

24. Yabuuchi H, Tamai I, Morita K, Kouda T, Miyamoto K, Takeda E, Tsuji A (1998) Hepatic sinusoidal membrane transport of anionic drugs mediated by anion transporter Npt1. J Pharmacol Exp, 286:1391–1396.

25. Jutabha P, Kanai Y, Hosoyamada M, Chairoungdua A, Kim DK, Iribe Y, Babu E, Kim JY, Anzai N, Chatsudthipong V, Endou H (2003) Identification of a novel voltage-driven organic anion transporter present at apical membrane of renal proximal tubule. J Biol Chem, 278:27930–27938.

26. Custer M, Lotscher M, Biber J, Murer H, Kaissling B (1994) Expression of Na–Pi cotransport in rat kidney: localization by RT-PCR and immunochemistry. Am J Physiol, 266:F767–F774.

27. Segawa H, Kaneko I, Takahashi A, Kuwahata M, Ito M, Ohkidol, Tatsumi S, Miyamoto K (2002) Growth-related renal type II Na/Pi cotransporters. J Biol Chem, 277:19665–19672.

28. Hilfiker H, Hattenhauer O, Traebert M, Forster I, Murer H, Biber J (1998) Characterization of a murine type II sodium-phosphate cotransporters expressed in mammalian intestine. Proc Natl Acad Sci USA, 95:14564–14569.

29. Hattenhauer O, Traebert M, Murer H, Biber J (1999) Regulation of small intestinal Na–P(i) type IIb cotransporters by dietary phosphate intake. Am J Physiol Gastrointest Liver Physiol, 277: G756–G762.

30. Xu H, Bau I, Collins JF, Ghishan FK (2002) Age dependent regulation of rat intestinal type IIb sodium phosphate cotransporters by 1,25(OH)$_2$ vitamin D$_3$. Am J Physiol Cell Physiol, 282:C487–C493.

31. Katai K, Miyamoto K, Kishida S, Segawa H, Nii T, Tanaka H, Tanai Y, Arai H, Tatsumi S, Morita K, Taketani Y, Takeda E (1999) Regulation of intestinal Na$^+$-dependent phosphate cotransporters by a low-phosphate diet and 1,25-dihydroxyvitamin D$_3$. Biochem J, 343 (Pt3): 705–712.

32. Levine BS, Ho LD, Pasiecznik K, et al. (1986) Renal adaptation to phosphorus deprivation; characteristics of early events. J Bone Minerl Res, 1: 33–40.

33. Haas JA, Berndt T, Knox FG (1978) Nephron heterogeneity of phosphate reabsorption. Am J Physiol, 234:F287–F290.

34. Taketani Y, Segawa H, Chikamori M, et al. (1998) Regulation of type II renal Na$^+$-dependent inorganic phosphate transporters by 1,25-dihydroxyvitamin D$_3$- identification of a vitamin D- responsive element in the human NAPI-3 gene. J Biol Chem, 273: 14575–14581.

35. Hammerman MR, Karl IE, Hruska KA (1980) Regulation of canine renal vesicle Pi transport by growth hormone and parathyroid hormone. Biochem Biophys Acta, 603: 322–355.

36. Mulroney SE, Lumpkin MD, Haramati A (1989) Antagonist to GH-releasing factor inhibits growth and renal Pi reabsorption in immature rats. Am J Physiol, 257:F29–F34.

37. Woda CB, Halaihel N, Wilson PV, Haramati A, Levi M, Mulroney SE (2004) Regulation of renal NaPi-2 expression and tubular phosphate reabsorption by growth hormone in the juvenile rat. Am J Physiol Renal Physiol, 287:F117–F123.

38. Cai Q, Hodgson SF, Kao PC, Lennon VA, Klee GG, et al. (1994) Brief report: inhibition of renal phosphate transport by a tumor product in a patient with oncogenic osteomalacia. N Engl J Med, 330:1645–1649.

39. Berndt TJ, Schiavi S, Kumar R (2005) "Phosphatonins" and the regulation of phosphorus homeostasis. Am J Physiol Renal Physiol, 289:F1170–F1182.

40. ADHR Consortium (2000) Autosomal dominant hypophosphatemic rickets is associated with mutations in FGF23. Nat Genet, 26:345–348.

41. Rowe PS, de Zoysa PA, Dong R, Wang HR, White KE, et al. (2000) MEPE, a new gene expressed in bone marrow and tumors causing osteomalacia. Genomics, 67:54–68.

42. Rowe PS, Kumagai Y, Gutierrez G, Garrett IR, Blacher R et al. (2004) MEPE has the properties of an osteoblastic phosphatonin and minhibin. Bone, 34:303–319.

43. Berndt T, Craig TA, Bowe AE, Vassiliadis J, Reczek D, et al. (2003) Secreted frizzled-related protein 4 is a potent tumor-derived phosphaturic agent. J Clin Invest, 112:785–794.

44. De Beur SM, Finnegan RB, Vassiliadis J, Cook B, Barberio D, et al. (2002) Tumors associated with oncogenic osteomalacia express gene important in bone and mineral metabolism. J Bone Miner Res, 17:1102–1110.

45. Carpenter TO, Ellis BK, Insogna KI, Philbrick WM, Sterpka J, Shimkets R (2005) FGF7: an inhibitor of phosphate transport derived from oncogenic osteomalacia-causing tumors. J Clin Endocrinol Metab, 90: 1012–1020.

46. Schiavi SC, Kumar R (2004) The phosphatonin pathway; new insights in phosphate homeostasis. Kidney Int, 65: 1–14.

47. Schiavi SC, Moe OW (2002) Phosphatonins: a new class of phosphate regulating proteins. Curr Opin Nephrol Hypertens, 11: 423–430.

48. Bowe AE, Finnegan R, de Beur SM, Cho J, Levine MA, Kumar R (2001) FGF-23 inhibits renal tubular phosphate transport and is a PHEX substrate. Biochem Biophys Res Commun, 284: 977–981.

49. Shimada T, Mizutani S, Muto T, Yoneya T, Hino R, Takeda S, Takeuchi Y, Fujita T, Fukumoto S, Yamashita T (2001) Cloning and characterization of FGF-23 as a causative factor of tumor-induced osteomalacia. Proc Natl Acad Sci USA, 98:6500–6505.

50. Perwad F, Azam N, Zhang MY, Yamashita T, Tenenhouse HS, Portale AA (2005) Dietary and serum phosphorus regulate fibroblast growth factor 23 expression and 1,25-dihydroxyvitamin D metabolism in mice. Endocrinology, 146:5358–5364.

51. Saito H, Maeda A, Ohtomo S, Hirata M, Kusano K, et al. (2005) Circulating FGF-23 is regulated by 1α,25-dihydoxyvitamin D₃ and phosphorus in vivo. J Biol Chem, 280:2543–2549.

52. Kurosu H, Ogawa Y, Miyoshi M, Yamamoto M, Nandi A, Rosenblatt KP, Baum M, Schiavi S, Hu MC, Moe OW, Kuro-o M (2006) Regulation of fibroblast growth factor-23 signaling by klotho. J Biol Chem, 281:6120–6123.

53. Urakawa I, Yamazaki Y, Shimada T, Iijima K, Hasegawa H, Okawa K, Fujita T, Fukumoto S, Yamashita T (2006) Klotho converts canonical FGF receptor into a specific receptor for FGF23. Nature, 444:770–774.

54. Shiraki-Iida T, Aizawa H, Matsumura Y, Sekine S, Iida A, Anazawa H, Nagai R, Kuro-o M, Nabeshima, Y (1998) Structure of the mouse klotho gene and its two transcripts encoding membrane and secreted protein. FEBS Lett, 424:6–10.

55. Kuro-o M, Matsumura Y, Aizawa H, Kawaguchi H, Suga T, Utsugi T, Obyama Y, Kurabayashi M, Kaname T, Kume E, Iwasaki H, Iida A, Shiraki-Iida T, Nishikawa S, Nagai R, Nabeshima YI (1997) Mutation of mouse klotho gene leads to syndrome resembling ageing. Nature, 390:45–51.

56. Kato Y, Arakawa E, Kinoshita S, Shirai A, Furuya A, Yamano K, Nakamura K, Iida A, Anazawa H, Koh N, Iwana A, Imura A, Fujimori T, Kur-o M, Hanai N, Takeshige K, Nabeshima Y, (2000) Establishment of anti-klotho monoclonal antibodies and detection of Klotho protein in kidneys. Bichem Biophy Res Commun, 267:597–602.

57. Torres PU, Prie D, Molina-Bletry V, Beck L, Silve C, Friedlander G (2007) Klotho: an antiaging protein involved in mineral and vitamin D metabolism. Kidney Int, 71:730–737.

58. Spitzer A, Barac-Nieto M (2001) Ontogeny of renal phosphate transport and the process of growth. Pediatr Nephrol, 16:763–771.

59. Russo JC, Nash MA (1980) Renal response to alterations in dietary phosphate in the young beagle. Biol Neonate, 38:1–10.

60. Caverzasio J, Bonjour J-P, Fleisch J (1982) Tubular handling of Pi in young, growing, and adult rates. Am J Physiol, 242:F705–F710.

61. Johnson V, Spitzer A (1986) Renal reabsorption of Pi during development: whole kidney events. Am J Physiol, 251:F251–F256.

62. Kaskel FJ, Kumar AM, Feld LG, Spitzer A (1988) Renal reabsorption of phosphate during development: tubular events. Pediatr Nephrol, 2:129–134.

63. Woda C, Mulroney SE, Halaihel N, Sun L, Wilson PV, Levi M, Haramati A (2001) Renal tubular sites of increased phosphate transport and NaPi-2 expression in the juvenile rat. Am J Physiol Regulatory Integrative Comp Physiol, 280:R1524–R1533.

64. Neiberger RE, Barac-Nieto M Spitzer A (1989) Renal reabsorption of phosphate during development: transport kinetics in BBMV. Am J Physiol, 257:F268–F274.

65. Bonjour JP, Fleish H (1980) Tubular adaptation to the supply and requirement of phosphate. In: Massry SG, Fleisch H (eds.) Renal Handling of Phosphate. Plenum Press, New York, pp. 243–264.

66. Barac-Nieto M, Dowd TL, Gupta RK, Spitzer A (1991) Changes in NMR visible kidney cell phosphate with age and diet: relationship to phosphate transport. Am J Physiol, 261: F153–F162.

67. Segawa H, Kaneko I, Takahasgi A, Kuwahata M, Ito M, Ohkido I, Tatsumi S, Miyamoto K (2002) Growth-related renal type II Na/Pᵢ Cotransporter. J Biol Chem, 277:19665–19672.

68. Ohkido I, Segawa H, Yanagida R, Nakamura M, Miyamoto K (2003) Cloning, gene structure and dietary regulation of the type-IIc Na Pi cotransporters in the mouse kidney. Pflugers Archiv, 446: 106–115.

69. Silverstein DM, Barac-Nieto M, Murer H, Spitzer A (1997) A putative growth-related renal Na⁺–Pi cotransporters. Am J Physiol Regul Integr Comp Physiol, 273:R928–R933.

70. Linarelli LG (1972) Nephron urinary cyclic AMP levels and developmental renal responsiveness to parathyroid hormone. Pediatrics, 50:14–32.

71. Woda C, Mulroney SE, Levi M, Halaihel N, Haramati A (1999) Nephron sites of phosphate (Pi) reabsorption in the juvenile rat (Abstract). J Am Soc Nephrol, 10:614A–615A.

72. Moe SM, Sprague SM (2008) Mineral bone disorders in chronic kidney disease. In: Brenner BM Levine SA (eds.) Brenner and Rector's The Kidney. Saunders, Elsevier, Philadelphia, pp. 1784–1813.

73. Bijvoet OLM (1969) Relation of plasma phosphate concentration to renal tubular reabsorption of phosphate. Clin Sci, 37:23–36.
74. Walton RJ, Bijvoet OLM (1975) Nomogram for the derivation of renal tubular threshold phosphate concentration. Lancet, 2:309–310.
75. McCrory WW, Forman CW, McNamara H, Barnett HL (1952) Renal excretion of inorganic phosphate in newborn infants. J Clin Invest, 31:357–366.
76. Arant BS (1978) Developmental patterns of renal functional maturation compared in the human neonate. J Pediatr, 92:705–712.
77. Brodehl J, Krause A, Hoyer PF (1988) Assessment of maximal tubular phosphate reabsorption: comparison of direst measurement with the nomogram of Bijvoet. Pediatr Nephrol, 2: 183–189.
78. Stark H, Eisenstein B, Tieder M, Rachmel A, Alpert, G. (1986) Direct measurement of TP/GFR: a simple and reliable parameter of renal phosphate handling. Nephron, 44:125–128.
79. Gupta A, Tenenhouse HS, Hoag HM, Wang D, Khadeer MA, Namba N, Feng X, Hruska KA (2001) Identification of the type II Na$^+$–Pi cotransporters (Npt2) in the osteoclast and the skeletal phenotype of Npt2$^{-/-}$. Bone, 29:467–476.
80. Shimada T, Mizutani S, Muto T, Yoneya T, Hino R, et al. (2001) Cloning and characterization of FGF23 as a causative factor of tumor-induced osteomalacia. Proc Natl Acad Sci USA, 98: 6500–6505.
81. Hesse E, Moessinger E, Rosenthal H, et al. (2007) Oncogenic osteomalacia: exact tumor localization by co-registration of position emission and computed tomography. J Bone Miner Res, 22:158–162.
82. Geller JL, Khosravi A, Kelly MH, Riminucci M, Adams JS, Collins MT (2007) Cinacalcet in the management of tumor-induced osteomalacia. J Bone Miner Res, 22:931–937.
83. Econs M, McEnery P (1997) Autosomal dominant hypophosphatemic rickets/osteomalacia: clinical characterization of a novel renal phosphate wasting disorder. J Clin Endocrinol Metab, 82:674–681.
84. Econs M, McEnery P, Lennon F, Speer M (1997) Autosomal dominant hypophosphatemic rickets is linked to chromosome 12p13. J Clin Invest, 100: 2653–2657.
85. Imel EA, Hui SL, Econs MJ (2007) FGF23 concentrations vary with disease status in autosomal dominant hypophosphatemic rickets. J Bone Mineral Res, 22:520–526.
86. ADHR Consortium T, White KE, Evans WE, O'Riordan JLH, Speer MC, Econs MJ, et al. (2000) Autosomal dominant hypophosphatemic rickets is associated with mutations in FGF23. Nat Genet, 26:345–348.
87. Kruse K, Woelfel D, Strom T (2001) Loss of renal phosphate wasting in a child with autosomal dominant hypophosphatemic rickets caused by a FGF23 mutation. Horm Res, 55:305–308.
88. White KE, Carn G, Lorenz-Depieteux B, Benet-Pages A, Strom TM, Econs MJ (2001) Autosomal-dominant hypophosphatemic rickets (ADHR) mutations stabilize FGF-23. Kidney Int, 60: 2079–2086.
89. Imel EA, Econs MJ (2005) Fibroblast growth factor 23: roles in health and disease. J Am Soc Nephrol, 16:2565–2575.
90. Meyer RA Jr, Meyer MH, Gray RW (1989) Parabiosis suggests a humoral factor is involved in X-linked hypophosphatemia in mice. J Bone Miner Res, 4:493–500.
91. Meyer RA Jr, Tenenhouse HS, Meyer MH, Klugerman AH (1989) The renal phosphate transport defect in normal mice parabiosed to X-linked hypophosphatemic mice persists after parathyroidectomy. J Bone Miner Res, 4:523–532.
92. Nesbitt T, Coffman TM, Griffiths R, Drezner MK (1992) Cross-transplantation of kidneys in normal and Hyp mice. Evidence that the Hyp mouse phenotype is unrelated to an intrinsic renal defect. J Clin Invest, 89:1453–1459.
93. Tenenhouse HS, Martel J, Gauthier C, Segawa H, Miyamoto K (2003) Differential effects of *Npt2a* gene ablation and the X-linked *Hyp* mouse mutation on renal expression of type IIc Na/Pi cotransporters. Am J Physiol, 285:F1271–F1278.
94. Jonsson K, Zahradnik R, Larsson T, White K, Sugimoto T, Imanishi Y, et al. (2003) Fibroblast growth factor 23 in oncogenic osteomalacia and X-linked hypophosphatemia. N Engl J Med, 348: 1656–1662.
95. Weber T, Liu S, Indridason O, Quarles L (2003) Serum FGF23 levels in normal and disordered phosphorus homeostasis. J Bone Miner Res, 18:1227–1234.

96. Liu S, Brown T, Zhou J, Xiao Z, Awad H, Guilak F, et al. (2005) Role of matrix extracellular phosphoglycoprotein in the pathogenesis of X-linked hypophosphatemia. J Am Soc Nephrol, 16: 91645–91653.

97. Sitara D, Razzaque MS, Hesse M, Yoganathan S, Taguchi T, Erben RG, et al. (2004) Homozygous ablation of fibroblast growth factor-23 results in hypophosphatemia and impaired skeletogenesis and reverses hypophosphatemia in Phex-deficient mice. Matrix Biol, 23:421–432.

98. Liu S, Zhou J, Tang W, Jiang X, Rowe DW, Quarles LD, (2006) Pathogenic role of Fgf23 in Hyp mice. Am J Physiol Endocrinol Metab, 291:E38–E49.

99. Aono Y, Shimada T, Yamazaki Y, Hino R, Takeuchi M, Fujita T, et al. (2003) The neutralization of FGF-23 ameliorates hypophosphatemia and rickets in Hyp mice. Meeting of the American Society for Bone and Mineral research. Minneapolis, Minnesota, p. 1056.

100. Benet-Pages A, Lorenz-Depiereux B, Zischka H, White K Econs M, Strom T (2004) FGF23 is processed by proprotein convertases but not by PHEX. Bone, 35:455–462.

101. Lorenz-Depiereux B, Bastepe M, Benet-Pages A, Amyere M, Wagenstaller J, Muller-Barth U, Badenhoop K, Kaiser SM, Rittmaster RS, Shlossberg AH, Oliveras JL, Loris C, Ramos FJ, Glorieux F, Vikkula M, Juppner H, Strom TM (2006) DMP1 mutations in autosomal recessive hypophosphatemia implicate a bone matrix protein in the regulation of phosphate homeostasis. Nat Genet, 38: 1248–1250.

102. Feng JQ, Ward LM, Liu S, Lu Y Xie Y, Yuan B, Yu X, Rauch F, Davis SI, Zhang S, Rios H, Drezner MK, Quarles LD, Bonewald LF, White KE (2006) Loss of DMP1 causes rickets and osteomalacia and identifies a role for osteocytes in mineral metabolism. Nat Genet, 38:1310–1315.

103. Borzani M, Mauri I, Roggero P, Auriti I Facchini R (1983) Non-rachitic hypophosphatemic osteopathy. Pediatr Med Chir, 5:99–102.

104. Scriver CR, MacDonald W, Reade T, et al. (1977) Hypophosphatemic nonrachitic bone disease; an entity distinct from X-linked hypophosphatemia in the renal defect, bone involvement, and inheritance. Am J Med Genet, 1:101–117.

105. Scriver CR, Reade T, Halal F, et al. (1981) Autosomal hypophosphatemic bone disease responds to 1,25(OH)2D3. Arch Dis Child, 56:203–207.

106. Frymoyer JW, Hodgkin W (1977) Adult-onset vitamin D-resistant hypophosphatemic osteomalacia. J Bone Joint Surg, 59: 101–106.

107. Hoffman W, Juppner H, Deyung B, O'dorisio M, Given K (2005) Elevated fibroblast growth factor-23 in hypophosphatemic linear nevus sebaceous syndrome. Am J Genet, 134: 233–236.

108. Heike C, Cunningham M, Steiner R, Wenkert D, Hornung R, Gruss J, et al. (2005) Skeletal changes in epidermal nevus syndrome: does focal bone disease harbor clues concerning pathogenesis? Am J Med Genet, 139:67–77.

109. Hoshino C, Satoh, N, Sugawara S, Kurivama C, Kikuchi A, Ohta M (2008) Sporadic adult-onset hypophosphatemic osteomalacia caused by excessive action of fibroblast growth factor 23. Intern Med, 47:453–457.

110. Cockerill FJ, Hawa NS, Yousaf N, et al. (1997) Mutations in the vitamin D receptor gene in three kindreds associated with hereditary vitamin D resistant rickets. J Clin Endocrinol Metab, 82: 3156–3160.

111. Malloy, PJ, Hochberg Z, Tiosano D, et al. (1990) The molecular basis of hereditary $1,25(OH)_2$ vitamin D_3 resistant rickets in seven families. J Clin Invest, 86:2071–2079.

112. Griffin E, Zerwekh JE (1983) Impaired stimulation of 25(OH) vitamin D-24-hydroxylase in fibroblasts from a patient with vitamin D-dependent rickets type II: form of receptor positive resistance of 1,25-dihydroxyvitamin D_3. J Clin Invest, 72:1190–1199.

113. Haussler MR, Haussler CA, Jurutka PWL (1997) The vitamin D hormone and its nuclear receptor, molecular action and disease states. J Endocrinol, 154 Suppl:557–573.

114. Silver J, Popovtzer MM (1984) Hypercalcemia with elevated dihydroxycholecalciferol levels and hypercalciuria. Arch Intern Med, 144:162–163.

115. Beighton P, Cremin BJ, Kozlowski K (1980) Osteoglophonic dwarfism. Pediatr Radiol, 10:46–50.

116. Beighton P (1989) Osteoglophonic dysplasia. J med Genet, 26:572–576.

117. White K, Cabral J, Evans W, Ichikawa S, Davis S, Ornitz D, et al. (2003) A missense mutation in FGFR1 causes a novel syndrome: craniofacial dysplasia with hypophosphatemia (CFDH). J Bone Miner Res, 18 Suppl 2:S4.

118. Farrow E, Davis S, Mooney S, Beighton P, Mascarenhas L, Gutierrez Y, et al. (2006) Extended mutational analysis of FGFR1 in osteoglophonic dysplasia. Am J Med Genet, 140:537–539.

119. Roberts TS, Stephen L Beighton P (2006) Osteoglophonic dysplasia; dental and orthodontic implications. Orthod Craniofac Res, 9:153–156.

120. Topaz O, Shurman DL, Bergman R, Indelman M, Ratajczak P, Mizrachi M, Khamaysi Z, Behar D, Petronius D, Friedman V, Zelikovic I, Raimer S, Metzker A, Richard G, Sprecher E (2004) Mutations in GALNT3, encoding a protein involved in o-linked glycosylation, cause of familial tumoral calcinosis. Nat Genet, 36:579–581.

121. Ichikawa S, Lyles K, Econs M (2005) A novel GALNT3 mutations in a pseudoautosomal dominant form of tumoral calcinosis: evidence that the disorder is autosomal recessive. J Clin Endocrinol Metab, 90:2420–2423.

122. Berndt TJ, Craig TA, McCormick DJ, Lanske B, Sitara D, Razzaque MS, Pragnell M, Bowe AE, O'Brien SP, Schiavi SC, Kumar R (2007) Biological activity of FGF-23 fragments. Pflugers Arch, 454:615–623.

123. Araya K, Fukomoto S, Backenroth R, Takeuchi Y, Nakayama K, Ito N, Yoshii N, Yamazaki Y, Yamashita T, Silver J, Igarashi T, Fujita T (2005) A novel mutation in fibroblast growth factor (FGF)23 gene as a cause of tumoral calcinosis. J Endocrinol Metab, 90:5523–5527.

124. Larsson T, Davis SI, Garringer HJ, Mooney SD, Dramann MS, Cullen MJ, White KE (2005) Fibroblast growth factor-23 mutants causing familial tumoral calcinosis are differently processed. Endocrinology, 146:3883–3891.

125. Ichikawa S, Imel EA, Kreiter ML, Yu X, Mackenzie DS, Sorenson AH, Goetz R, Mohammadi M, White KE, Econs MJ (2007) A homozygous missence mutation in human KLOTHO causes severe tumoral calcinosis. J Clin Invest, 117:2684–2691.

126. Garringer HJ, Fisher C, Larsson TE, et al. (2006) The role of mutant UDP-*N*-acetyl-alpha-D-galactosamine-polypeptide *N*-acetylgalactosaminyltransferase 3 in regulating serum intact fibroblast growth factor 23 and matrix extracellular phosphoglycoprotein in heritable tumoral calcinosis. J Clin Endocrinol Metab, 91:4037–4042.

127. Narchi H (1997) Hyperostosis with hyperphosphatemia: evidence of familial occurrence and association of tumoral calcinosis. Pediatrics, 99:745–748.

128. Clarke E, Swischuk LE, Hayden CK Jr (1984) Tumoral calcinosis, diaphysitis and hyperphosphatemia. Radiology, 151:643–646.

129. Wilson MP, Lindsley CB, Warady BA, Johnson JA (1989) Hyperphosphatemia associated with cortical hyperostosis and tumoral calcinosis. J Pediatr, 114:1010–1013.

130. Pande S, Ritter CS, Rothstein M, Wiesen K, Vassiliadis J, Kumar R, Schiavi SC, Slatapolskt E, Brown AJ (2006) FGF-23 and sFRP-4 in chronic kidney disease and post-renal transplantation. Nephron Physiol, 104:23–32.

131. Imanishi Y, Inaba M, Nakatsuka, Nagasue K, Okuno S, Yoshihara A, Miura M, Miyauchi A, Kobayashi K, Miki T, Shoji T, Ishimura E, Nishizawa Y (2004) FGF-23 in patients with end-stage renal disease on hemodialysis. Kidney Int, 65:1943–1946.

132. Larsson T, Nisbeth U, Ljunggren O, Juppner H, Jonsson KB (2003) Circulating concentration of FGF-23 increases as renal function declines in patients with chronic kidney disease, but does not change in response to variation in phosphate intake in healthy volunteers. Kidney Int, 64: 2272–2279.

133. Block GA, Port FK (2000) Re-evaluation of risks associated with hyperphosphatemia and hyperparathyroidism in dialysis patients: recommendations for a change in management. Am J Kidney Dis, 35:1226–1237.

134. Wagner CA (2007) Novel insights into the regulation of systemic phosphate homeostasis and renal phosphate excretion. J Nephrol, 20:130–134.

135. Fukumoto S (2008) Physiological regulation and disorders of phosphate metabolism-pivotal role of fibroblast growth factor 23. Inter Med, 47:337–343.

136. Bonnardeaux A, Bichet DG (2008) Inherited disorders of the renal tubule. In: Brenner BM LevineSA (eds.) Brenner and Rector's The Kidney. Saunders Elsevier. Philadelphia, pp. 1390–1427.

III DISORDERS OF ACID–BASE HOMEOSTASIS

7 Acid–Base Physiology

Shefali Mahesh and Victor L. Schuster

Key Points

1. How acid is buffered by blood and cells?
2. How filtered bicarbonate is reclaimed by the proximal tubule?
3. How the daily acid load is excreted?
4. How new bicarbonate is regenerated after metabolic acidosis?
5. How various factors modulate tubular acid–base handling?

Key Words: Henderson–Hasselbalch equation; extracellular buffers; intracellular buffers; bone buffers; acid–base homeostasis; acidification

1. INTRODUCTION

Acids and alkali are ingested as part of the diet. The metabolism of carbohydrates and fats generates approximately 15,000 mmol of CO_2 per day. Under normal circumstances, the lungs are able to effectively eliminate this large quantity of CO_2 so as not to affect the acid–base balance of the body. Cellular metabolism produces substances that have an impact on total body H^+ and pH. Yet, the pH, CO_2, and H^+ concentration are maintained within narrow limits. The normal extracellular H^+ ion concentration is approximately 40 nmol/L, which is roughly one millionth the millimole per liter concentrations of Na^+, K^+, Cl, and HCO_3^-. It is important to maintain this low level of H^+ ion concentration because all cellular functions are very sensitive to pH.

2. HENDERSON–HASSELBALCH EQUATION

Traditionally the Henderson–Hasselbalch equation has been used to describe the acid–base balance of the blood. In order to do this, we must define acid and base.

Acid is a substance that can donate a proton

$$HA \leftrightarrow H^+ + A^-$$

From: *Nutrition and Health: Fluid and Electrolytes in Pediatrics*
Edited by: L. G. Feld, F. J. Kaskel, DOI 10.1007/978-1-60327-225-4_7,
© Humana Press, a part of Springer Science+Business Media, LLC 2010

Base is a substance that can accept a proton

$$B + H^+ \leftrightarrow BH^+$$

The general reaction is

$$H^+ + A^- \leftrightarrow HA \text{ where } pH = -\log[H^+]$$

The ionization/dissociation coefficient is

$$Ka \equiv \frac{[H^+][A^-]}{[HA]} \quad [H^+] = Ka\frac{[HA]}{[A^-]}$$

The *pH* of a solution can be defined as $pH = -\log[H^+]$. Similarly $pKa = -\log Ka$

The pH varies inversely with the H^+ concentration. The range of H^+ concentrations that is compatible with life is 16–160 nmol/L (pH = 7.8–6.8)

Taking minus logs

$$-\log[H^+] = -\log[Ka] - \frac{\log[HA]}{[A^-]}$$

$$pH = pKa + \log\frac{[A^-][base]}{[HA][acid]}$$

This is the Henderson–Hasselbalch equation.

3. BUFFER SYSTEMS

Buffering is an important defense mechanism in minimizing the impact of changes in the amount of acids or bases in solution on the hydrogen ion concentration. Buffers can be extracellular or intracellular.

Extracellular Buffers: HCO_3^- is the most important extracellular buffer. Other buffers are plasma phosphates and plasma proteins.

Intracellular Buffers: Proteins, organic, and inorganic phosphates and hemoglobin in the red blood cells are the intracellular buffers.

Bone Buffers: Acid loads can result in uptake of excess H^+ by the bone, in exchange for surface Na^+ and K^+ and dissolution of bone minerals, releasing $Na\,HCO_3$, $K\,HCO_3$, $CaCO_3$, and $CaHPO_4$ into extracellular fluid. Bone buffering plays a particularly important role in chronic acid retention as seen in chronic kidney disease.

The contribution of any buffer to maintain the body pH depends on two factors; firstly, the quantity of buffer available, the higher the concentration, the better the buffering capacity. Secondly, how close the pK of the buffer is to the body fluid pH. A buffer is most efficient when the pH of the solution is within ±1.0 pH unit of its pKa. Example, HPO_4^{2-} is an important urinary buffer due to its high urinary excretion and pKa of 6.8. Creatinine (pKa = 4.97) and uric acid (pKa = 5.75) are comparatively weaker urinary buffers.

The time course of buffering an acid load varies with each system. The plasma HCO_3^- system buffers immediately, in seconds to minutes. Respiratory compensation takes minutes to hours to lower the pCO_2. Intracellular and bone buffering takes 2–4 h. Renal defense and generation of new HCO_3^- takes hours to days.

Strong acids completely dissociate in biological solutions releasing H^+ and the anion. Thus they have a high dissociation constant. Example NaOH or HCl.

Weak acids are those that do not completely dissociate in solution. They form good buffers since addition of strong acids and base results in less change in H ion concentration than would occur in pure water. They establish equilibrium between H^+ and the anion in biological solution. Weak acids form the principal buffers in the body. Example of a weak acid is H_2PO_4.

Volatile Acid: Acids with a potential to generate H^+ after hydration with H_2O; example CO_2.

Nonvolatile acid OR Fixed acids: Those not derived from the hydration of CO_2. Examples of nonvolatile acids are metabolism of dietary amino acids, organic anions, anaerobic metabolism and lactate, organic acids in diabetes mellitus.

The common acid–base buffer systems in the body include

Plasma	$H^+ + HCO_3^- \leftrightarrow H_2CO_3$	$pKa = 6.1$
Urine	$H^+ + NH_3 \leftrightarrow NH_4$	$pKa = 9.0$
Urine	$H^+ + HPO_4^{2-} \leftrightarrow H_2PO_4^-$	$pKa = 6.8$
Cell	$H^+ + Protein - \leftrightarrow Protein \bullet H$	$pKa = 7.0$

The bicarbonate system is the most important buffer in the plasma

$$H^+ + HCO_3^- \leftrightarrow H_2CO_3 \leftrightarrow CO_2 + H_2O \text{ "lumped" } pKa = 6.1$$

$$pH = pKa + \log\frac{[HCO_3^-]}{[H_2CO_3]}$$

Since the relationship between solubility of CO_2 and H_2CO_3 is known to be $[H_2CO_3] = 0.03 \times [pCO_2 \text{ in mmHg}]$, then

$$pH = 6.1 + \log\frac{[HCO_3^-]}{[0.03 \times pCO_2]}$$

The kidneys cannot excrete free acids; instead they excrete the salts of these acids. The PO_4 buffer system is important in urinary excretion of acid.

$$H^+ + HPO_4^{2-} \leftrightarrow H_2PO_4^- \text{ where } pKa = 6.8$$

At physiological pH

$$7.4 = 6.8 + \log\frac{HPO_4^{2-}}{H_2PO_4^-} \text{ So } \frac{HPO_4^{2-}}{H_2PO_4^-} = 4$$

Thus at physiological pH PO_4 tends to be in the proton acceptor form.

Although buffers are the first line of defense against changes in pH, they are present in limited quantities. Therefore, it is necessary to be able to eliminate the excess acid or base by the lungs or kidney and restore the buffer capacity.

4. ROLE OF THE RESPIRATORY SYSTEM

Respiratory rate is regulated by the pCO_2 and pH. Peripheral (carotid and aortic bodies) and central chemoreceptors (medulla) sense the change in pH and alter ventilatory rate. The medulla cannot sense changes in plasma H^+ concentration due to its impermeability to the blood–brain barrier. On the other hand CO_2 can cross the blood–brain barrier, get hydrated to H_2CO_3 and then dissociate to H^+ and HCO_3^-. Thus elevated plasma pCO_2 lowers CSF pH, which in turn stimulates the respiratory rate, decreases the plasma pCO_2, and returns the plasma and CSF pH to normal. Decreased plasma pCO_2 has the opposite effect on respiratory rate.

5. ACID–BASE HOMEOSATSIS BY THE KIDNEY

The kidney must excrete 50–100 mEq of non-carbonic/non-volatile acids generated per day. It uses three processes in the maintenance of acid–base homeostasis.

1) Reabsorption of all filtered HCO_3, mainly in the proximal tubule (high-capacity system): Normally all the filtered bicarbonate is reabsorbed. Eighty percent of filtered bicarbonate is reabsorbed by the proximal tubule, the thick ascending limb of loop of Henle reabsorbs another 10–15%, and distal tubule and collecting duct reabsorb the remaining 5–10%, so that no bicarbonate is left in the urine.

    Proximal tubular reabsorption of HCO_3^- requires a luminal carbonic anhydrase, which converts the filtered HCO_3^- and secreted H^+ to CO_2 and H_2O. CO_2 readily diffuses into the cell, is rehydrated with cytosolic carbonic anhydrase to generate HCO_3^- and H^+ HCO_3^- enters the blood stream on the basolateral side via an electrogenic Na/HCO_3^- co-transporter that couples the efflux of 1 Na^+ with 3 HCO_3^-. Additional Na is provided by the basolateral Na–K-ATPase pump. H^+ is secreted into urine via Na/H antiporter/exchanger and H^+ pumps (Fig. 1).

    Daily proximal tubule HCO_3^- reclamation ~180 L/d $\times$ 25 mEq/L = 4500 mEq/day
    This Na/H antiporter also mediates the HCO_3^- reabsorption that takes place in the thick ascending limb of the loop of Henle accounting for reclamation of 15% of the filtered HCO_3^- load.

2) Secretion of acid by the collecting duct: Low capacity, high gradient

    Daily acid load = $\sim$1 mEq/kg BW/day H^+ secretion occurs via the intercalated cell. In the intercalated cells $CO_2 + H_2O \rightarrow HCO_3^- + H$. H^+ is secreted into the tubular fluid by two mechanisms. The α-intercalated cells express H-ATPase on the luminal membrane, excreting protons into the urine. Secondly, H^+–K^+-ATPase couples the secretion of H^+ with reabsorption of K^+. The HCO_3^- is released into the blood stream by the basolateral Cl/HCO_3^- exchanger (Fig. 2).

    The collecting duct apical membrane is not readily permeable to H^+, thus the tubular fluid can be rendered quite acidic. The most acidic tubular fluid along the nephron is produced in the collecting duct, with a minimum pH of 5. This is in contrast to the

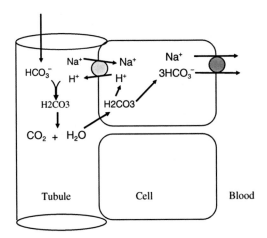

Fig. 1. Proximal tubule bicarbonate reclamation.

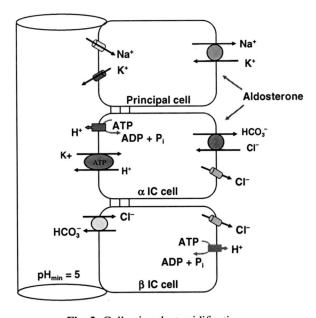

Fig. 2. Collecting duct acidification.

proximal tubule, which is leaky, and permits H^+ to cross into the blood stream. Thus the minimum obtainable pH at the end of the proximal tubule is 6.8.

3) Generation of new HCO_3^- and synthesis of titratable acids (Proton acceptors) like ammonia and phosphate to excrete protons:

The daily acid load adds H^+ to the system. The H^+ combines with HCO_3^- and forms CO_2 and H_2O. Thus new HCO_3^- is needed to handle this additional H^+ load. New HCO_3^- is formed by the secretion of H^+ that reacts with the non-bicarbonate buffers present in the glomerular filtrate.

5.1. Proton Acceptor #1: NH₃

In the proximal tubule, glutamine is metabolized to ammonium.

$$\text{Glutamine} \xrightarrow{\text{glutaminase}} 2NH_4^+ + \text{Glutamate} \rightarrow 2\,HCO_3^-$$

$$+ 2NH_4^+ \rightarrow NH_3 + CO_2 + H_2O$$

This requires extraction of glutamine from the blood across the basolateral membrane. The amino acid transporter responsible for the uptake of glutamine into the proximal tubule cells is up-regulated during metabolic acidosis (Fig. 3). The NH_3 thus formed can readily diffuse out of the cell across the basolateral or luminal membrane; on the other hand, NH_4^+ can only be secreted into the tubular lumen because the transporters are only present on the luminal membrane.

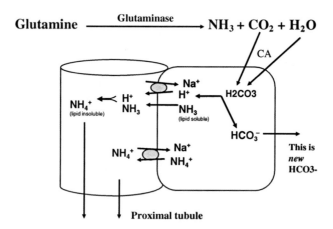

Fig. 3. Generation of new HCO_3^-.

Intracellular carbonic anhydrase in the proximal tubular cell hydrates CO_2 to form H_2CO_3, which then dissociates into H^+ and HCO_3^-. The NH_3 in the tubular cells combine with H^+ to form NH_4^+, which is secreted into the tubular lumen by the Na–H exchanger, which then acts like a Na–NH_4^+ exchanger. The newly formed HCO_3^- exits the cell at the basolateral membrane and enters the blood circulation. Thus H^+ in the form of NH_4^+ has been secreted and newly formed HCO_3^- has been reabsorbed and added to the system.

NH_4^+ undergoes counter-current multiplication. After NH_4^+ is secreted into the proximal tubule via the Na–H antiporter, the medullary thick ascending limb via the Na–K–2Cl symporter reabsorbs it, where it is converted into NH_3 and H^+. Here the H^+ is secreted into the lumen via the Na–H^+ exchanger and combines with HCO_3^- from the proximal tubule to enhance HCO_3^- reabsorption. NH_3 permeates through the basolateral membrane to accumulate in the medullary interstitium, finally to be secreted into the medullary collecting ducts. The collecting duct cells are not permeable to NH_4^+, but NH_3 can freely cross from the medullary interstitium to the tubular lumen. Here it binds the H^+ ions secreted by the intercalated cells to form NH_4^+.

$$H^+ + NH_3 \rightarrow NH_4^+$$

Since NH_4^+ cannot cross back into the collecting duct cells it gets "trapped" in the tubular lumen and excreted in the urine (Fig. 4).

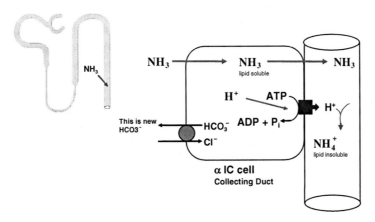

Fig. 4. Excretion of ammonium, generation of new HCO_3^-.

NH_4^+ excretion depends on H^+ secretion by the collecting duct. If H^+ is not secreted, the NH_4^+ reabsorbed by the thick ascending limb will not be excreted into the urine. It will enter the systemic circulation and be metabolized by the liver to produce urea and consume HCO_3^- in doing so. Thus, even though the metabolism of glutamine produces HCO_3^-, this new HCO_3^- is not added to the system unless NH_4^+ is excreted in the urine.

NH_4^+ excretion is regulated by the blood and urine pH. The more acidic the blood pH, the more NH_4^+ is produced in the proximal tubule from glutamine metabolism. Similarly, the more acidic urine pH increases the gradient for NH_3 secretion from the collecting duct cells into the medullary collecting duct lumen, resulting in formation of NH_4^+ and its excretion in urine. In states of chronic acidosis, the NH_4^+ excretion can be up-regulated to increase acid excretion. The reverse occurs in chronic alkalosis.

5.2. Proton Acceptor #: PO_4^-

Phosphate is another important urinary buffer, derived mainly from the diet. Therefore, it cannot be relied upon to generate enough new bicarbonate to handle the daily acid load. Also, its excretion is not controlled by the pH but by the phosphate balance of the body.

In the proximal tubule, $H_2CO_3^-$ formed from the hydration of CO_2 dissociates into HCO_3^- and H^+. H^+ is secreted into the tubular lumen and buffered by the HPO_4^{2-} to form $H_2PO_4^-$ (titratable acid). The HCO_3^- from the cell moves into the bloodstream adding new HCO_3^- to the system.

6. REGULATION OF ACID–BASE BALANCE

Under normal circumstances, the H^+ concentration is maintained relatively constant. The body maintains the acid–base balance of the body by maintaining the pH between 7.35 and 7.45, pCO_2 of 35–45 mmHg and HCO_3^- between 23 and 27 mEq/L. Acid–base disturbances occur when an acid load or alkali load causes the blood pH to fall out of this range. When the primary change is in the HCO_3^-, it results in a metabolic disorder; when the primary change is the pCO_2, it results in a respiratory disorder. When these disorders occur, the body has a series of defense mechanisms to protect itself against changes in the blood pH. It is important to note that these defense mechanisms do not correct the acid–base disturbance itself, but merely minimizes changes in the pH in order for cellular machinery to work at its optimum. The body does this by three important defense mechanisms:

1) Extracellular and Intracellular Buffering: Extracellular buffering is the first line of defense. HCO_3^- is the most important extracellular buffer that works almost instantaneously. A volatile acid load is counteracted by consumption of HCO_3^- in the buffering process. Other extracellular buffers like phosphates and plasma proteins provide additional buffering. Intracellular buffering does not occur as instantaneously since it involves the movement of H^+ into the cells with subsequent buffering by HCO_3^-, phosphates and proteins.
2) Respiratory Defense: This is the second line of defense to adjust pCO_2. A change in ventilatory rate regulates the pCO_2, which in turn alters the pH. Central and peripheral chemoreceptors are sensitive to changes in the pCO_2 and pH; when metabolic acidosis ensues, they sense the decreased pH and in turn increase the ventilatory rate to compensate. This compensation may take minutes to hours.
3) Renal Defense: This is third line of defense to adjust ECF HCO_3^-. Even though buffering may minimize changes in extracellular pH, the excess H^+ need to be excreted in order to prevent depletion of buffers and ultimate development of metabolic acidosis. Net acid excretion is inversely proportional to the acid load. When there is metabolic acidosis, the kidneys adjust proximal HCO_3^- reabsorption and distal acid secretion to compensate for the acid load. This usually takes several days to occur since the kidney has to upregulate enzymes in order to produce more NH_4 and add new HCO_3^- to the system.

Proximal and distal acidification is driven by the extracellular pH. In states of acid load, the proximal tubule enhances the activities of the Na–H exchanger and luminal H-ATPase, increases activity of the Na: 3 HCO_3^- cotransporter in the basolateral membrane, and increases NH_4^+ production from glutamine. In the event of an acid load, the distal tubule inserts the preformed H^+ ATPase pumps into the luminal membrane of the intercalated cells to increase acid excretion.

Under normal circumstances, by increasing the plasma HCO_3^- concentration, the reabsorption of HCO_3^- plateaus off to maintain serum HCO_3^- level close to 25 mEq/L. All excess HCO_3^- is filtered into the urine. The "tubular maximum" of the proximal tubule is plastic, thus the HCO_3^- reabsorption can be altered accordingly. In states of volume contraction the Tm of the proximal tubule is increased.

Other factor that can increase the Tm of HCO_3^- in the proximal tubule is Angiotensin II, a potent stimulator of luminal Na–H exchanger and Na–3 HCO_3^- cotransporter.

Hypokalemia causes the intracellular K to move into extracellular space in exchange for H and Na. This intracellular acidosis simulates H^+ secretion, HCO_3^- reabsorption, and NH_4^+ excretion.

SUGGESTED READING

1. Cogan MG, Maddox DA, Lucci MS, Rector FC Jr.: Control of proximal bicarbonate reabsorption in normal and acidotic rats. J Clin Invest 64:1168–1180, 1979
2. Bichara M, Paillard M, Leviel F, Gardin JP: Hydrogen transport in rabbit kidney proximal tubules – $Na^+/^+H$ exchange. Am J Physiol 238:F445–F451, 1980.
3. Sasaki S, Shiigai T, Takeuchi J: Intracellular pH in the isolated perfused rabbit proximal tubule. Am J Physiol 249:F417–F423, 1985.
4. Rector FC Jr, Carter NW, Seldin DW: The mechanism of bicarbonate reabsorption in the proximal and distal tubules of the kidney. J Clin Invest 44:278–290, 1965.
5. Murer H, Hopfer U, Kinne R: Sodium/proton antiport in brush-border membrane vesicles isolated from rat small intestine and kidney. Biochem J 154:597–604, 1976.
6. Alpern RJ: Mechanism of basolateral membrane $H^+/OH^-/HCO_3^-$ transport in the rat proximal convoluted tubule. J Gen Physiol 86:613–636, 1985.
7. Collins JF, Honda T, Knobel S, et al.: Molecular cloning, sequencing, tissue distribution, and functional expression of a Na^+/H^+ exchanger (NHE-2). Proc Natl Acad Sci USA 90:3938–3942, 1993.
8. Biemesderfer D, Reilly RF, Exner M, et al.: Immunocytochemical characterization of $Na^+–H^+$ exchanger isoform NHE-1 in rabbit kidney. Am Physiol 263:F833–F840, 1992.
9. Schuster VL, Bonsib SM, Jennings ML: Two types of collecting duct mitochondria-rich (intercalated) cells: Lectin and band 3 cytochemistry. Am J Physiol 251:C347–C355, 1986.
10. Pitts RF: Production and excretion of ammonia in relation to acid–base regulation. In: Orloff J, Berliner RW (eds.): Handbook of Physiology, Section 8, Renal Physiology American Physiological Society, Washington DC, 1973, pp. 455–496.

8 Metabolic Acidosis

Howard E. Corey and Uri S. Alon

Key Points

1. Normal acid–base balance is crucial for proper cell function and integrity.
2. Metabolic acidosis is due to either the loss of blood buffers, or the gain of non-volatile strong acids.
3. An organized, step-wise approach (the "ABCDE toolkit") is crucial in determining both the magnitude and the cause of a metabolic acidosis and deciding upon appropriate therapy.
4. Base excess is a measure of the *magnitude* (extent) of the deviation from normal acid–base balance.
5. Ion "gaps" give important clues as to the possible *cause* of the metabolic derangement.

Key Words: Metabolic acidosis; base excess; anion gap; strong ion gap; urine anion gap; renal tubular acidosis

1. INTRODUCTION

Acid–base balance is regulated carefully to maintain optimal cellular integrity and function. Metabolic acidosis may depress myocardial contractility, over-stimulate sympathetic activity, blunt the effect of catecholamines, and vasoconstrict pulmonary arteries. In the critically ill patient, the accumulation of "unmeasured anions" (lactic acid, keto acids, by-products of intermediate metabolism, and intoxicants) is associated with a poor outcome *(1)*. Therefore, extracellular pH is kept within a narrow physiologic range through the coordinated action of blood buffers and homeostatic mechanisms.

Acidosis, the addition of an acid load, is countered immediately by the buffering action of extracellular bicarbonate, intracellular proteins, and intracellular phosphorus (a total capacity of 12–15 mEq/kg body weight). Afterwards, the lungs and the kidneys act to restore normal homeostasis by excretion of the acid load and re-generation of the buffer stores. The most important excretion of acid occurs via the lungs, amounting to approximately 13,000 mEq/day of CO_2. The kidneys excrete an additional $\sim$1 mEq/kg body weight per day in the form of titratable acid, in a process directly linked to the formation of "new" bicarbonate *(2)*. According to the law of electroneutrality, the gain and loss of plasma protons and buffers must be counter-balanced by a similar gain and losses

From: *Nutrition and Health: Fluid and Electrolytes in Pediatrics*
Edited by: L. G. Feld, F. J. Kaskel, DOI 10.1007/978-1-60327-225-4_8,
© Humana Press, a part of Springer Science+Business Media, LLC 2010

of electrolytes. The electroneutrality principle is used to devise algebraic descriptions of plasma acid–base balance and also to provide an alternative explanation of acid–base physiology *(3)*.

When the defensive mechanisms become overwhelmed, the acid–base balance of the body is disturbed. The term "acidemia" refers to a plasma pH < 7.4, and the more general term "acidosis" refers to the imposition of an acid load. Conceptually, acidosis may be classified as either "respiratory" (arising from the retention of CO_2) or "metabolic" (arising from the net loss of buffer base or the gain of a strong acid). Although the definition of metabolic acidosis is based on plasma pH, in practice acidosis usually suspected based upon the discovery of a low plasma bicarbonate concentration.

2. CAUSES OF METABOLIC ACIDOSIS

Through metabolism, the liver generates ~1 mM per kg BW per day of endogenous acid and accompanying anion. In the growing infant and child, daily acid generation can reach up to 3 mM per kg BW. The kidneys play an important role in the maintenance of systemic acid–base balance due to their ability to regulate the ions involved. To defend against metabolic acidosis, the proximal renal tubule absorbs bicarbonate, while the distal tubule secretes protons and generates new bicarbonate ions. The latter replaces bicarbonate ions lost in the process of buffering the protons that have been generated during metabolism. The hydrogen ion secreted into the distal tubule combines with ammonium and titratable acids (TA), comprised mostly in the form of phosphates. As secretion of diet-dependent TA is more or less fixed, it is mostly ammonia secretion that increases during metabolic acidosis. The process requires several days to achieve its maximum ability. Although urine pH is an important factor in assessing acid–base balance and in some diseases like uric acid lithiasis where it plays an important pathophysiologic role, "free" urine hydrogen ion concentration represents only a miniscule amount of the total protons that are excreted.

Metabolic acidosis can arise from renal or extra-renal etiologies. The extra-renal causes may result from the addition of non-volatile acid (lactic anion acidosis) or from a loss of base (diarrhea). The renal causes may result from abnormalities in the structure and function of the kidneys (renal tubular acidosis) or from the physiologic response of the kidneys to excessive or insufficient extra-renal stimuli (hyperparathyroidism and hypoaldosteronism, respectively). An "ABCDE toolkit" compiles the information needed to unravel the different possible mechanisms.

3. ABCDE TOOLKIT

The diagnosis of metabolic acidosis can be made by application of an "ABCDE toolkit," a compendium of useful equations, rules of thumb, and physiological approximations:

A is "assessment"
B is "base excess" and "blood gas"
C is "creatinine" and "compensations"
D is "deltas" or gaps
E = "extras"

An explanation of the toolkit is as follows:

Assessment: The clinical setting, be it sepsis, shock, dehydration, stool losses, growth retardation, intoxication, or uremia, provides important clues that are necessary for arriving at a correct differential diagnosis.

Blood gas and Base Excess: A blood gas (arterial or venous) provides essential information for the evaluation of acid–base disorders, including the pH, pCO_2, bicarbonate concentration, and base excess (BE). The hallmark of metabolic acidosis is a low plasma bicarbonate concentration (in a child and adult <24 mEq/L; a low value in a newborn or infant is <20–22 mEq/L) in the setting of a low pCO_2 measurement (<40 mmHg). Base excess (BE), defined as the milli-equivalents of a strong acid or strong base that is needed to titrate 1 L of blood to pH 7.4 when pCO_2 is held constant at 40 mmHg, provides the magnitude of the metabolic (non-respiratory) portion of an acidosis. In general, the larger the negative BE, the more severe the disturbance.

Creatinine and Compensation: Renal failure is an important cause of metabolic acidosis and the plasma creatinine concentration is an important index of renal function. In the absence of a specific defect in renal tubular function, the plasma creatinine concentration is inversely proportional to the ability of the kidney to "handle" an acid load. *Teaching Point:* Patients in renal failure with hypocalcemia may develop tetany due to the shift in ionized calcium from free to albumin-bound with the change in blood pH when there is too rapid correction of the acidosis.

For any disturbance causing a metabolic acidosis, there is an expected renal and respiratory compensation. A simple test for the adequacy of the renal response in patients with normal renal function is the "urine anion gap" (UAG = Na^+ + K^+ – Cl^-), a misnomer for an indirect estimate of urine NH_4^+. In compensation of metabolic acidosis, the normal kidney increases its production of ammonia and secretion of H^+, thus increasing urine ammonium secretion and with that chloride secretion. Consequently urine Cl^- will exceed the sum of urine Na^+ plus K^+, thus creating a negative (–) gap. In patients with distal renal tubular acidosis, interstitial renal disease, or renal insufficiency, ammoniagenesis is inadequate, thus creating a positive (+) gap. It should be pointed out that the UAG gap test is invalid in dehydrated patients, such as children with gastroenteritis and a low urine Na^+ < 20 mEq/L. Avid reabsorption of Na^+ by the proximal renal tubular results in low delivery of Na^+ to the distal nephron and diminished Na^+–H^+ exchange.

The adequacy of the respiratory response is assessed by Winter's formula, a "rule of thumb" or pearl that relates the measured plasma bicarbonate concentration to the expected, "compensated" pCO_2:

$$pCO_2 = (1.5 \times [HCO_3^-]) + 8 \pm 2$$

The measurement of a pCO_2 greater than calculated from Winter's formula indicates an inadequate ventilatory response, and the presence of a mixed metabolic-respiratory disorder.

Additional Pearls: For each 1 mM decrement in plasma bicarbonate (due to metabolic acidosis), respiratory compensation lowers the plasma pCO_2 by 1.25 mmHg.

As a rough guide, pCO_2 is equal approximately to the last 2 digits of the pH.

Example: Ammonium chloride is administered to normal volunteer, lowering the plasma bicarbonate from 24.25 mM to 14.25 mM. Using the "pearls," one would expect the plasma pCO_2 to decrease from 40 mmHg to $\sim$29 mmHg, as the plasma pH decreases from 7.4 to $\sim$7.29. Deviations from the expected compensation suggest presence of a second, concomitant acid–base process.

On the other hand, primary respiratory alkalosis blunts the reabsorption of bicarbonate by the proximal tubule, lowering the plasma pH by 0.008 units per mmHg change in pCO_2 acutely, and 0.003 units per mmHg change in pCO_2 chronically. In practice, compensation in mixed acid–base disorders may be difficult to interpret, as commingled processes may occur.

Deltas or Gaps: The plasma anion gap (AG) serves as a simple and effective tool in the evaluation of the etiology of metabolic acidosis. The anion gap indicates anions that are not routinely measured when plasma electrolytes are assessed. According to the law of electroneutrality, the sum of the charges of the plasma cations must equal the sum of the charges of the anions:

$$\text{Anion gap} (AG, mEq/L) = (Na^+ + K^+) - (Cl^- + HCO_3^-)$$

The use of the term strong ion gap (SIG) improves upon the AG by accounting for the charge contribution of weak acids, such as albumin and phosphate *(4)*.

$$SIG = AG - [\text{albumin g/dl}](1.2 \times pH - 6.15) + [\text{phosphate mg/dl}] (0.097 \times pH - 0.13)$$

Under normal conditions, the AG is $\sim$12 mEq/L $\pm$4, while the SIG is $\sim$0. A high AG may be due to a low plasma albumin concentration or an "unmeasured" anion such as lactate, while a high SIG is always due to an "unmeasured" anion *(2, 5)*.

Metabolic acidosis may be divided conveniently into disorders that present with a normal AG/SIG (high plasma chloride) and those with an elevated AG/SIG (normal or low plasma chloride) (Table 1).

The osmol gap, the difference between the measured and calculated plasma osmolality, may be useful if intoxicants such as ethylene glycol are suspected. In normal subject the main constituents of plasma osmolality are sodium salts of chloride and bicarbonate, glucose, and blood urea nitrogen (BUN). Under normal circumstances, the measured plasma osmolality is equal to the calculated value:

$$\text{Calculated plasma osmolality} (Posm, mOsm/kg) = 2[Na^+] + [\text{Glucose in mg/dL}]/18 + [\text{BUN in mg/dL}]/2.8$$

In the above equation, plasma sodium concentration is doubled to account for its accompanying anions, and glucose and BUN are divided by 18 and 2.8, respectively, to convert their units from mg/dL to mOsm/kg. An exogenous substance may be present if the measured osmolality exceeds the calculated value by >10 mOsm/kg.

Extras: Alkaline urine per se does not necessarily indicate an impaired renal acidification mechanism, as it may result from dietary factors or physiological proton trapping of urinary ammonia/ammonium. Several tests have been devised to more effectively test

Table 1
Causes of Metabolic Acidosis by Type of Anion Gap

Normal anion gap (hyperchloremic)	Elevated anion gap	Low anion gap
Renal (loss of bicarbonate) Renal tubular acidosis – Type 1 (distal) –, 2 (proximal) and 4 (mineralocorticoid) – (see Table 5 below) Renal failure (early) Carbonic anhydrase inhibitors – acetazolamide Potassium sparing diuretics Mineralocorticoid deficiency	Renal failure – acute and chronic	Dilution Hypoalbuminemia Severe hypernatremia Hypercalcemia Hypermagnesemia Lithium
Gastrointestinal (loss of bicarbonate) Diarrhea, drainage (small bowel, pancreatic, biliary, fistula, etc.), anion exchange resins	Poisoning – carbon monoxide or cyanide	
Miscellaneous Rapid intravenous expansion with bicarbonate or isotonic/hypertonic solutions Recovery from ketoacidosis Post-hypocapnia Exogenous chloride administration ($CaCl_2$, $MgCl_2$, arginine HCl, HCl) Hyperalimentation	Circulatory failure/tissue hypoxia	
	Lactic acidosis – hypoxia, glycogen storage disease (type 1), pancreatitis, leukemia, seizures Ingestions or overdose – ethanol, methanol, ethylene glycol, salicylate, isoniazid Ketoacidosis – diabetes mellitus, starvation Inborn errors in metabolism, organic acidosis Paraldehyde – organic anions	

Reproduced with permission from Feld *(9)*.

the acidification capacity of the kidney. As an example, the administration of ammonium chloride acidifies the urine, except in patients with distal renal tubular acidosis who are unable to excrete the "acid load." These tests are quite cumbersome and currently used infrequently. A test developed recently is based on the simultaneous dosing of furosemide (to increase the delivery of sodium to the distal tubule) and fludrocortisone (to promote reabsorption of sodium by principal cells and the secretion of protons by alpha-intercalated cells) *(6)*. Patients with distal renal tubular acidosis fail to lower the urine pH < 5.8, indicating an abnormality in H^+ secretion. Another test assessing distal tubule H^+ secretion is to measure the (urine–blood) pCO_2. This elegant test (although difficult to obtain in most centers) is based on the fact that when bicarbonate reaches the distal tubule it combines with the secreted H^+ to form carbonic acid, which then splits to H_2O and CO_2. At this part of the nephron and all the way further down to the urethral meatus CO_2 cannot diffuse back, thus its tension in the urine is the same as in the distal tubule. In different laboratories normal values range between 20 and 30 mmHg. It is important to make sure that the urine is sufficiently alkaline (pH > 7.4) and contains sufficient HCO_3^- (>40 mEq/L) as substrate. To achieve that goal, most studies in adults use $NaHCO_3$ given orally or intravenously. Oral acetazolamide administration has several advantages including being more palatable, causing mild metabolic acidosis that stimulates H^+ secretion, and being a diuretic shortens the time of the test *(7)*. It is also recommended to analyze the second and third voids after the drug administration, with the venous blood sample to be obtained between these voids.

The fractional excretion of bicarbonate is extremely helpful for the diagnosis of proximal RTA (pRTA). The test should be conducted after serum bicarbonate concentration is corrected to its normal range with alkali treatment. Under such circumstances, patients with pRTA will have $FE_{HCO3} > 15\%$. In infants with distal RTA, there may be large quantities of bicarbonate in the urine due to the greater role of the distal tubule in bicarbonate reabsorption in this age group. Consequently treatment of these infants will require large doses of alkali that decreases over time when expressed in mg/kg body weight. The latter condition used to be called RTA type III, a condition now reserved for patients with carbonic anhydrase II deficiency (vide infra). Another reason for the need of higher doses of alkali in younger patients is the increased metabolic rate and build-up of bone (storing alkali), generating more non-volatile acids.

4. DIAGNOSIS OF METABOLIC ACIDOSIS: APPLICATION OF THE ABCDE TOOLKIT (TABLE 2, FIG. 1)

Table 2

Application of ABCDE Toolkit in Cases of Metabolic Acidosis (pH < 7.4, HCO_3^- < 24 mEq/L, BE > –3 mEq/L)

	Compensations	*Deltas*
Diarrhea	Urine anion gap negative	SIG/AG normal osmol gap normal
Renal tubular acidosis	Urine anion gap positive	SIG/AG normal osmol gap normal
Diabetic ketoacidosis	Urine anion gap negative	SIG/AG high osmol gap normal
Methanol ingestion	Urine anion gap negative	AG/SIG normal osmol gap high

5. HIGH AG/SIG

In the setting of normal renal and pulmonary function, these disorders are characterized by significant acidosis (pH < 7.4, HCO_3^- < 24 mEq/L, BE > –3 mEq/L), a high plasma SIG, and adequate renal (urine anion gap negative) and respiratory (pCO_2 < 40 mmHg, according to Winter's formula) responses. The differential diagnosis includes lactic anion acidosis, ketoacidosis, and a variety of intoxications (Table 1).

Lactic Anion Acidosis: Lactic anion acidosis occurs whenever production of lactic anion exceeds consumption or clearance. First, glucose enters the muscle cells by facilitative diffusion through the Glut-1 transporter and is then oxidized by a sequence of enzymatic reactions to form 2 molecules each of pyruvate, NADH, ATP and H^+. Pyruvate is then reduced by the cytosolic enzyme dehydrogenase (LDH) to form lactate anion. Lactate anion, along with H^+ derived from the hydrolysis of ATP, may enter the circulation by way of the membrane-bound lactate-H^+ co-transporter *(8)*.

Lactic Acidosis (plasma concentration > 1 mM) has been divided into 2 categories. Type A lactic anion acidosis caused by dysoxia, or the inability of cells to generate sufficient ATP to meet metabolic demand when mitochondrial P_{O2} is low. Dysoxia is most often due to hypoxia and ischemia secondary to pulmonary disease, cardiac disease, hemoglobin deficiency, or carbon monoxide poisoning. In turn, mitochondrial dysfunction results in the accumulation of pyruvate and lactic anion (often with a high plasma lactate/pyruvate ratio).

Type B lactic anion acidosis is due to *cytopathic* hypoxia, or the inability of pyruvate to enter the tricarboxylic acid cycle (TCA) or the electron transport chain (ETC). Cytopathic hypoxia may occur secondary to drugs (biguanides, isoniazid, salicylates, propofol, linezolid, nucleoside reverse transcriptase inhibitors), toxins (ethanol, methanol, ethylene glycol, propylene glycol, cyanide), or errors of metabolism (congenital lactic acidosis, thymine deficiency). In addition, *accelerated glycolysis* in well-oxygenated patients with sepsis may result in hyperlactemia due to a high production rate. *Poor lactate "shuttling"* in patients with severe liver and/or renal failure may result in hyperlactemia due to low consumption or clearance.

Other *endogenous* causes of metabolic acidosis with a high AG include inborn errors of metabolism and diabetic ketoacidosis. *Exogenous etiologies include* salicylate ingestion, pyroglutamic acidosis, D-lactic acidosis, propylene and ethylene glycol poisoning, methanol ingestion, alcoholic ketoacidosis, and arsenic poisoning *(2)*.

Salicylates stimulate respiratory drive, initiating a mixed metabolic acidosis and respiratory alkalosis. Patients present with vomiting, fever and central nervous system disturbance, which progresses to pulmonary edema and renal failure. Hypermetabolism results in an additional lactic anion acidosis, which increases the permeability of the blood–brain barrier to salicylates. Alkalinization of the urine greatly aids the renal excretion of salicylate and is the key to effective treatment. In some severe cases, hemodialysis may be indicated.

Pyroglutamic Acidosis. Pyroglutamic acidosis may occur in malnourished patients who have received acetaminophen or the antibiotic flucloxacillin. The diagnosis is confirmed by the finding of an elevated blood or urine 5-oxoproline level.

D-*Lactic Acidosis.* Patients with the short gut syndrome may develop encephalopathy. An associated D-lactic acidosis may arise due to the overgrowth of intestinal bacteria that ferment dietary carbohydrate. The diagnosis of D-lactic acidosis is made by a specific enzymatic test. Treatment consists of restriction of oral feeds while providing intravenous dextrose for calories.

Alcohols. In the early stages of propylene glycol, ethylene glycol or methanol poisoning, metabolic acidosis with a high AG is accompanied by a high plasma "osmol gap." Later in the clinical course, the osmol gap returns to normal as these active osmolytes are *metabolized by hepatic alcohol dehydrogenase* to osmotically – inactive but highly toxic by-products.

Propylene Glycol. A vehicle to deliver topical (e.g., silver sulfadiazine cream) and intravenous (e.g., diazepam) medications, propylene glycol that is not excreted by the kidneys is metabolized to lactic anion. Lactic anion acidosis may develop if the lactate–pyruvate–acetyl-CoA pathway is sluggish, as in thiamine deficiency.

Ethylene Glycol. Ethylene glycol, used commonly as an anti-freeze agent, is oxidized by the liver to glycolic acid and oxalate. Patients with ethylene glycol poisoning present with metabolic acidosis, flank pain, hypocalcemia, vomiting, ataxia, seizure and coma, progressing to cardiac, renal, and respiratory failure.

Unreliable indicators of ethylene glycol poisoning include a discrepancy between breath alcohol analyzer and ethanol blood levels, a high serum osmol gap, urinary calcium oxalate crystals, and urine that fluoresces under Wood's lamp. These non-specific tests cannot substitute for direct measurement of plasma ethylene glycol and glycolic acid.

Methanol. Methanol, used commonly in antifreeze, paint thinner, and rubbing alcohol, is metabolized to formaldehyde and formic acid. Formic acid accumulates in the optic nerve, and patients with methanol poisoning present with metabolic acidosis, blindness, cardiovascular instability, pancreatitis, and optic disc edema.

Treatment of all three poisonings centers on inhibition of alcohol dehydrogenase with either fomepizole or ethanol, and in some cases removal of toxins and their toxic-by-products with hemodialysis. As with other poisonings an important key to successful treatment is early diagnosis and intervention.

CASE SCENARIO 1

A 17-year-old girl is brought to the emergency department because of hyperpyrexia, vomiting, and confusion. Recently, she had been diagnosed with a hepatitis C infection but was otherwise well. On examination, the temperature is 40°C, the respirations are 32/min, and the pulse is 120/min. The lung examination is normal. The initial treatment consists of intravenous normal saline.

An arterial blood gas (analyzed at 37°C) is obtained. The pH and pCO_2 are 7.4 and 25 mmHg, respectively, and base excess (BE) is –11 mM. An additional blood sample has been sent to the laboratory for determination of plasma electrolytes.

What is the underlying acid–base disorder? What additional information is needed to make this determination? What is the diagnosis and proper treatment?

Case Scenario Discussion: A BE of −11 mM indicates a significant metabolic acidosis. The clinical examination and low pCO_2 suggest a compensatory respiratory alkalosis. The plasma electrolytes are reported: Na 140 mM, K 3.8 mM, chloride 115 mM, HCO_3^- 15 mM, and albumin 1.5 g/dL. The normal anion gap of 14 mM suggests a hyperchloremic, metabolic acidosis, perhaps due to the rapid infusion of crystalloids. However, the SIG (*SIG = AG − [albumin g/dL](1.2xpH−6.15) + [phosphate mg/dL](0.097xpH−0.13)*) of −9 mM reveals an "unmeasured" plasma anion as the major cause of the acidosis.

6. NORMAL AG/SIG

In the setting of normal renal and pulmonary function, these disorders are characterized by significant acidosis (pH < 7.4, HCO_3^- < 24 mEq/L, BE > −3 mEq/L), normal plasma SIG, and an adequate (urine anion gap negative) or inadequate (urine anion gap positive) renal response (Table 1, Fig. 1). The differential diagnosis includes diarrhea, dilutional acidosis, total parenteral nutrition, and renal tubular acidosis.

As an example, a positive urine anion gap in well-hydrated patient with normal renal function suggests the possibility of a renal tubular acidosis (Tables 3 and 4).

Proximal renal tubular acidosis. Proximal renal tubular acidosis (Type II) is characterized by a low threshold for bicarbonate reabsorption, due to a genetic defect in the SLC4A4 gene encoding NBC-1, a mutation in the CAII gene encoding carbonic anhydrase II or the use of carbonic anhydrase inhibitors such as acetazolamide or topiramate. SLC4A4 gene mutation is associated with cataracts and glaucoma, while CAII gene mutation is associated with osteopetrosis, as well as acidification defect in the distal tubule, making the latter the only true RTA type III.

Characterized by phosphaturia, aminoaciduria, glucosuria, and proximal renal tubular acidosis, Fanconi syndrome is a generalized defect in proximal tubular function that may be due to heavy metal poisoning, cystinosis, Lowe syndrome, Chinese Herb Nephropathy, mitochondrial disorder, Wilson disease, fructose intolerance, and monoclonal IgG light chain disease. Clinically only the phosphaturia and metabolic acidosis have metabolic consequences. In the young child with Fanconi syndrome the first potential diagnosis to be considered is cystinosis. Untreated children with Fanconi syndrome suffer from severe failure to thrive and rickets. The acidosis is often difficult to treatment as the treatment does not change the low bicarbonate threshold and the more bicarbonate is taken the more is found in the urine.

The finding of positive urinary anion gap (Cl^- < (Na^+ + K^+)), namely inappropriately low ammonium ion secretion automatically focuses the attention on the kidney (although positive anion gap is also observed in toluene ingestion due to the excretion of hippurate salts, but these conditions are not easily confused).

Distal Renal Tubular Acidosis. Distal renal tubular acidosis (Type I) is due to low net acid excretion in the distal nephron, and may be secondary to an autosomal dominant mutation in the SLC4A1 gene with aberrant trafficking of AE1 or an autosomal

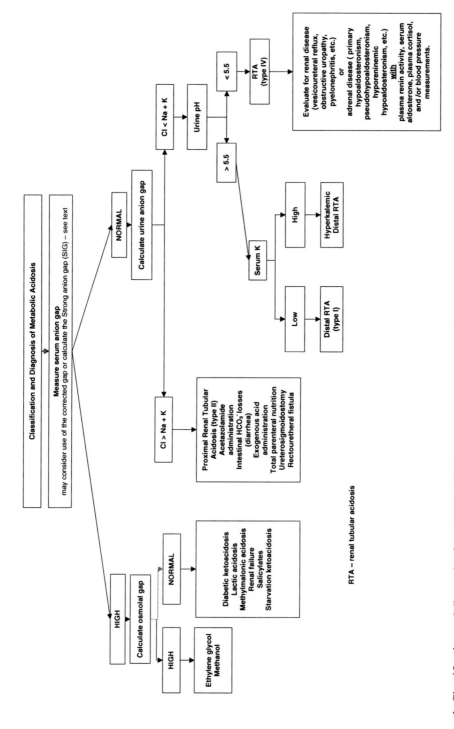

Fig. 1. Classification and diagnosis of metabolic acidosis.

Table 3
Selected Causes of Renal Tubular Acidosis (RTA)

Proximal RTA	Distal RTA	Type IV RTA
Isolated	*Primary*	*Mineralocorticoid deficiency*
Sporadic, transient in infancy	Transient in infancy	Aldosterone disorders
Hereditary	Persistent	Addison disease
	Adult type	Congenital adrenal hyperplasia
Fanconi syndrome	Incomplete	Primary hypoaldosteronism
	With bicarbonate wasting	Hyporeninemic hypoaldosteronism
Primary	With nerve deafness	
Secondary		*Other causes*
Inherited	*Secondary*	
Carbonic anhydrase II deficiency		Chloride shunt syndrome
Cystinosis	Interstitial nephritis	Diabetes mellitus
Galactosemia	Lupus nephritis	Idiopathic
Glycogen storage disease type I	Medullary sponge kidney	Interstitial nephritis
Hereditary fructose intolerance	Nephrocalcinosis	Nephrosclerosis
Leigh syndrome	Obstructive uropathy	Obstructive uropathy
Lowe syndrome	Pyelonephritis	Pseudohypoaldost-eronism
Medullary cystic disease	Reflux nephropathy	Pyelonephritis
Metachromatic leukodystrophy	Sickle cell nephropathy	Transient in infancy
Mitochondrial cytopathies	Transplant rejection	Unilateral kidney diseases
Tyrosinemia		
Wilson disease	*Other causes*	
Acquired		
Cyclosporine	Carbonic anhydrase II deficiency	
Gentamicin	Chronic active hepatitis	
Heavy metals	Ehlers–Danlos syndrome	
Hyperparathyroidism	Elliptocytosis	
Interstitial nephritis		
Nephrotic syndrome	*Toxin or drug induced*	
Vitamin D deficiency rickets	Amphotericin B	
	Analgesics	
	Lithium	

Rodriquez Soriano *(10)*; Adrogue and Madias *(11)*.

Table 4
Features of Renal Tubular Acidosis in Childhood

Features	Type I (distal)	Type II (proximal)	Type IV (hyperkalemic)
Urine pH during acidosis	>5.5	<5.5	<5.5
Urine anion gap	Positive	Negative	Positive
FEHCO$_3^-$ at normal serum HCO$_3$	<15%*	>15%	<15%
(Urine–blood) pCO$_2$	<20 mmHg	>20 mmHg	?
Serum potassium	Normal or low	Normal or low	Increased
Calcium excretion	Increased	Normal or ↑	Normal (?)
Citrate excretion	Decreased	Normal	Normal
Nephrocalcinosis	Common	Rare	Absent
Associated tubular defects	Rare	Common	Rare
Rickets	Rare	Common	Absent
Daily alkali requirement (mEq/kg/day)	1–4*	10–15	2–3
Potassium supplementation	No	Yes	No

* Often higher in infants.
Modified with permission from Rodriquez-Soriano and Vallo (12).

recessive mutation in the ATP6B1 gene encoding the B1 subunit of the vacuolar H$^+$-ATPase. The recessive form may be associated with growth retardation and hearing loss, whereas the dominant form is usually milder. Hypokalemia is common, and hypercalciuria and hypocitraturia predispose to nephrocalcinosis and nephrolithiasis. Distal renal tubular acidosis may also be observed with Sjogren's syndrome, hypergammaglobulinemia, amphotericin, and HIV infection.

Pathophysiologically, several mechanisms are responsible to dRTA. Among them (a) a secretory defect due to genetic or acquired abnormalities in the H$^+$-ATPase pump of the alpha intercalated cell (b) a gradient defect in which there is a backleak of luminal H$^+$ as seen in patients treated with amphotericin.

Renal Tubular Acidosis Type IV. This is the most common type of RTA. Contrary to RTA type II and most cases of RTA type I, which are associated with hypokalemia, RTA type IV is associated with hyperkalemia (Table 4). While the patients are able to lower their urine pH in response to systemic acidosis their ammonia generation is impaired. It is unclear to what extent it is the hyperkalemia itself causing the interference in ammonia metabolism. The hyperkalemia is due to either low serum aldosterone or to tubular defects. Based on the various abnormalities in the axis renin–aldosterone–kidney, RTA type IV is divided into 5 subtypes (Fig. 1). The rationale in this classification is in both in defining the pathophysiologic mechanism and the optimal treatment.

In order to identify the sub-type it is needed to assess the patient's blood pressure, obtain blood samples for renin, aldosterone, and cortisol and evaluate the urinary tract anatomy by ultrasound. Only pseudohypoaldosteronism type II is characterized by hypervolemia and hypertension. This autosomal dominant disorder is due to a genetic mutation resulting in increased NaCl reabsorption in the distal tubule. Secondary to the hypervolemia plasma renin activity and serum aldosterone are suppressed. In all other sub-types patients is hypo- or euvolemic and hypo- or normotensive. They result from either primary or secondary lack of aldosterone or decreased responsiveness of the renal tubule to aldosterone, namely end-organ resistance.

Chronic Renal Failure. In advanced chronic renal failure, low net acid excretion is due to global loss of functioning renal mass, resulting in progressive inability of the kidneys to clear phosphates, sulfate, and organic acids, combined with tubular damage lowering the ability to secrete H^+ lead to either normal anion gap (hyperchloremic) or high anion gap metabolic acidosis.

CASE SCENARIO 2

A 6-month-old Israeli boy is evaluated for failure to thrive, associated with vomiting, diarrhea, lethargy, and abdominal distention. He was the full-term product of a normal vaginal delivery, with height and weight initially at the 50th percentile. On examination, the weight is now 7 kg (9th percentile) and the height is 63 cm (2nd percentile). Laboratories revealed

Na 140 mmol/L; K 3.2 mmol/L, Cl 110 mmol/L; HCO_3 16 mmol/L, BUN 3 mg/dL, Pcr 0.3 mg/dL;
Venous pH 7.28; urine pH 8, ketones negative; anion gap 14 mmol/L

Suspecting renal tubular acidosis (RTA) on the basis of a normal anion gap and an alkaline urine pH, bicarbonate (Bicitra) 3 mEq/kg/day was prescribed. However, the infant deteriorated neurologically, developing ophthalmoplegia and upward gaze nystagmus. A head CT scan was normal.

Case Scenario Discussion:

1. Is the diagnosis of RTA correct?
   ANSWER: In this case, RTA may be an incorrect diagnosis. Urine pH is alkaline in many forms of chronic acidosis, due to "proton-trapping" by high concentrations of urinary ammonia. Furthermore, the anion gap may be misleading in patients with hypoalbuminemia.
2. What additional information do you need to make the diagnosis?
   ANSWER: The urine anion gap, the plasma osmol gap, and the plasma strong ion gap may be helpful to make diagnosis.

In this case, the urine anion gap (Na + K − Cl) is negative, suggesting a high concentration of urinary ammonium and pointing away from the diagnosis of RTA. The plasma albumin is 1.5 g/dL and the plasma osmolality is 285 mOsm/kg, so the plasma osmol gap is normal while the albumin-corrected anion gap is 21 nM and plasma strong ion gap (SIG) is also elevated at 11 mM.

3. What further diagnostic test lead to the correct diagnosis?

The alkalinizing effect of hypoalbuminemia may "mask" the metabolic acidosis due to an "unmeasured" anion. In this case, the blood lactate level was found to be elevated. The differential diagnosis of lactate anion acidosis includes dysoxia (due to sepsis or shock), inborn errors of metabolism, a variety of drugs, and several intoxications.

On reviewing the history, the infant was fed a soy-based formula (Remedia Super Soya 1) that was specifically manufactured for the Israeli market. An erythrocyte transketolase activity assay revealed significant thiamine deficiency as the cause of the lactate anion acidosis.

Treatment with thiamine reversed the clinical symptoms and lead to a complete recovery.

7. TREATMENT

In general, treatment centers on the correction of the disordered pathophysiology (Table 5). For example, maneuvers that improve ventilation and perfusion will benefit critically ill patients with lactic anion acidosis due dysoxia. Bicarbonate therapy is helpful in children with renal tubular acidosis, but is of unclear benefit or harmful in patients with lactic anion or ketoacidosis. Hemodialysis may be indicated in severe intoxication and some of the metabolic disorders, but is of uncertain benefit in other conditions. Future investigations that link mitochondrial function, intracellular pH, and blood buffers may provide additional insight to the optimal treatment.

Table 5
Treatment of Some Forms of Metabolic Acidosis

Anion	Cause	Treatment	Unclear benefit or possibly harmful
Chloride	Acute diarrhea, renal tubular acidosis, acute, and chronic renal failure,	Bicarbonate (see Table 4)	Careful administration in hypocalcemic patients
Lactic anion	Dysoxia	Improve ventilation and perfusion	Hemodialysis/ hemofiltration
Keto acids	Diabetes mellitus	Insulin	Bicarbonate, Carbicarb
Salicylate	Ingestion	Alkalinization of urine	Over-aggressive fluid administration
Alcohols (propylene glycol, ethylene glycol, methanol)	Ingestion	Fomepizole, ethanol, hemodialysis	

The treatment of the various types of RTA type IV depends on the pathophysiology. In the case of chloride shunt, a thiazides diuretic is the drug of choice. In hypoaldosteronism, either primary or secondary, a mineralocorticoid will be the drug of choice. However in patients with chronic renal failure who are also hypertensive the drug should be replaced by furosemide. In patients with end-organ resistance a combination treatment with NaCl and NaHCO₃ is often required. In children with RTA type IV due to obstructive uropathy alleviation of the obstruction results in normalization of function of the tubule. A similar situation may be observed in patients with pyelonephritis especially when superimposed on an anatomic abnormality in the urinary tract.

REFERENCES

1. Rixen D, Raum M, Bouillon B, Lefering R, Neugebauer E. Arbeitsgemeinschaft "Polytrauma" of the Deutsche Gesellschaft fur Unfallchirurgie. Base deficit development and its prognostic significance in posttrauma critical illness: an analysis by the trauma registry of the Deutsche Gesellschaft fur unfallchirurgie. Shock. 2001 Feb;15(2):83–89.
2. Boron WF. Acid–base transport by the renal proximal tubule. J Am Soc Nephrol. 2006 Sep;17(9): 2368–2382
3. Corey HE. Stewart and beyond: new models of acid–base balance. Kidney Int. 2003 Sep;64(3): 777–787.
4. Kraut JA, Madias NE. Serum anion gap: its uses and limitations in clinical medicine. Clin J Am Soc Nephrol. 2007 Jan;2(1):162–174.
5. Corey HE. Bench-to-bedside review: Fundamental principles of acid–base physiology. Crit Care. 2005 Apr;9(2):184–192.
6. Walsh SB, Shirley DG, Wrong OM, Unwin RJ. Urinary acidification assessed by simultaneous furosemide and fludrocortisone treatment: an alternative to ammonium chloride. Kidney Int. 2007;71:1310–1316
7. Alon U, Hellerstein S, Warady BA. Oral acetazolamide in the assessment of (urine–blood) pCO₂. Pediatric Nephrology 1991;5:307–311.
8. Gladden LB. Lactate metabolism: a new paradigm for the third millennium. J Physiol. 2004 Jul 1;558 (Pt 1):5–30
9. Feld LG. Nephrology. In: Feld LG, Meltzer AJ., eds. Fast Facts in Pediatrics. 1st ed. Elsevier, Amsterdam, 2006:p.434.
10. Rodriquez Soriano J. Renal tubular acidosis: the clinical entity. J Am Soc Nephrol 2002;13:2160–2170.
11. Adrogue HJ, Madias NE. Disorders of acid-base balance. In Berl T., ed. Disorders of Water, Electrolytes, Blackwell Science. Philadelphia, 1999:6.17–6.19.
12. Rodriquez-Soriano J, Vallo A. Renal tubular acidosis, Peds Nephrol 19990;4268–275.

9 Diagnosis and Treatment of Metabolic Alkalosis

Wayne R. Waz

Key Points

1. Primary metabolic alkalosis should be distinguished from metabolic compensation to respiratory acidosis.
2. Measurement of urine chloride concentration is essential for diagnosis and treatment.
3. Metabolic alkalosis with low urine chloride (chloride responsive) represents an appropriate renal response to H^+ and Cl^- losses from non-renal sites (GI, skin).
4. Metabolic alkalosis with high urine chloride (chloride unresponsive) should prompt an evaluation for renal and endocrine disorders and can be further evaluated by the presence or absence of hypertension, renal and adrenal imaging, and the relative concentrations of plasma renin activity and serum aldosterone.

Key Words: Metabolic alkalosis; urine chloride; hypokalemia; hypochloremia; bicarbonate; Bartter syndrome; Gitelman syndrome; aldosterone; loop diuretic; thiazide diuretic

1. DEFINITION

Metabolic alkalosis is defined as a primary increase in both plasma pH and plasma bicarbonate concentration. It is associated with a compensatory decrease in ventilation and increased $PaCO_2$ (Table 1). Typically, $PaCO_2$ increases 0.5–0.7 mmHg to compensate for each 1 mM increase in plasma HCO_3^-. For example, in a patient whose serum $[HCO_3^-]$ has increased from 22 to 30 mEq/L, the expected respiratory compensation will be approximately 0.7 times the difference between the normal serum $[HCO_3^-]$ and the alkalotic serum $[HCO_3^-]$, in this case 0.7×8, or 5.6. When added to a normal $PaCO_2$ of 40 mmHg, the expected $PaCO_2$ is 45.6 mmHg. A more rapid method to estimate the expected respiratory compensation to metabolic alkalosis is to add 15 to the patient's serum bicarbonate level for bicarbonate values ranging from 25 to 40 *(1)*. For example, for a patient with a serum $[HCO_3^-]$ of 30, add 15 to give an estimated $PaCO_2$ of 45 mmHg. If the actual respiratory compensation is less than estimated, consider a mixed respiratory and metabolic disorder. Also, remember that an increased serum $[HCO_3^-]$ also occurs in metabolic compensation to respiratory acidosis, but this can be

From: *Nutrition and Health: Fluid and Electrolytes in Pediatrics*
Edited by: L. G. Feld, F. J. Kaskel, DOI 10.1007/978-1-60327-225-4_9,
© Humana Press, a part of Springer Science+Business Media, LLC 2010

Table 1
Estimated Respiratory Compensation to Primary Metabolic Alkalosis

Method 1:
    Compensated $PaCO_2 = 40 + [0.7$ (patient $[HCO_3^-]$ – normal $[HCO_3^-])]$
    Example: a patient's serum $[HCO_3^-]$ has increased from 22 to 30 mEq/L:
    Compensated $PaCO_2 = 40 + [0.7 (30–22)]$
    Compensated $PaCO_2 = 40 + 5.6$
    Compensated $PaCO_2 = 45.6$
Method 2:
    Compensated $PaCO_2 =$ patient $[HCO_3^-] + 15$
    Example: a patient has a serum $[HCO_3^-] = 30$
    Compensated $PaCO_2 = 30 + 15$
    Compensated $PaCO_2 = 45$

distinguished from metabolic alkalosis by looking at plasma pH. In this case, the pH will generally be <7.35, as the metabolic compensation is not sufficient to over-correct the respiratory acidosis into the alkalotic range.

2. ETIOLOGY

How might you make someone alkalotic? While most of the disease states that lead to metabolic alkalosis result from varying combinations of the mechanisms discussed below, it is helpful to consider the influence of specific single perturbations and their impact on the generation and maintenance of alkalosis. This section will discuss primarily net effects of the various mechanisms, with more specific details of the physiology found in several comprehensive reviews (1–4).

Because the kidney can normally excrete large bicarbonate loads, the finding of persistent metabolic alkalosis requires first an initial insult (generation phase), followed by a maintenance phase. Initial insults that contribute to the generation of alkalosis include HCl depletion, potassium depletion, volume depletion, or mineralocorticoid excess (described below). The maintenance phase occurs when renal mechanisms perpetuate the alkalotic state. These renal mechanisms include decreased glomerular filtration rate, development of intracellular acidosis, increased proximal tubule H^+ secretion (with subsequent HCO_3^- reabsorption), and increased distal tubule H^+ secretion, again with subsequent distal HCO_3^- reabsorption, and generation.

Infuse Bicarbonate or Other Alkali: Exogenous bicarbonate infusion is not an effective method of generating metabolic alkalosis. The kidney responds quickly and effectively to large bicarbonate loads. As long as the ECF volume (and the accompanying glomerular filtration rate) is adequate, the proximal tubule threshold for bicarbonate reabsorption is exceeded, and distal nephron mechanisms are inadequate to handle the load. However, in patients with significantly decreased glomerular filtration rates (GFR), either due to severe volume depletion or intrinsic renal disease, renal excretion of bicarbonate is impaired and exogenous loads can cause significant alkalosis. Examples of bicarbonate or other alkali administration causing metabolic alkalosis in patients with decreased GFR include milk–alkali syndrome (often discussed but rarely seen), oral or IV $NaHCO_3$ administration, acetate loads in parenteral nutrition solutions, citrate from blood transfusions or from regional anticoagulation during continuous renal replacement or other extracorporeal therapies, and the combination of antacids plus cation exchange resins.

Remove HCl from the Gastrointestinal Tract: As both H^+ and Cl^- are lost from the GI tract or other sites, plasma $[HCO_3^-]$ increases, increasing the renal filtered load. The net negative charge in the distal nephron caused by excess bicarbonate leads to increased tubular sodium and potassium losses, with accompanying water loss. Chloride, on the other hand, is avidly retained by the kidney to compensate for the high amount of GI (or other non-renal) loss. The resulting electrolyte profile is one of a hypochloremic (from GI loss) hypokalemic (from renal loss) metabolic alkalosis, with a decreased ECF volume because of both GI and renal volume losses. This state is also referred to as a contraction alkalosis, because the ECF volume is relatively contracted, with HCO_3^- as a more significant contributor to the overall anion concentration than in the normal state. The renin–angiotensin–aldosterone axis becomes more active, with a net effect of increasing sodium and water reabsorption, improving ECF volume but with a cost of contributing further to hypokalemia.

At this point, even if HCl losses stop, alkalosis is maintained until total body chloride content is replenished and ECF volume is restored. As long as the plasma chloride concentration is low, very little will show up in the distal nephron, and the primary anion in the distal nephron will be HCO_3^-, thus any tubular reabsorption of anion necessary to maintain electroneutral plasma will be of HCO_3^-. In addition, increased aldosterone activity and the high $[HCO_3^-]$ in the tubular lumen will promote Na^+–H^+ exchange and even further H^+ loss into the urine. During the initial period of GI HCl losses, the urine pH is typically alkaline (6.5–7), but as HCl losses stop but renal mechanisms maintain the alkalosis, the urine pH can decrease (5.5–6). Once plasma Cl^- is restored and some appears in the lumen of the distal nephron, selective reabsorption of Cl^-, with subsequent excretion of HCO_3^- can occur, and alkalosis can be corrected. As ECF volume improves, aldosterone effects diminish, and net H^+ loss decreases, further contributing to the resolution alkalosis.

Create a State of Hypokalemia: Hypokalemia contributes to the generation and maintenance of alkalosis through several mechanisms:

– At the glomerulus, hypokalemia produces a reduction in glomerular filtration rate, although precise mechanisms have not been described.
– In the proximal nephron, hypokalemia increases net proximal tubule bicarbonate reabsorption. This proximal net bicarbonate reabsorption probably occurs when hypokalemia causes proximal tubule cells to develop an intracellular acidosis, created by exchange of extracellular H^+ for intracellular K^+ in an effort to maintain normal plasma potassium levels.
– Also, in the proximal nephron, hypokalemia enhances renal ammoniagenesis, increasing the amount of NH_3 in the tubule lumen available to bind secreted H^+, with net acid subsequently lost in the urine.

- In the distal nephron, hypokalemia impairs renal chloride reabsorption in a way that enhances secretion of H^+ into the tubular lumen.
- Additionally, hypokalemia creates intracellular acidosis in the distal nephron, which results in mechanisms similar to those seen in the proximal tubule.
- Finally, hypokalemia increases H^+–K^+ ATPase activity in the collecting duct.

Create a State of Hyperaldosteronism: The physiologic effect of mineralocorticoids, primarily aldosterone, is to respond to conditions of decreased intravascular volume by stimulating the apical sodium channel and the basolateral Na, K-ATPase of the principal cell of the cortical collecting duct, resulting in increased sodium reabsorption and increased urinary potassium secretion. Furthermore, mineralocorticoids directly increase tubular H^+ excretion through stimulation of Na^+–H^+ exchange. The systemic result is the development of increased intravascular volume (from Na retention), with hypokalemia and metabolic alkalosis. When mineralocorticoid effects go unchecked, as in states of mineralocorticoid excess, volume-overload hypertension, hypokalemia, and metabolic alkalosis are generated and maintained. Hypokalemia is particularly important for the maintenance of metabolic alkalosis in mineralocorticoid excess states. Note that while there is a phenomenon of escape from the Na-retaining effects of excess mineralocorticoid, permitting diuresis and natriuresis, no such mechanisms exist to prevent chronic loss of potassium. So, while generation of alkalosis occurs because of increased tubular excretion of both H^+ and K^+, the maintenance of alkalosis is driven by hypokalemia (discussed above).

3. CLINICAL PRESENTATION

Clinically relevant metabolic alkalosis arises from various combinations of the physiologic perturbations discussed above. The relative contributions of decreased intravascular volume, hypokalemia, Cl^- and H^+ loss, exogenous or endogenous HCO_3^-, and mineralocorticoids can be difficult to sort out, and one is often unsure what caused what. Fortunately, both the diagnosis and treatment can be pinned down with a careful history and physical exam and a few simple and inexpensive laboratory tests (Fig. 1).

Metabolic alkalosis is typically seen in patients with serious illness, either acute or chronic, at times making it difficult to separate symptoms specific to alkalosis from those of underlying illnesses. Significant alkalosis may manifest with serious CNS and cardiac complications; patients may develop stupor, confusion, lethargy, muscle weakness, and/or cramping. The frequent finding of hypokalemia with alkalosis predisposes patients to cardiac arrhythmias and sudden death. EKG findings include QT interval prolongation, ST segment depression, a flat or low amplitude T-wave, prominent U-wave, AV dissociation, torsade de pointes, ventricular tachycardia, and ventricular fibrillation *(5)*. Cardiac arrhythmias can be life threatening and refractory to treatment unless alkalosis and, equally importantly, hypokalemia are corrected. An alkalosis-induced shift of the oxygen-hemoglobin dissociation curve to the left, combined with relative hypoxia related to compensatory hypoventilation, can lead to decreased tissue delivery of oxygen. Also seen are decreased ionized calcium concentrations, increased lactate production, elevated anion gap, and decreased urinary calcium excretion *(6)*.

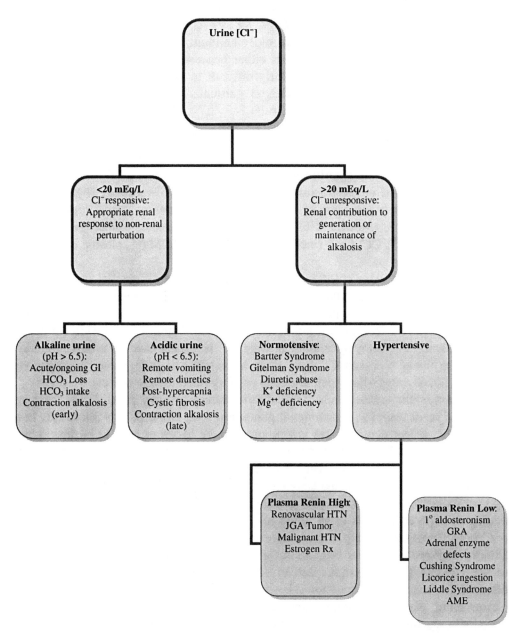

Fig. 1. Diagnostic algorithm for metabolic alkalosis (HTN: hypertension, JGA: juxtaglomerular appa-ratus, GRA: glucocorticoid remediable aldosteronism, AME: apparent mineralocorticoid excess).

In the acute care setting, it is important to review the patient's history for significant sources of GI loss, including nasogastric suction, surgical drains, and ostomies. Current and past history of diuretic use should also be obtained. Careful evaluation of enteral and parenteral nutrition may reveal potential sources of exogenous alkali administration. In the chronic setting, an evaluation for failure to thrive should include investigation for alkalosis and hypokalemia. For infants, an assessment of feeding, particularly in formula-fed infants, may contribute. In older children, particularly adolescents, eating disorders may present with alkalosis either because of diuretic abuse or chronic vomiting. This history may be particularly difficult to elicit, and index of suspicion should be high. Patients with chronic fatigue, particularly muscle weakness or muscle spasm, should also be evaluated for alkalosis.

4. EVALUATION

Figure 1 is a diagnostic algorithm for patients with metabolic alkalosis. In addition to patient history and physical exam findings, key factors in guiding diagnosis and treatment include measurement of urine [Cl⁻], assessment of blood pressure and intravascular volume, assessment of renal function, and assessment of plasma electrolytes including K^+, Cl^-, Ca^{++} (including ionized Ca), and Mg^{++}, plasma renin activity, and serum aldosterone.

Most importantly, urine chloride measurement simplifies differential diagnosis and guides treatment. Metabolic alkalosis can be divided into chloride responsive and chloride unresponsive types. If urine Cl^- is less than 20 mEq/L, the kidneys are responding appropriately to HCl losses from non-renal sites [most commonly GI, skin (in cystic fibrosis patients) or posthypercapnia]. If urine Cl^- is greater than 20 mEq/L, the kidneys are the site of excessive Cl^- loss, either in response to endogenous or exogenous hormone effects, drugs (diuretics), or due to primary renal tubular defects.

Urine potassium measurement helps differentiate a primary renal defect from an appropriate renal response to extrarenal potassium loss. Urine $[K^+] > 30$ mEq/L in a hypokalemic patient demonstrates inappropriate renal losses as seen in intrinsic renal defects (Bartter and Gitelman syndromes), diuretic use, or high circulating aldosterone levels. A urine $[K^+] < 20$ mEq/L denotes an appropriate renal response to extrarenal loss.

For patients with chloride unresponsive alkalosis, renal and adrenal imaging studies, particularly ultrasound or CT imaging, may aid in differential diagnosis. A finding of nephrocalcinosis in an infant may point to a diagnosis of neonatal Bartter syndrome. Renal size discrepancy or, more specifically, asymmetrical blood flow to the kidneys may prompt further evaluation for renal artery stenosis. A finding of a renal or adrenal mass may suggest, respectively, a renin-producing or aldosterone-producing tumor. While a complete discussion is beyond the scope of this section, measurement of plasma renin, plasma aldosterone, and calculation of a plasma aldosterone to plasma renin ratio can assist in sorting through the differential diagnosis of chloride unresponsive alkalosis (7). Rarely, evaluation for congenital adrenal enzymatic defects or parathyroid hormone function may be required.

5. CAUSES

Table 2 summarizes the differential diagnosis of metabolic alkalosis. Most cases of metabolic alkalosis are acquired in the hospital setting, including prolonged nasogastric suctioning, contraction alkalosis from aggressive diuresis, posthypercapnia, recovery from lactic acidosis or ketoacidosis, or carbohydrate refeeding after starvation. These

Table 2
Differential Diagnosis of Metabolic Alkalosis

Mechanism	Disorder	Urine [Cl⁻]
Exogenous alkali	Acute alkali administration	↓
	Regional citrate anticoagulation	?
	Milk–alkali syndrome	↓
Intravascular volume	*Gastrointestinal or other (non-renal)*	
contraction,	Pyloric stenosis	↓
Normotension,	Vomiting	↓
K⁺ deficiency,	Bulimia	↓
2° Hyperreninemic	Gastric aspiration	↓
hyperaldosteronism	Gastrocystoplasty	↑
	Congenital chloride diarrhea	↓
	Villous adenoma	↓
	Cystic fibrosis (sweat Cl⁻) loss	↓
	Renal	
	Diuretics (especially thiazide and loop diuretics)	↑ or ↓
	Edematous states	↓
	Posthypercapnia	↓
	Hypercalcemia–hypoparathyroidism	?
	Recovery from lactic acidosis or ketoacidosis	↓
	Nonreabsorbable anions such as penicillin, carbenicillin	↓
	Mg^{2+} deficiency	↑
	K⁺ depletion	↑ or ↓
	Bartter Syndrome	↑
	Gitelman Syndrome	↑
	Carbohydrate refeeding after starvation	?
Intravascular volume	*Associated with high renin*	
expansion, hypertension,	Renal artery stenosis	↑
K⁺ deficiency, hypermin-	Accelerated hypertension	↑
eralocorticoidism	Renin-secreting tumor	↑
	Estrogen therapy	↑
	Associated with low renin	
	Primary aldosteronism	
	Adenoma	↑
	Hyperplasia	↑
	Carcinoma	↑
	Glucocorticoid suppressible	↑
	Adrenal enzymatic defects	
	11β-Hydroxylase deficiency	↑
	17α-Hydroxylase deficiency	↑

Table 2
(Continued)

Mechanism	Disorder	Urine [Cl⁻]
	Cushing syndrome or disease	
	Ectopic corticotropin	↑
	Adrenal carcinoma	↑
	Adrenal adenoma	↑
	Primary pituitary	↑
	Other	
	Licorice	↑
	Carbenoxolone	↑
	Chewing tobacco	↑
Intravascular volume	Liddle syndrome	↑
expansion	Apparent mineralocorticoid excess syndrome	↑
hypertension		
K⁺ deficiency		
hyporeninemic		
hypoaldosteronism		

presentations will respond to early recognition and treatment of alkalosis and resolve with improvement in the underlying disease process.

Critical Care: Circumstances unique to the critical care setting may lead to alkalosis and contribute significantly to morbidity in critically ill patients. In patients recovering from respiratory acidosis, an appropriate renal response to acidosis may persist for several days after hypercapnia has resolved. The resulting avid retention of bicarbonate by the kidneys, often exacerbated by decreased intravascular volume and hypokalemia created by the necessary use of diuretics, creates a state of metabolic alkalosis. Once recognized, attention to restoring intravascular volume, potassium and chloride stores is usually sufficient to correct alkalosis. Alkalosis is a frequent complication of cardiac surgery and is strongly associated with younger age, cardiopulmonary bypass, preoperative ductal dependency, and perioperative hemodilution *(8)*. The use of regional citrate anticoagulation in patients requiring continuous renal replacement therapies can lead to alkalosis through its metabolism in Krebs cycle to bicarbonate *(9)*. This phenomenon is often referred to as citrate loc or citrate gap. Citrate-induced alkalosis responds to decreased citrate infusion rates, increased clearance rates, and/or saline infusion *(10, 11)*.

Chloride Responsive Alkalosis: While most cases of chloride responsive alkalosis are acquired in the hospital setting as a result of nasogastric suctioning, drainage, or emesis, several diseases should be considered in the differential diagnosis. Alkalosis is a classic presentation of pyloric stenosis in infants. Infants with a recent history of emesis and presence of alkalosis should be evaluated by abdominal ultrasound, and fluid resuscitation with correction of alkalosis should precede surgical correction when possible to minimize surgical and anesthetic morbidity *(12–15)*. Cystic fibrosis is unique among diseases that may present with chloride responsive alkalosis because chloride loss is through the skin, via excessive sweat chloride loss, rather than through the GI tract *(16–18)*. Patients with eating disorders frequently present with alkalosis as a result of bulimia. However, measurement of urine chloride is particularly important. If urine chloride is excessive in a patient with a history of eating disorder, diuretic abuse should be considered *(19)*. Congenital chloride diarrhea is frequently listed in the differential diagnosis, but rarely seen. While congenital chloride diarrhea can be fatal if not recognized, once identified treatment consists of NaCl and KCl replacement, with an excellent long-term prognosis *(20, 21)*. Villous adenoma is often listed in the differential diagnosis of alkalosis, but no reports of this association were found in a review of the pediatric literature.

Chloride Unresponsive Alkalosis: A finding of chloride unresponsive alkalosis should prompt studies for primary renal and endocrine disorders once acquired alkalosis from diuretic use/abuse or glycyrrhizic acid (licorice, licorice root) *(22)* has been ruled out. The differential diagnosis of chloride unresponsive alkalosis can be refined by consideration of blood pressure. Disorders in which the primary defect is renal chloride wasting such as Bartter syndrome, Gitelman syndrome, and diuretic abuse present with hypotension and secondary (compensatory) increases in aldosterone activity. Alternatively, disorders in which increased mineralocorticoid production or renal tubular activity mimicking increased mineralocorticoid activity present with hypertension.

Three renal tubular disorders account for most cases of renal-mediated alkalosis: Bartter syndrome, Gitelman syndrome, and Liddle's syndrome. Both Bartter and Gitelman syndromes present with normotension or hypotension, while Liddle syndrome presents with hypertension. While molecular diagnostic techniques continue to clarify the transport mechanisms involved in these disorders, considering each by its site of action in the nephron can help us understand the various clinical presentations and guide therapy. Bartter syndrome and its variants arise from mutations in electrolyte transporters in the thick ascending limb (TAL) of the loop of Henle, Gitelman syndrome from electrolyte transport defects in the distal convoluted tubule, and Liddle syndrome from a defective transporter in the collecting duct.

Bartter Syndrome: To date, four types of Bartter syndrome have been identified based on molecular identification of mutations in TAL transmembrane proteins *(23–25)*. These defective proteins include an electroneutral bumetanide-sensitive luminal Na–2Cl–K cotransporter (NKCC2) (type 1), a luminal potassium channel: ROMK (type 2), a basolateral membrane chloride channel: CLCNKB (type 3), and a subunit of two basolateral chloride channels (CLCNKA and CLCNKB): Barttin (type 4 also associated with sensorineural deafness). Molecular characterization has significantly improved our understanding of these disorders but has not, to date, led to specific therapies. Description of Bartter-like or Gitelman-like syndromes whose physiology and genetics have not yet been described *(26)* suggests that additional mutations might be found. A rare genetic Bartter-like syndrome with hypocalcemia due to activation of the calcium sensing receptor *(27)* and an acquired Bartter-like syndrome following the use of gentamicin *(28)* have been reported.

Despite the various mutations, it is helpful to think of all Bartter syndrome types as a genetic model resembling loop diuretic abuse. All the mutations above lead to urine chloride wasting, with resulting hypovolemia and hypotension. Secondary aldosterone release to compensate for the hypovolemia leads to further potassium and proton loss and maintenance of a chronic hypokalemic, hypochloremic metabolic alkalosis. Types 1, 2, and 4 typically present in newborns (neonatal Bartter), often with a history of polyhydramnios and premature birth. Classic Bartter syndrome (Type 3) may present at birth, but can also present later in infancy. On occasion, patients with neonatal Bartter (usually type 2) may present initially with a hyperkalemic metabolic acidosis and hyponatremia before developing the classic picture of hypokalemic metabolic alkalosis *(29)*. Clinical and laboratory features of Bartter syndrome include: polydipsia, polyuria, salt craving, growth retardation, dehydration, nephrocalcinosis (in neonatal types), high urine NaCl excretion, increased urine calcium excretion (in most cases), impaired urine concentrating ability, hyperreninism/hyperaldosteronism with normo- to hypotension, increased prostaglandin production, and hypertrophy of the juxtaglomerular apparatus.

Gitelman Syndrome: If loop diuretic abuse serves as a pharmacologic analogy for Bartter syndrome, Gitelman syndrome can be understood as analogous to thiazide diuretic abuse. Distal convoluted tubule (DCT) mutations account for the clinical findings. In particular, impaired sodium reabsorption by a thiazide-sensitive NaCl cotransporter (NCCT) is responsible. While both Bartter syndrome and Gitelman syndrome present with metabolic alkalosis, patients with Gitelman syndrome typically present later in childhood or adolescence, usually complaining of fatigue, weakness, muscle cramps, seizures, or tetany. Other features that help to distinguish Gitelman from Bartter include the absence of polyuria/polydipsia, the absence of growth retardation, the absence of nephrocalcinosis and associated hypercalciuria, and the presence of hypomagnesemia.

Liddle syndrome: Unlike the tubular defects in Bartter and Gitelman syndromes, which cause chronic salt-wasting and hypotension, the defect in Liddle syndrome causes sodium and volume retention, and hypertension, mimicking states of aldosterone excess. The disease is caused by mutations in the distal tubule amiloride-sensitive epithelial Na channel (ENaC), resulting in a sodium channel that is essentially "always open." The resulting excess reabsorption of sodium leads to volume overload, with secondary increased loss of potassium and protons in the urine, leading to hypokalemic metabolic alkalosis. Liddle syndrome is often found during evaluations for secondary hypertension, with initial findings of hypokalemic alkalosis, very low plasma renin activity and serum aldosterone, and a family history of hypertension in younger individuals following an autosomal dominant pattern.

Apparent Mineralocorticoid Excess Syndrome (AME): AME is a rare inherited disorder that, like Liddle syndrome, presents with hypokalemic metabolic alkalosis and low-renin, low aldosterone hypertension mimicking hyperaldosteronism. It is caused by a deficiency of a renal isozyme of 11β-hydroxysteroid dehydrogenase. In the absence of this enzyme, cortisol is not being oxidized to cortisone. Cortisol, unlike cortisone, binds to the renal mineralocorticoid receptors. Since cortisol binds as avidly as aldosterone to the mineralocorticoid receptor but its serum level is 100 times higher than that of aldosterone, the end result is very excessive mineralocorticoid activity, causing sodium retention, hypertension, and hypokalemic alkalosis *(30)*. The pharmacologic analog to AME is chronic glycyrrhizic acid (licorice, licorice root) ingestion, which competitively inhibits the 11β-hydroxysteroid dehydrogenase.

AME is usually transmitted as an autosomal recessive trait. It is characterized by low birth weight, failure to thrive, very early onset of hypertension, and damage to end organs. Those with the more severe form of AME also exhibit hypercalciuria, nephrocalcinosis, and renal failure. A milder phenotype was reported in adults with compound heterozygous mutations.

Glucocorticoid-Remediable Aldosteronism (GRA): GRA is typically diagnosed during evaluations for low-renin hypertension in families with a strong history of childhood hypertension in an autosomal-dominant pattern. Nevertheless, it may present additionally with laboratory features of hypokalemia and metabolic alkalosis. The somewhat awkward (but physiologically appropriate) name of this disorder provides insight into the pathophysiology: patients with GRA have a chimeric gene in the adrenal zona fasciculata linking the promoter sequence of the 11β-hydroxylase gene (which normally promotes cortisol synthesis in response to ACTH) to the coding sequence of aldosterone synthase. With this mutation, aldosterone is produced in response to ACTH (instead of by angiotensin II and potassium in the zona glomerulosa, as in unaffected individuals), resulting in adrenal hyperplasia and excessive aldosterone production. Glucocorticoid administration reduces ACTH production, thus decreasing aldosterone production by the chimeric gene *(31)* and improvement in hypertension, hypokalemia, and alkalosis. Interestingly some patients with GRA are normokalemic probably due to the circadian rhythm of ACTH secretion and lack of effect of dietary potassium on aldosterone secretion. Patients with GRA respond by profound hypokalemia to thiazide administration. GRA has also been called Familial Hyperaldosteronism Type I. A form of Familial Hyperaldosteronism (Type II) that is not responsive to glucocorticoids has also been described, and its genomics and proteomics are currently being investigated *(32)*.

Mineralocorticoid Receptor Gain of Function: A recently described mutation adds to the mechanisms related to increased aldosterone activity and chloride-resistant hypertensive metabolic alkalosis *(33)*. In this disorder, the aldosterone receptor itself is mutated and is activated by not only aldosterone, but also by cortisol, cortisone, and progesterone.

Primary hyperreninemia: States of primary renin overproduction leading to significant hypertension and metabolic alkalosis are rare in children, and usually are secondary to renal artery stenosis. Several types of renin-producing tumors have been described in children and adults, including tumors of the juxtaglomerular apparatus, Wilms' tumor, and a rhabdoid tumor of the kidney *(34, 35)*.

Primary Aldosteronism: In adults, increasing attention is being paid to states of increased aldosterone activity as a cause of hypertension *(7, 36)*. In children, adrenocortical adenoma, adrenocortical carcinoma, and bilateral nodular hyperplasia have been described *(37–41)*, but are quite rare. Renal and adrenal imaging, along with measurement of plasma renin and aldosterone levels (see "Section 4") can aid in the diagnosis.

Adrenal Enzyme Defects: Although one usually thinks of congenital adrenal hyperplasia (CAH) presenting as classic 21-hydroxylase deficiency (salt wasting, hypotension, hyperkalemia), two autosomal recessive rare variants of CAH may present with hypertension, hypokalemia, metabolic alkalosis, and low plasma renin activity: 11β-hydroxylase deficiency and 17α-hydroxylase deficiency *(42)*. 11β-Hydroxylase deficiency is the second most common form of CAH, accounting for 5–8% of cases of CAH. Virilization secondary to excess adrenal androgen secretion is a characteristic finding. 17α-Hydroxylase deficiency accounts for approximately 1% of CAH. Underproduction of testosterone leads to undervirilized genitalia in males, and in girls who fail to develop secondary sex characteristics at puberty. In both disorders, overproduction of deoxycorticosterone (DOC), an aldosterone precursor, is responsible for hyperreninemic, hypervolemic hypertension, hypokalemia, and metabolic alkalosis.

Cushing Syndrome: Hypertension is common in patients receiving exogenous corticosteroids and in those with Cushing's disease. The mechanisms contributing to metabolic alkalosis in patients with states of glucocorticoid excess probably include the mineralocorticoid effects of glucocorticoids and, in patients with endogenous overproduction of glucocorticoids, the concomitant overproduction of aldosterone precursors with mineralocorticoid effects.

6. TREATMENT

6.1. Chloride Responsive Alkalosis

Chloride responsive alkalosis is characterized by intravascular volume contraction, hypo- or normotension, chloride deficiency, potassium deficiency, and secondary hyperreninemic hyperaldosteronism. Once alkalosis is established, correction of intravascular volume, chloride deficit, and potassium deficit is necessary to reverse the alkalosis. In severe, symptomatic, or life-threatening cases, urgent correction of alkalosis with acid administration may be required. Ultimately, identification and, if possible, removal or treatment of the underlying cause is the goal.

Restoring Intravascular Volume: Assessment of intravascular volume and calculation of fluid deficit has been addressed elsewhere in this volume. To facilitate correction of alkalosis, the fluid deficit should be replaced with isotonic saline: the administered chloride is necessary to facilitate renal tubular exchange of bicarbonate for chloride, and the correction of volume deficit is necessary to reverse the secondary hyperaldosteronism, which contributes to ongoing potassium and proton loss if not corrected. Once intravascular volume is restored and additional maintenance and ongoing losses are provided for, attention can then focus on whether chloride and potassium deficits still exist.

Restoring Chloride Deficit: Once euvolemia has been restored, total body chloride deficit can be calculated using the formula

$$Cl^- \, deficit\,(mEq) = 0.2 \times Body\,Weight\,(kg) \times (100 - patient\,[Cl^-])$$

For example, for a 20 kg patient with a $[Cl^-] = 90$ mEq/L,

$$Cl^- \, deficit\,(mEq) = 0.2 \times 20 \times (100 - 90)$$
$$= 4 \times 10$$
$$= 40\,mEq$$

Thus, for the above example, an additional 40 mEq of Cl⁻ should be added to calculations of the patient's maintenance and ongoing losses (if any). Whether to give the Cl⁻ as NaCl or as KCl will depend on whether the patient also has an accompanying potassium deficit. When in doubt, assume that patients with metabolic alkalosis have a total body potassium deficit unless there is decreased GFR and provide the bulk of chloride deficit replacement as KCl.

Restoring Potassium Deficit: Correction of intravascular volume with isotonic saline and subsequent correction of chloride deficit with KCl is usually sufficient to correct total body potassium deficit. After initial fluid resuscitation, KCl in concentrations of 10–20 mEq/L should be added to maintenance fluids. In cases of severe hypokalemia, particularly those associated with cardiac arrhythmias or neuromuscular complications, additional oral or intravenous potassium may be needed.

Urgent Correction of Alkalosis: When alkalosis contributes to deteriorating clinical status in critically ill patients (for example, cardiac arrhythmia, digitalis cardiotoxicity, altered mental status, hepatic encephalopathy), typically when serum pH > 7.55, intravenous administration of acid, either as HCl or NH_4Cl may be considered. HCl, administered as an isotonic solution (150 mEq/L HCl) must be given through a central venous catheter with demonstrated good flow. The infusion rate should not exceed 25 mEq/h. The dose of HCl, in mEq, is calculated as follows:

$$HCl\, dose\, (mEq) = 0.5 \times Body\, Weight\, (kg) \times (patient\, [HCO_3^-] - 24\, mEq/L)/2$$

Note (at the end of the equation) that for an initial correction, the difference between the patient $[HCO_3^-]$ and a normal $[HCO_3^-]$ (24 mEq/L) is divided by 2 to provide a "1/2" correction. The goal is to decrease symptoms of sever alkalosis, and rapid correction to a "normal" value may increase the risk of complications, particularly in patients whose course is complicated by chronic respiratory acidosis. For example, for a 20 kg patient with an $HCO_3^- = 34$ mEq/L,

$$
\begin{aligned}
HCl\, dose &= 0.5 \times 20\, kg \times (34\, mEq/L - 24\, mEq/L)2 \\
&= 10 \times 10/2 \\
&= 50\, mEq
\end{aligned}
$$

HCl should be infused over 8–24 h. In this example, 50 mEq of a 150 mEq/L solution of HCl yields a volume of 333 ml. For an 8 h infusion, the rate would be 42 ml/h (6.3 mEq/h), and for a 24 h infusion, the rate would be 14 ml/h (2.25 mEq/h). The expected $[HCO_3^-]$ from this "1/2 correction" would be 29–30 mEq/L.

NH_4Cl has been used as an alternative to HCl particularly when no central venous access is available, as it may be given through a peripheral line. NH_4Cl is contraindicated in patients with severe hepatic or renal disease. There is little pediatric experience with this therapy, and use should be limited to the critical care setting. Dose (in mEq) is calculated using the same formula as that for HCl. Typical administration is to prepare a 200 mEq/L solution and infuse over 3–6 h, with a maximum infusion rate of 1 mEq/kg/h. Monitor serum electrolytes and ammonia levels during therapy.

In patients with edematous states, particularly those with decreased GFR and oliguria, administration of NaCl or KCl may be contraindicated. NaCl administration
can contribute to volume overload and edema, while KCl administration may lead
to life-threatening hyperkalemia. If some residual renal function is present (GFR >
20–30 ml/min), acetazolamide, a carbonic anhydrase inhibitor, may increase urinary
bicarbonate losses in exchange for increased acid reabsorption. Careful attention should
be paid to serum electrolytes, as acetazolamide may contribute to hypovolemia and
hypokalemia. Chronic use of carbonic-anhydrase inhibitors can result in nephrocalcinosis and urolithiasis.

In patients with renal failure (GFR < 20 ml/min) dialysis against a high-chloride
dialysis bath will exchange bicarbonate for chloride and correct alkalosis.

Correcting the Underlying Cause: If ongoing gastric loss of HCl is identified, gastric
HCl production can be decreased with H_2-receptor blockers or proton pump inhibitors.
If possible, diuretics particularly loop or thiazide diuretics should be decreased or discontinued and if their use is obligatory, it should be supplemented by KCl or K-sparing
diuretics.

6.2. Chloride Unresponsive Alkalosis

Chloride unresponsive forms of alkalosis are less common than chloride responsive
types. With the exception of diuretic abuse and licorice ingestion, which resolve with
discontinuation of the offending substance, treatment of other forms of chloride unresponsive alkalosis requires recognition of the underlying diagnosis and specific treatment for that disorder.

Bartter Syndrome: No mechanism-specific treatment for Bartter syndrome has yet
been identified. Treatment consists of decreasing the fluid and electrolyte losses as much
as possible and replacement of remaining deficits. Current therapy consists primarily
of prostaglandin synthesis inhibition and potassium replacement. Most clinical experience is with indomethacin (2–5 mg/kg daily) or ibuprofen (30 mg/kg daily). A specific
COX-2 inhibitor, rofecoxib, has also been used with good results *(24)*, but experience
is limited and further trials needed. With chronic use of any NSAID, careful attention
should be paid to symptoms suggestive of toxicity. In addition to prostaglandin synthesis inhibition, potassium supplementation, in the form of KCl, is usually required, with
patients typically requiring 1–5 mEq/kg daily. Spironolactone and amiloride have also
been used; they have the advantage of Mg-sparing but also carry the risk of worsening
intravascular volume depletion, particularly in infants and young children.

Spironolactone may be superior to amiloride, as it blocks the effect of high serum
levels of aldosterone *(43)*. Enalapril and other angiotensin converting enzyme inhibitors
have also been used with some success, but no clear recommendation has yet emerged.
Their introduction should be gradual due to the risk of hypotension. No treatment for
nephrocalcinosis has been described. The use of thiazide diuretics to reduce urinary
calcium excretion is contraindicated, as thiazides exacerbate the tubule defects seen in
Bartter syndrome. Children with Bartter syndrome are particularly sensitive to dehydration during acute illnesses, and early evaluation for fluid and electrolyte problems
should occur during times of decreased oral intake or increased GI losses.

Gitelman Syndrome: For Gitelman syndrome, like Bartter syndrome, no defect-specific therapy has yet been identified, and therapy consists of potassium and magnesium replacement. The roles of prostaglandin synthesis inhibitors and K-sparing diuretics need further investigation.

Liddle Syndrome: Early descriptions of Liddle syndrome, before the molecular mechanisms were identified, demonstrated that patients responded to amiloride, but not to spironolactone, suggesting that the defect was directly in the tubule, and not a tubular response to mineralocorticoid. Amiloride remains the drug of choice. Hypertension in Liddle syndrome is particularly salt sensitive, and dietary sodium restriction is also an important part of therapy.

Apparent Mineralocorticoid Excess Syndrome: Spironolactone, a mineralocorticoid receptor blocker, targets the defect in AME and is an effective treatment.

Glucocorticoid Remediable Aldosteronism (GRA): As the name implies, hypertension and hypokalemia in GRA respond to ACTH suppression with glucocorticoids. However, because of the side effects of chronic glucocorticoid use, spironolactone or amiloride may also be used.

Aldosterone Excess States: Inhibition of mineralocorticoid effects with spironolactone is useful as initial therapy in states of primary mineralocorticoid or glucocorticoid excess, but definitive diagnosis and treatment (beyond the scope of this section) are often curative.

CASE SCENARIOS

(a) Easy Fix or a Life-Long Problem?

A 3-month-old infant presents with a 1 week history of poor oral intake, vomiting, and increasing lethargy. Parents note decreased tears, one wet diaper over the past 24 h, and four to five episodes of emesis over the past 24 h. There is no history of diarrhea, no fever, and there are no ill contacts. On presentation, the heart rate is 140/min, the blood pressure is 80/45 mmHg, respiratory rate is 18/min, and temperature is 37°F. On physical exam, the child is difficult to arouse, the anterior fontanel is sunken, there are decreased tears, mucus membranes are sticky, eyes are slightly sunken, capillary refill is >2 s.

A. Initial therapy: Regardless of our ultimate findings, the child in this vignette is severely dehydrated, with a fluid deficit of 10–15%. Initial evaluation should include assessment of renal function, acid–base status, and electrolyte status. Because of the severe degree of dehydration, intravenous fluid resuscitation should begin immediately with 20 ml/kg boluses of isotonic saline.

B. Initial laboratory values: Just before a fluid bolus has been given, the initial laboratory values are as follows:

Na =	132 mEq/L
K =	2.5 mEq/L
Cl =	88 mEq/L
BUN =	30 mg/dL
Creatinine =	0.9 mg/dL

pH =   7.50
pCO$_2$ =   47 mmHg
HCO$_3^-$ =   36 mEq/L

A pH of 7.5 reflects alkalosis, not a typical finding since most infants with severe dehydration present with metabolic acidosis. Using the equations in Table 1 to determine if the alkalosis is primary metabolic with an appropriate respiratory compensation, or instead represents a mixed acid–base disorder:

Method 1: Compensated PaCO$_2$ = 40 + [0.7 (patient [HCO$_3^-$] – normal [HCO$_3^-$])]
In this case the patient's serum [HCO$_3^-$] has increased from normal for age of 22 mEq/L to 32 mEq/L:

Compensated PaCO$_2$ = 40 + [0.7 (32–22)]
Compensated PaCO$_2$ = 40 + 7
Compensated PaCO$_2$ = 47

Method 2: Compensated PaCO$_2$ = patient [HCO$_3^-$] + 15
In this case, the patient has a serum [HCO$_3^-$] = 32

Compensated PaCO$_2$ = 32 + 15
Compensated PaCO$_2$ = 47

Either equation can be used to demonstrate that the patient has a primary metabolic alkalosis with an appropriate respiratory compensation (decrease in ventilation to raise pCO$_2$).

C. Further diagnosis and treatment are guided by measurement of urine electrolytes, particularly urine [Cl$^-$] (Fig. 1). We will consider two likely diagnostic possibilities based on the patient's urine [Cl$^-$]:

Case Scenario 1: The patient's urine [Cl$^-$] is <5 mEq/L and urine pH is >6.5. The urine results reflect an appropriate renal response to HCl loss from a non-renal site, or exogenous HCO$_3^-$ administration. The history of vomiting and poor oral intake point to gastric HCl loss (rather than alkali administration) as the alkalosis-generating step, with maintenance of alkalosis promoted by a decreased GFR from dehydration, and hypokalemia from both decreased oral intake and increased urine loss from secondary hyperaldosteronism (an appropriate response to volume depletion, but one which has an unintended consequence of maintaining alkalosis). The increased aldosterone activity also contributes to alkalosis by increasing urinary H$^+$ loss.

Investigation of causes for vomiting in a 3-month-old should include abdominal imaging, with ultrasound being the study of choice. In this case, a finding of pyloric stenosis explains the metabolic alkalosis. Pyloric stenosis is a surgically treatable lesion, but to minimize the chance of anesthetic and intraoperative complications, fluid deficit and alkalosis should be corrected prior to surgery. After initial fluid resuscitation, fluid deficit should again be estimated, with a goal to replace the fluid deficit over 24 h with isotonic saline. Potassium can be added to maintenance fluids at concentration of 10–20 mEq/L. If either potassium or chloride fails to correct with initial fluid therapy, additional KCl can be added to replace the chloride deficit:

$$Cl^- \text{deficit} \, (mEq) = 0.2 \times \text{Body Weight} \, (kg) \times (100 - \text{patient} \, [Cl^-])$$

In this case, for patient with a $[Cl^-] = 90$ mEq/L and weight $= 6$ kg,

$$
\begin{aligned}
Cl^- \text{deficit} \, (mEq) &= 0.2 \times 6 \times (100 - 88) \\
&= 1.2 \times 12 \\
&= 14.4 \, mEq, \text{or approximately } 2 - 3 \, mEq/kg \text{ of KCl in addition} \\
&\quad \text{to maintenance KCl.}
\end{aligned}
$$

Case Scenario 2: While metabolic alkalosis secondary to gastric loss in pyloric stenosis is a classic presentation in pediatrics, measurement of urine $[Cl^-]$ can sometimes reveal surprises. In this scenario, urine $[Cl^-] = 35$ mEq/L. In a patient with a serum $[Cl^-] = 88$ mEq/L, this is an inappropriate renal loss, and reflects an underlying problem with renal mechanisms to preserve chloride. Since the patient is relatively hypotensive, with evidence of severe intravascular volume depletion, reference to Fig. 1 points to renal tubular defects, diuretic abuse, or severe K^+ or Mg^+ deficiency. The history in this case is not suggestive of dietary deficiency or medication administration, and the most likely diagnosis is Bartter syndrome or Gitelman syndrome. An ultrasound finding of nephrocalcinosis would suggest neonatal Bartter syndrome, but is not seen in all cases. To further differentiate Bartter from Gitelman syndromes, measurement of urine calcium excretion (usually high in Bartter, low in Gitelman is helpful). Serum magnesium is typically low in Gitelman, and normal in Bartter. While initial fluid resuscitation should follow guidelines for all dehydrated patients, once euvolemia has been established, disease-specific therapy must be initiated to prevent further serious decompensation.

(b) When metabolic alkalosis is combined with hypertension

A 3-year-old is brought to the Emergency Department for an ear infection. Vital signs show blood pressure of 150/100 mmHg, confirmed by repeat measurements. The family history is positive for the biological father having hypertension who since young age was treated by a medicine unknown to the mother. Besides the ear infection the rest of the physical examination is unremarkable. Blood work shows Na 136, K 2.8, Cl 86, HCO_3 34 mEq/l, creatinine 0.5, Ca 9.6, P 4.2 mg/dL. Urinalysis is normal.

What is your next step in evaluating the metabolic alkalosis?

As always, the first step is assessment of urine chloride, which is 38 mEq/L.

The child has chloride resistant metabolic alkalosis with hypertension.

As shown in Fig. 1 and Table 1, in such cases assessment of PRA and serum aldosterone is crucial in establishing the diagnosis. In this case, both were very low. The family history in this case indicates Liddle syndrome rather than AME. In the future, genetic studies will provide the definitive diagnosis.

Contrary to most cases of metabolic alkalosis, which are associated with hypovolemia, the rare situation of metabolic alkalosis combined with hypertension is caused by hypervolemia. Therefore, there is no indication to treat with NaCl, which may aggravate the hypertension. Treatment of Liddle syndrome requires the use of K-sparing diuretics as discussed above.

REFERENCES

1. DuBose TD. Acid–Base Disorders. In: Brenner BM, ed. Brenner and Rector's The Kidney. 7 ed. Philadelphia: W.B. Saunders Company; 2003:969–976.
2. Laski ME, Sabatini S. Metabolic alkalosis, bedside and bench. Seminars in Nephrology 2006;26: 404–421.
3. Galla JH. Metabolic alkalosis. American Journal of Nephrology 2000;11:369–375.
4. Rose BD, Post TW. Metabolic Alkalosis. In: Clinical Physiology of Acid–Base and Electrolyte Disorders. 5 ed. New York: McGraw Hill Medical Publishing Division; 2001:551–572.
5. Malafronte C, Borsa N, Tedeschi S, et al. Cardiac arrhythmias due to severe hypokalemia in a patient with classic Bartter disease. Pediatric Nephrology 2004;19:1413–1415.
6. Toto RD, Alpern, R.J. Metabolic acid–base disorders. In: Kokko JP, Tannen R.L., ed. Fluids and Electrolytes. 3 ed. Philadelphia: W.B. Saunders Company; 1996:241–256.
7. Pimenta E, Calhoun DA. Primary aldosteronism: diagnosis and treatment. Journal of Clinical Hypertension 2006;8:887–893.
8. van Thiel RJ, Koopman SR, Takkenberg JJM, Ten Harkel ADJ, Bogers AJJC. Metabolic alkalosis after pediatric cardiac surgery. European Journal of Cardio-Thoracic Surgery 2005;28:229–233.
9. Barletta G-M, Bunchman TE. Acute renal failure in children and infants. Current Opinion in Critical Care 2004;10:499–504.
10. Morgera S, Scholle C, Voss G, et al. Metabolic complications during regional citrate anticoagulation in continuous venovenous hemodialysis: single-center experience. Nephron 2004;97: c131–136.
11. Gabutti L, Marone C, Colucci G, Duchini F, Schonholzer C. Citrate anticoagulation in continuous venovenous hemodiafiltration: a metabolic challenge. Intensive Care Medicine 2002;28:1419–1425.
12. Blumer SL, Zucconi WB, Cohen HL, Scriven RJ, Lee TK. The vomiting neonate: a review of the ACR appropriateness criteria and ultrasound's role in the workup of such patients. Ultrasound Quarterly 2004;20:79–89.
13. MacMahon B. The continuing enigma of pyloric stenosis of infancy: a review [see comment]. Epidemiology 2006;17:195–201.
14. Dinkevich E, Ozuah PO. Pyloric stenosis. Pediatrics in Review 2000;21:249–250.
15. Hernanz-Schulman M. Infantile hypertrophic pyloric stenosis. Radiology 2003;227:319–331.
16. Bates CM, Baum M, Quigley R. Cystic fibrosis presenting with hypokalemia and metabolic alkalosis in a previously healthy adolescent. Journal of the American Society of Nephrology 1997;8: 352–355.
17. Fustik S, Pop-Jordanova N, Slaveska N, Koceva S, Efremov G. Metabolic alkalosis with hypoelectrolytemia in infants with cystic fibrosis. Pediatrics International 2002;44:289–292.
18. Salvatore D, Tomaiuolo R, Abate R, et al. Cystic fibrosis presenting as metabolic alkalosis in a boy with the rare D579G mutation. Journal of Cystic Fibrosis 2004;3:135–136.
19. Woywodt A, Herrmann A, Eisenberger U, Schwarz A, Haller H. The tell-tale urinary chloride [see comment]. Nephrology Dialysis Transplantation 2001;16:1066–1068.
20. Hihnala S, Hoglund P, Lammi L, Kokkonen J, Ormala T, Holmberg C. Long-term clinical outcome in patients with congenital chloride diarrhea. Journal of Pediatric Gastroenterology & Nutrition 2006;42:369–375.
21. Lok K-H, Hung H-G, Li K-K, Li K-F, Szeto M-L. Congenital chloride diarrhea: a missed diagnosis in an adult patient. American Journal of Gastroenterology 2007;102:1328–1329.

22. Lin S-H, Yang S-S, Chau T, Halperin ML. An unusual cause of hypokalemic paralysis: chronic licorice ingestion. American Journal of the Medical Sciences 2003;325:153–156.
23. Ellison DH. Divalent cation transport by the distal nephron: insights from Bartter's and Gitelman's syndromes. American Journal of Physiology - Renal Physiology 2000;279:F616–625.
24. Kleta R, Bockenhauer D. Bartter syndromes and other salt-losing tubulopathies. Nephron Physiology 2006;104:73–80.
25. Shaer AJ. Inherited primary renal tubular hypokalemic alkalosis: a review of Gitelman and Bartter syndromes. American Journal of the Medical Sciences 2001;322:316–332.
26. Laine J, Jalanko H, Alakulppi N, Holmberg C. A new tubular disorder with hypokalaemic metabolic alkalosis, severe hypermagnesuric hypomagnesaemia, hypercalciuria and cardiomyopathy. Nephrology Dialysis Transplantation 2005;20:1241–1245.
27. Watanabe S, Fukumoto S, Chang H, et al. Association between activating mutations of calcium-sensing receptor and Bartter's syndrome. Lancet 2002;360:692–694.
28. Chou C-L, Chen Y-H, Chau T, Lin S-H. Acquired Bartter-like syndrome associated with gentamicin administration. American Journal of the Medical Sciences 2005;329:144–149.
29. Rodriguez-Soriano J. Tubular Disorders of Electrolyte Regulation. In: Avner ED, Harmon WE, Niaudet P, ed. Pediatric Nephrology. 5 ed. Philadelphia: Lippincott Williams & Wilkins; 2004: 729–741.
30. Moudgil A, Rodich G, Jordan SC, Kamil ES. Nephrocalcinosis and renal cysts associated with apparent mineralocorticoid excess syndrome. Pediatric Nephrology 2000;15:60–62.
31. Williams SS. Advances in genetic hypertension. Current Opinion in Pediatrics 2007;19:192–198.
32. So A, Duffy DL, Gordon RD, et al. Familial hyperaldosteronism type II is linked to the chromosome 7p22 region but also shows predicted heterogeneity. Journal of Hypertension 2005;23:1477–1484.
33. Geller DS, Farhi A, Pinkerton N, et al. Activating mineralocorticoid receptor mutation in hypertension exacerbated by pregnancy [comment]. Science 2000;289:119–123.
34. Friedman K, Wallis T, Maloney KW, Hendrickson RJ, Mengshol S, Cadnapaphornchai MA. An unusual cause of pediatric hypertension. Journal of Pediatrics 2007;151:206–212.
35. Markey RB, MacLennan GT. Juxtaglomerular cell tumor of the kidney. Journal of Urology 2006;175:730.
36. Mulatero P, Morello F, Veglio F. Genetics of primary aldosteronism. Journal of Hypertension 2004;22:663–670.
37. Abasiyanik A, Oran B, Kaymakci A, Yaar C, Calikan U, Erkul I. Conn syndrome in a child, caused by adrenal adenoma. Journal of Pediatric Surgery 1996;31:430–432.
38. Abdullah N, Khawaja K, Hale J, Barrett AM, Cheetham TD. Primary hyperaldosteronism with normokalaemia secondary to an adrenal adenoma (Conn's syndrome) in a 12 year-old boy. Journal of Pediatric Endocrinology 2005;18:215–219.
39. Baranwal AK, Singhi SC, Narshimhan KL, Jayashree M, Singhi PD, Kakkar N. Aldosterone-producing adrenocortical adenoma in childhood: a case report. Journal of Pediatric Surgery 1999;34:1878–1880.
40. Boushey RP, Dackiw AP. Adrenal cortical carcinoma. Current Treatment Options in Oncology 2001;2:355–364.
41. Rogoff D, Bergada I, Venara M, Chemes H, Heinrich JJ, Barontini M. Intermittent hyperaldosteronism in a child due to an adrenal adenoma. European Journal of Pediatrics 2001;160:114–116.
42. New MI, Ghizzoni, Lucia. Congenital Adrenal Hyperplasia. In: Lifshitz F, ed. Pediatric Endocrinology. 4 ed. New York: Marcel Dekker, Inc.; 2003:175–178.
43. Colussi G, Rombola G, De Ferrari ME, Macaluso M, Minetti L. Correction of hypokalemia with antialdosterone therapy in Gitelman's syndrome. American Journal of Nephrology 1994;14:127–135.

10 Diagnosis and Treatment of Respiratory Acidosis

Edwin Young

Key Points

1. Infants and children have limited pulmonary reserve.
2. Hypoventilation and hypoxemia are consequences of respiratory acidosis.
3. Supplemental oxygen can mask worsening respiratory acidosis.
4. Respiratory acidosis treatment is directed toward each specific cause.
5. Respiratory acidosis requires rapid assessment and stepwise treatment.

Key Words: Respiratory acidosis; acidosis; hypoventilation; hypoxemia; compliance

1. INTRODUCTION

Respiratory acidosis is a common problem of childhood. Respiratory acidosis involves ventilation difficulties and is always accompanied by oxygenation impairment. Infants and children can be compromised quickly and treatment decisions must be made rapidly.

Functional immaturity of the respiratory system places infants and children at greater risk for respiratory acidosis. Disadvantages include mechanics of the rib cage and upper airways, ventilation, gas exchange, and control of ventilation.

The adult ribs extend downward allowing more elevation during inspiration to improve mechanical efficiency; this configuration results in an oval-shaped thorax (1). Adults may obtain approximately 60% of their tidal breathing volumes from rib cage movements. In contrast infant ribs are in a parallel position oriented at right angles to the thoracic vertebrae. This forms a circular thorax creating mechanical inefficiency by preventing the ribs from elevating and increasing tidal volume Therefore infants may obtain as little as one-third of their normal tidal volume from rib cage contributions.

Infant chest wall compliance is greater than lung compliance. This compliance difference creates a greater load for the chest wall muscles (1). Any pulmonary pathology that further decreases lung compliance may exceed the infant's respiratory muscle reserve and progress to respiratory acidosis and ventilation abnormalities.

From: *Nutrition and Health: Fluid and Electrolytes in Pediatrics*
Edited by: L. G. Feld, F. J. Kaskel, DOI 10.1007/978-1-60327-225-4_10,
© Humana Press, a part of Springer Science+Business Media, LLC 2010

In infancy, the upper airway is delineated by a cephalad position of the larynx, a large epiglottis, and a horizontal tongue position, all contributing to obligatory nasal breathing. Mouth breathing can occur when the nose becomes obstructed; however, this is associated with increased work of breathing. Over the first 2 years of life, the configuration of the oropharynx takes on the adult orientation, and oropharyngeal dynamics make mouth breathing more efficient (2). Baseline airway resistances are increased in infants and small children because of the smaller diameters of proximal airways. Airway resistance may be ten times higher than the adult at rest. Any pathologic narrowing of the infant or child's upper airway can significantly increase airway resistance placing them at greater risk for respiratory acidosis.

Ventilation disturbances, including apnea and periodic breathing, are much more common in infancy. Apnea and periodic breathing can occur at various stages of sleep. Apnea can be elicited or aggravated in infants and small children by many factors. They include gastroesophageal reflux, hypothermia, hypoxia, CNS abnormalities, respiratory infections, metabolic disorders, and certain drugs. Gas exchange may be limited by a number of factors. Adults have ten times as many functional alveoli as a term infant (500 million versus 50 million) (3). This decrease in alveolar surface area puts infants at risk for lower oxygen tension in the face of a higher metabolic rate (O_2 consumption). This becomes especially important due to the newborns' ventilatory response to hypoxia producing only a transient increase in respiratory rate followed by a decrease in rate. This biphasic response is aggravated by sleep states, which can comprise up to 80% of an infant or small child's day.

Developmental factors of the respiratory system have a large impact on the clinical problems seen in pediatric respiratory acidosis. Infants and children have limited pulmonary reserve requiring alert observation and early intervention for children with respiratory difficulties.

2. DEFINITION

Respiratory acidosis results from an abnormal control of ventilation. Carbon dioxide (CO_2) production exceeds CO_2 elimination. This is a direct result of alveolar hypoventilation. Elevations of CO_2 react with H_2O to form carbonic acid (H_2CO_3). This increases the denominator in the Henderson–Hasselbalch equation resulting in lower plasma pH (see chapter on acid–base physiology) (4).

$$pH = pKa + \log\frac{[HCO_3^-]}{[H_2CO_3]}$$

Under normal conditions CO_2 is eliminated quickly because of a high diffusion gradient. Equilibrium between alveolar and arterial CO_2 is 97% complete at rest. There is <1 mmHg difference between alveolar (the number approaches a person's baseline arterial CO_2) and arterial CO_2. During exercise this difference can approach 6 mmHg (5). If control of ventilation is impaired, CO_2 elevations of 10 mmHg or more can occur quickly and respiratory acidosis will result (6).

Persistent respiratory acidosis results from chronic hypoventilation. The kidneys begin immediately to restore pH by generating HCO_3^-. The renal tubular cells recognize increased CO_2 and excrete a more acidic urine. H^+ ions are eliminated as ammonia (NH_4^+) or phosphate ($H_2PO_4^-$). Bicarbonate ions are generated in the process. Renal compensation for chronic respiratory acidosis may take several days but does not bring pH quite back to 7.4 *(7–9)*.

3. ETIOLOGY

Under normal conditions CO_2 levels are maintained in tight control by central and peripheral chemoreceptors and upper airway receptors. Central chemoreceptors in the medulla respond quickly to changes in H^+ concentration. Minute ventilation is increased to eliminate CO_2 and normalize pH. Peripheral chemoreceptors in the carotid bodies are stimulated by hypoxemia to increase ventilation *(10, 11)*. Three mechanisms can impair control of breathing and result in hypoventilation *(12)*:

1. Central decrease in respiratory drive
2. Lung and chest wall abnormalities
3. Respiratory muscle weakness

Respiratory acidosis from respiratory drive impairment occurs when lung function is normal. Drugs and diseases of the brain and spinal cord are examples of respiratory impairment causing hypoventilation. Lung and chest wall deformities by definition result in abnormal lung function *(13)*. Either decreased pulmonary compliance or increased airway resistance can result in decreased alveolar ventilation and cause respiratory acidosis. Respiratory muscle weakness may or may not be associated with normal lungs. If muscle weakness is chronic, decreased lung compliance is usually present *(11, 14, 15)*. Table 1 is an extensive list of the etiologies of respiratory acidosis.

Table 1
Causes of Respiratory Acidosis

Respiratory Drive Inhibition
    Drugs – opiates, anesthetics, sedatives, alcohol
    Head trauma
    Brain stem lesions
    Sleep apnea
    Apnea of prematurity
    Severe obesity – (Pickwickian syndrome)
Neuromuscular disease
    Cervical cord trauma
    Neuromuscular junction disorders
        Botulism
        Tetanus
        Myasthenia gravis
        Paralyzing drugs

(Continued)

Table 1
(Continued)

Demyelinating disease
    Guillain–Barre syndrome?
    Multiple sclerosis
    Amyotrophic lateral sclerosis
    Poliomyelitis
    Transverse myelitis
Skeletal muscle abnormalities
    Electrolyte disorders
        Hypokalemia
        Hypophosphatemia
    Myxedema
    Myositis
    Dermatomyositis
    Lupus
    Myopathies
        Muscular dystrophy
        Spinal muscle atrophy
    Respiratory muscle fatigue
    Mechanical ventilation (permissive hypercapnia)
Obstructive disorders
    Upper airway obstruction
        Aspiration
        Laryngotracheobronchitis
        Laryngomalacia
        Vocal cord paralysis
        Foreign body aspiration
        Vascular ring
        Laryngospasm
        Subglottic stenosis
Asthma
Bronchopulmonary dysplasia (BPD)
Chronic obstructive pulmonary disease (COPD)
Restrictive disorders:
    Pneumonia/empyema
    Surfactant deficiency
    Acute lung injury/adult respiratory distress syndrome
    Cardiogenic pulmonary edema
    Interstitial fibrosis
    Phrenic nerve paralysis
    Kyphoscoliosis
    Pneumothorax

Hemothorax
Chylothorax
Pulmonary contusion
Flail chest
Pulmonary embolus
Cardiac arrest/cardiopulmonary resuscitation
Near drowning

Permission granted from Swenson and Hlastla *(5)*.

4. CLINICAL PRESENTATION AND EVALUATION

Patient presentation varies with etiology, duration, and severity of the underlying disease. Degree of associated hypoxemia also impacts symptoms. Supplemental oxygen while valuable can mask increasingly severe respiratory acidosis. Mild symptoms of acute respiratory acidosis include tachycardia, tachypnea, increased work of breathing, stridor, anxiety, and headache. More severe symptoms are blurred vision, confusion, hallucinations, shock, and coma *(4, 16, 17)*.

Chronic respiratory acidosis may present with sleep abnormalities, headache, daytime sleepiness, tremor, myoclonic jerks, and cor pulmonale. Patients with normally functioning CNS are agitated by moderate to severe acute respiratory acidosis. The body's defense of normal pH is strong. Respiratory work and tachypnea will mirror severity of respiratory acidosis until high levels of CO_2 are reached. Profound hypercapnia (>80) can be a CNS depressant, slowing minute ventilation and worsening respiratory acidosis *(4, 17)*. Without supplemental oxygen (O_2), the hypoxemia associated with respiratory acidosis will cause oxygen-starved tissues to switch to anaerobic metabolism resulting in metabolic acidosis. While the symptoms of respiratory acidosis may be obvious early, respiratory acidosis with high CO_2 levels may cause sufficient CNS depression to result in the loss of work of breathing and other signs of distress. This is a deceptive premorbid situation, which must be recognized and treated quickly. CNS-depressing medications can mimic high CO_2 levels and should be used with extreme caution in patients with respiratory acidosis to prevent worsening hypoventilation.

Patients with chronic respiratory acidosis have had sufficient time for renal conservation of HCO_3^- and restoration of near-normal pH. These patients are less dependent on CO_2 as a respiratory stimulant. Hypoxemia becomes a more important respiratory control. Supplemental O_2 in patients with chronic respiratory acidosis can worsen hypoventilation *(16, 18, 19)*.

Long-term consequences of chronic respiratory acidosis also occur. Elevated CO_2 directly causes increased cerebral blood flow (CBF) and cerebral blood volume (CBV) *(20)*. Over time this can raise intracranial pressure (ICP) causing headache, pseudotumor cerebri, and papilledema *(21)*. Hemoglobin (Hgb) levels rise gradually, pulmonary hypertension develops, and right heart failure may result (Fig. 1).

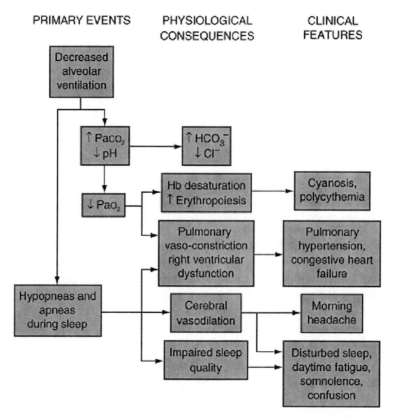

Fig. 1. Diagram showing the primary events, physiologic responses, and clinical features resulting from alveolar hypoventilation. Permission granted from Phillipson and Duffin *(68)*.

Arterial blood gas (ABG) analysis is the gold standard for assessing severity and chronicity of respiratory acidosis. The Henderson–Hasselbalch equation allows us to predict pH changes with CO_2 elevations *(22)*.

$$pH = 6.1 + \log [HCO_3^-]/(0.03 \times PCO_2)$$

Arterial CO_2 levels of greater than 44 mmHg and pH less than 7.36 are associated with respiratory acidosis. Importantly children less than 3 years of age may have a slightly lower normal CO_2 (33–37mmHg) *(23)*. The lower normal CO_2 is primarily a result of less efficient kidney reabsorption of HCO_3^- and a slightly lower baseline level.

Both HCO_3^- and pH change with CO_2 elevations. With acute respiratory acidosis CO_2 increases of 10 mmHg are accompanied by a 1 mEq/L rise in HCO_3^- and a 0.08 unit fall in pH. For chronic respiratory acidosis CO_2 increases of 10 mmHg reflect 4 mEq/l elevations in HCO_3^- and a 0.03 unit fall in pH *(24, 25)* (Fig. 2).

Hypoxemia is an additional consequence of respiratory acidosis. Alveolar O_2 determines arterial O_2. If alveolar O_2 is decreased by respiratory acidosis/hypoventilation, then arterial O_2 must decrease (Fig. 3)

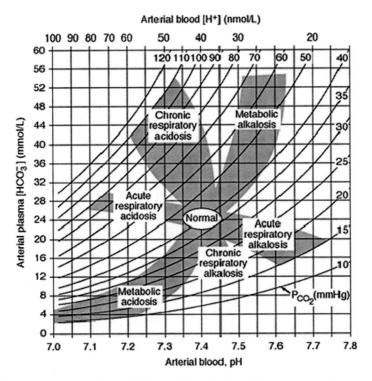

Fig. 2. Acid–base nomogram. It shows 95% confidence limits of the normal respiratory and metabolic compensations for primary acid–base disturbances. Permission granted from Dubose *(69)*.

Chapter 2: Gas Exchange

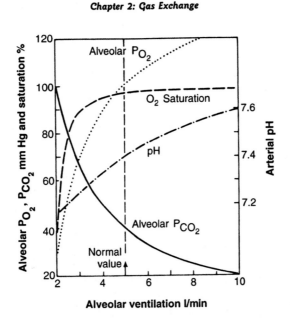

Fig. 3. Gas exchange during hypoventilation. Permission granted from West *(70)*.

This figure shows there are only small drops in pO_2 despite moderate respiratory acidosis. If supplemental O_2 is given, the hypoxemia of hypoventilation can be reversed. The ultimate clinical example of hypoxemia reversal can be seen during an apnea test for brain death determination. Determining brain death requires confirmation of the absence of brain stem reflexes including spontaneous respirations. An apnea test is performed, confirming loss of respiratory drive. Supplemental oxygen and adequate mean airway pressure are provided for the apnea test. During 5–10 min of apnea, the arterial partial pressure of oxygen (pO_2) is maintained greater than 100. The ABG values below were obtained from a 17-year-old after sustaining a fatal head injury in a motor vehicle accident. Without significant lung pathology, the pO_2 is easily maintained with an increase in FiO_2 from 0.4 to 1.0.

Baseline ABG before apnea:
pH 7.34; pCO_2 34; **pO_2 120**; HCO_3 18; FiO_2 0.40

ABG after 10 min of apnea:
pH 7.03; pCO_2 88; **pO_2 208**; HCO_3 23; FiO_2 1.00

Noninvasive monitoring of CO_2 is the standard in ventilated pediatric patients (26). End tidal CO_2 ($etCO_2$) is measured via capnography (27). Healthy patients show close correlation between $etCO_2$ and arterial partial pressure of CO_2 (pCO_2). In patients with increased dead-space ventilation the gap between $etCO_2$ and pCO_2 widens. $EtCO_2$ can be quite low in patients with large pulmonary embolus or inadequately resuscitated cardiopulmonary arrest and will poorly correlate with pCO_2 (28, 29). Wide gaps between $etCO_2$ and pCO_2 can be an early clue to increased dead-space ventilation.

Transcutaneous CO_2 (tCO_2) detectors are used in neonates and children when $etCO_2$ is unreliable, specifically during high-frequency oxygen ventilation (HFOV) (30). The early tCO_2 sensors required skin heating and could cause burns, especially in neonates. Improved technology has refined the probes to be more accurate and similar to pulse oximetry in safety. These devices will likely be used more frequently to detect respiratory acidosis/hypoventilation in spontaneously breathing and ventilated patients. It may prove to be a valuable noninvasive monitoring technique for sedation procedures, rapid assessment of respiratory failure, and any other patient situation where hypoventilation is a concern.

5. TREATMENT

Treatment for respiratory acidosis is directed toward each specific cause. The goal of therapy is improved ventilation and restoration of normal serum pH. Stepwise treatment is important and may prevent the need for mechanical ventilation or other rescue therapies.

Treatment of electrolyte deficiencies may improve patient ventilation. Severe hypophosphatemia, hypomagnesemia, hypokalemia, and hypocalcemia are the primary electrolyte disturbances that potentiate hypoventilation and should be supplemented to normal ranges.

Adequate nutrition is vital for recovery from disease. In patients with limited or fixed minute ventilation, nutritional formula choices can either moderate or exacerbate respiratory acidosis. High carbohydrate loaded formulas or overfeeding generate more CO_2 by product *(31)*. The excess production of CO_2 cannot easily be eliminated in hypoventilation syndromes. Carbohydrate calories may need to be reduced to decrease CO_2 production *(32)*.

Elevated temperature control may play an important role in respiratory acidosis. Every $1°$ Celsius (C) rise in temperature increases CO_2 production by 13% *(16)*. Thus $3°$ increase raises CO_2 production by 40%. In infants and children with limited pulmonary reserve and in disease states with pulmonary reserve limitations, elevated temperature may significantly exacerbate respiratory acidosis. Antipyretics and cooling techniques may be used but patient shivering should be avoided. Shivering increases both CO_2 production and O_2 consumption, thus complicating the treatment of respiratory acidosis.

Heliox therapy, first reported in 1934, has been shown to improve gas exchange in a variety of clinical problems *(33)*. Since the density of helium is one-seventh the density of air, laminar flow of helium through narrowed airways occurs at higher flow rates *(34)*. Helium is used as the carrier gas for O_2 to increase total flow and oxygen flow. The net result is decreased work of breathing, improved ventilation and oxygenation, and improvement in respiratory acidosis *(35, 36)*. Standard heliox ratios (He/O$_2$) are 80:20 or 70:30. If helium concentrations are reduced below these standard ratios, increased gas density results and the advantageous flow characteristics of helium are lost.

Clinical and laboratory evidence of sodium bicarbonate ($NaHCO_3$) benefits are lacking *(37)*. Significant risks of $NaHCO_3$ treatment include increased CO_2 production, tissue acidosis, and possible decreased respiratory drive related to pH correction *(37)*. If there is a superimposed metabolic acidosis causing severe pH lowering, sodium bicarbonate can be considered. Theoretical benefits of sodium bicarbonate include improved smooth muscle responsiveness to bronchodilators (beta agonists) and improved cardiovascular function. $NaHCO_3$ administration does not improve CNS acidosis because HCO_3^- does not cross the blood–brain barrier. Most sources do not recommend routine $NaHCO_3$ administration for respiratory acidosis *(38)*.

Noninvasive positive pressure ventilation (NPPV) is a first step in the treatment of respiratory acidosis before proceeding to mechanical ventilation *(39)*. NPPV has been used in neonates in the form of nasal CPAP (continuous positive airway pressure) for many years *(40)*. NPPV use has exploded with the treatment of obstructive sleep apnea, other forms of chronic respiratory acidosis, and short-term treatment of congestive heart failure *(41–43)*. Pediatric intensive care units have added NPPV primarily as nasal or face mask BiPAP (bidirectional positive airway pressure) as a treatment to avoid intubation *(44)*. BiPAP has been used for a variety of clinical problems involving hypoventilation, respiratory acidosis, and respiratory failure *(45, 46)*. BiPAP can be effective both acutely and chronically.

Positive pressure with mechanical ventilation may be necessary when respiratory acidosis is severe or develops quickly and other less invasive treatments have failed. Mechanical ventilation improves ventilation efficiency, oxygenation, and work of breathing *(47)*. If spontaneous breathing and supportive therapies no longer meet metabolic demands and respiratory acidosis is severe, endotracheal intubation is indicated. This decision should be made using clinical assessment, natural history of the suspected disease, and laboratory findings including arterial blood gas (ABG) analysis.

Decision for intubation and mechanical ventilation should be made before irreversible organ failure or cardiovascular collapse occurs. Mechanical ventilation can be life-saving but important potential complications should be considered (48–50). Direct trauma can occur at the time of intubation with injury to the oral cavity, posterior pharynx, or vocal cords. Airway reflexes are impaired during intubation and pulmonary aspiration can occur, damaging lung tissue and promoting subsequent pneumonia. The profound pressure changes from spontaneous (negative pressure) breathing to positive pressure ventilation dramatically affect cardiopulmonary function (51). Preload, stroke volume, and cardiac output may be compromised. Hyperinflation and the resultant increase in auto-PEEP (positive end expiratory pressure) increase pulmonary vascular resistance. This can impair left ventricular loading and results in hypotension. Worsening hyperinflation, higher auto-PEEP and over-distension of lung units may result in barotrauma and volutrauma. Examples of barotraumas include pneumomediastinum, pneumothorax, and pneumopericardium. Volutrauma results from over-distension of alveoli and precipitates an inflammatory cascade resulting in acute lung injury/ARDS (acute respiratory distress syndrome) (52). Aspiration, impaired pulmonary secretion clearance, and bacterial colonization increase the incidence of ventilator-associated pneumonia (VAP). Increased morbidity and prolonged hospital stays are seen when a VAP complicates a mechanical ventilation course (53).

Lung-protective ventilation techniques minimize over-distension and prevent or attenuate acute lung injury (54). Historically, mechanical ventilation was employed to normalize pCO_2 in severe respiratory acidosis. The benefit of this approach was near normalization of ABGs with the cost of excessive airway pressures in the diseased non-compliant lungs (47, 55). Barotrauma complications were common with this strategy. Morbidity and mortality have been significantly improved by reducing airway pressures (tidal volumes), allowing pCO_2 to rise, and tolerating lower pH initially until renal HCO_3^- conservation gradually normalizes pH (56). This lung-protective strategy is termed permissive hypercapnia (57, 58). Once lung function improves and respiratory acidosis resolves, normocapnia can be re-established.

6. RESCUE THERAPIES

The most severe cases of respiratory acidosis and respiratory failure may fail to improve with mechanical ventilation. High-frequency oscillatory ventilation (HFOV) is used with some success in these patients (59–61). HFOV employs very small tidal volumes of 1–3 ml/kg. These small volumes are generated by rates or frequencies of 2–15 Hz (Hertz). The tidal volumes are delivered by a power setting that determines the amplitude of each frequency. The potential benefits of this ventilation strategy are improved lung recruitment and lung expansion without unwanted barotrauma (62, 63).

Extracorporeal membrane oxygenation (ECMO) can be offered when the underlying etiology of respiratory acidosis/respiratory failure is thought to be reversible and all less invasive treatments have failed (64, 65). ECMO involves removal of patient blood volume from a central vein. The blood is oxygenated with a membrane oxygenator and returned either through central vein or large artery. This technique provides adequate tissue oxygenation until pulmonary function improves and ECMO can be stopped (66).

Bleeding complications are possible since blood must be anticoagulated to prevent clotting while traveling through the ECMO circuit *(67)*.

7. CONCLUSION

Infants have their first encounter with respiratory acidosis at birth during vaginal or cesarean section delivery. Infants and children continue to be at greater risk for respiratory acidosis until compensatory mechanisms and respiratory reserve reach maturity. Respiratory acidosis has an extensive list of causes. Best patient outcomes are achieved with rapid accurate assessment and stepwise treatment.

CASE SCENARIO #1

A 2-year-old with winter URI symptoms develops fever and a suspected febrile seizure. She is brought by ambulance to the hospital. Her seizure has stopped after a dose of lorazepam but her respiratory rate is decreased. Pulse oximetry reading is 100% on supplemental O_2. An ABG is obtained.

pH 6.95; pCO_2 99; pO_2 246; HCO_3 25; FiO_2 1.00

This is a common problem for pediatricians and emergency medicine physicians. Hypoventilation and respiratory acidosis is a frequent result of seizures and is exacerbated by CNS-depressing anticonvulsant therapy. Respiratory acidosis develops acutely with seizures. If a 0.08 pH change is predicted for every 10 mmHg increase in CO_2 with acute respiratory acidosis, the predicted pH is 6.93. This closely correlates to the measured pH of 6.95 and represents acute respiratory acidosis.

The treatment for this patient was supplemental O_2 and airway opening maneuvers until the lorazepam and postictal CNS clouding improved. An ABG 36 min after the initial sample showed

pH 7.30; pCO_2 45; pO_2 437; HCO_3 22; FiO_2 1.00

The predicted pH for a CO_2 of 45 is 7.36. The measured pH of 7.30 is slightly lower, representing a mixed acid–base problem with concurrent mild metabolic acidosis.

CASE SCENARIO #2

A 14-year-old boy with Duchenne's muscular dystrophy has been confined to a wheelchair and bed for 2 years. He has always been a good student, but is falling asleep in class. He no longer arouses to his alarm clock and complains of morning headaches. His mother is also worried that his scoliosis is worse. He is seen by his pediatrician. Findings include room air O_2 saturations of 93%, poor air movement with distant breath sounds, and increased weakness compared to previous office exams. He is referred to a pulmonologist for further evaluation. The pulmonologist orders an ABG as part of the work up.

pH 7.36; pCO_2 80; pO_2 65; HCO_3 38; FiO_2 0.21

The ABG confirms the healthcare team's fear of progressive deterioration with chronic respiratory acidosis. The predicted pH for a CO_2 of 80 with chronic hypoventilation is 7.28. This clinical case illustrates compensation with renal conservation of HCO_3^-, producing metabolic alkalosis, and consequent correction of pH toward normal.

Treatment options for this young man include low-flow oxygen therapy, initiation of nighttime BiPAP, and possible scoliosis repair to improve pulmonary reserve. Nighttime BiPAP was started with settings of 16/8 and 30% oxygen. Within a week, an ABG showed evidence of improved ventilation.

pH 7.43; pCO$_2$ 44; pO$_2$ 95; HCO$_3$ 28; FiO$_2$ 0.30

REFERENCES

1. Wohl ME: Developmental Physiology of the Respiratory System. In Chernick V, Boat TF (eds.): Kendig's Disorders of the Respiratory Tract in Children, 6th ed. Philadelphia, Saunders, 1998, Chapter 2, pp. 19–27.
2. Myer CM, Cotton RT, Shott SR: The Pediatric Airway, Philadelphia, Lippincott, 1995, Chapters 1 and 2, pp. 1–23.
3. O'Brodovich HM, Haddad GG: The functional basis of respiratory pathology and disease. In Chernick V, Boat TF (eds.): Kendig's Disorders of the Respiratory Tract in Children, 6th ed. Philadelphia, Saunders, 1998, Chapter 3, pp. 27–73.
4. Madias N, Cohen J: Respiratory acidosis. In Kassirer JP, Cohen JJ (eds.): Acid–Base. Boston, Little Brown, 1982, pp. 307–348.
5. Swenson ER, Hlastla MP: Carbon dioxide transport and acid–base balance: tissue and cellular. In Chernick V, Mellin R (eds.): Basic Mechanisms of Pediatric Respiratory Disease: Cellular and Integrative. Philadelphia. BC Decker Inc. 1991, Chapter 12, pp. 145–161.
6. Wasserman K, Hansen JE, Sue JY, et al.: Principles of Exercise Testing and Interpretation. Philadelphia, Lea and Febiger, 1987.
7. Madias NE, Wolf CJ, Cohen JJ: Regulation of acid–base equilibrium in chronic hypercapnia. Kidney Int 1985: 27 (3): 538–543.
8. Tannen RL, Hamid B: Adaptive changes in renal acidification in response to chronic respiratory acidosis. Am J Physiol 1985: 248(4 pt. 2): F492–499.
9. Madias N, Androgue H: Respiratory acidosis and alkalosis. In Tobin J (eds.): Respiratory Monitoring (Contemporary Management in Critical Care. Vol. 1. N. 4) Edinburgh, Churchill Livingstone, 1991, pp. 37–53.
10. Krachman S, Griner GJ: Hypoventilation syndromes. Clin Chest Med 1998:19(1): 139–155.
11. Caruana-Montaldo B, Gleeson K, Zwillich CW: The control of breathing in clinical practice. Chest 2000:117(1): 205–225.
12. Berger AJ: Control of breathing. In Murray JF, Nadel JA, Mason RJ Boushey HA (eds.): Textbook of Respiratory Medicine. 3rd ed. Philadelphia, Saunders, 2000, Chapter 8, pp. 179–196.
13. Goldstein RS: Hypoventilation: neuromuscular and chest wall disorders. Clin Chest Med 1992:13(3): 507–521.
14. Krachman S, Griner GJ: Hypoventilation Syndromes. Clin Chest Med 1998:19(1): 139–155.
15. Epstein SK: An overview of respiratory muscle function. Clin Chest Med 1994:15(4): 619–639.
16. Weinberger SE, Schwartzstein RM, Weiss JW: Hypercapnia. N Engl J Med 1989:321(19): 1223–1231.
17. Epstein SK, Singh N: Respiratory acidosis. Respiratory Care 2001:46(4): 366–383.
18. Heinemann HO., Goldring RM: Bicarbonate and the regulation of ventilation. Am J Med 1971: 51: 772.

19. Goldring RM, Turino GM, Heinemann HO: Respiratory-renal adjustments in chronic hypercapnia in man: Extracellular bicarbonate concentration and the regulation of ventilation. Am J Med 1974: 57: 361.
20. Alberti E, Hoyer S, Hamer J, et al.: The effect of carbon dioxide on cerebral blood flow and cerebral metabolism in dogs. Br J Anaesth 1975:47(9): 941–947.
21. Williams G, Roberts PA, et al.: The effect of apnea on brain compliance and intracranial pressure. Neurosurgery 1991:29(2): 242–246.
22. Androgue H, Madias N: Arterial blood gas monitoring: acid–base assessment. In Tobin J (ed.). Principles and Practice of Intensive Care Monitoring. New York, McGraw Hill, 1998, 217–241.
23. Gunnarsson L, Tokies L, Brismar B. Hedenstierna G: Influence of age on circulation and arterial blood gases in man. Acta Anaesthesiol Scand 1996:40(2): 237–243.
24. Bracket NC, Cohen JJ, Schwartz WB: Carbon dioxide titration curve of normal man: Effect of increasing degrees of acute hypercapnia on acid–base equilibrium. N Engl J Med 1965:6: 272.
25. Malley WJ: Clinical Acid–Base. Clinical Blood Gases: Assessment and Intervention. Philadelphia, Saunders 2005.
26. Hamel DS, Cheifetz IM: Do all mechanically ventilated pediatric patients require continuous capnography. Respir Care Clin 2006:12: 501–513.
27. Stock MC: Capnography for Adults. Critical Care Clin 1995:11(1): 219–232.
28. Gudipati CV, Weil MH, Bisera J, et al.: Expired carbon dioxide: A noninvasive monitor of cardiopulmonary resuscitation. Circulation 1988:77(1): 234–239.
29. Levine RL, Wayne MA, Miller CC: End-tidal carbon dioxide and outcome of out-of-hospital cardiac arrest. N Engl J Med 1997:337(5): 301–306.
30. Berkenbosch JW, Tobias JD: Transcutaneous carbon dioxide monitoring during high-frequency oscillatory ventilation in infants and children. Crit Car Med 2002:30(5): 1024–1027.
31. Covelli HD, Black JW, Olsen MS, et al.: Respiratory failure precipitated by high carbohydrate loads. Ann Intern Med 1981:95t(5): 579–581.
32. Efthimiou J, Mounsey PJ, Benson DN, et al.: Effect of carbohydrate rich versus fat rich loads on gas exchange and walking performance in patients with chronic obstructive lung disease. Thorax 1992:47(6): 451–456.
33. Barach AL: Use of helium as a new therapeutic gas. Proc Soc Exp Biol Med 1934:32: 462–464.
34. Papamoschou D: Theoretical validation of the respiratory benefits of helium-oxygen mixtures. Respir Physiol 1995:99: 183–190.
35. Wratney AT, Hamel DS, Cheifety IM: Inhaled Gases. In Nichols DG (ed.) Rogers Textbook of Pediatric Intensive Care. 4th ed. Philadelphia, Lippincott, Williams and Wilkins, 2008, Chapter 35, pp. 532–543.
36. Wolfson MR, Bhutani VK, Shaffer TH, et al.: Mechanics and energetics of breathing helium in infants with bronchopulmonary dysplasia. J Pediatr 1984:104: 752–757.
37. Kallet RH, Liu K, Tang J: Management of acidosis during lung-protective ventilation in acute respiratory distress syndrome. Respir Care Clin 2003:9: 437–456.
38. Forsyth SM, Schmidt GA: Sodium bicarbonate for the treatment of lactic acidosis. Chest 2000:117: 260–267.
39. Morly CJ, Davis PG, Doyle LW, et al.: Nasal CPAP or intubation at birth for very preterm infants. N Engl J Med 2008:358: 700–708.
40. Gitterman MK, Fusch C, Gitterman AR, et al.: Early nasal continuous positive airway pressure treatment reduces the need for intubation in very low birth weight infants. Eur J Pediatr 1997:156: 384–388.
41. Plant PK, Owen JL, Elliott MW: Early use of non-invasive ventilation for acute exacerbations of chronic obstructive pulmonary disease on general respiratory wards: A multicenter randomized controlled trial. Lancet 2000:35: 1931–1935.
42. Brochard L, Mancebo J, Wysoki M, et al.: Noninvasive ventilation for acute exacerbations of chronic obstructive pulmonary disease. N Eng J Med 1995:333: 817–822.
43. Lin M, Yang YF, Chiang HT, et al.: Reappraisal of continuous positive airway pressure therapy in acute cardiogenic pulmonary edema: Short term results and long term follow up. Chest 1995:107: 1379–1386.

44. Essouri S, Chevret L: Noninvasive positive pressure ventilation: Five years of experience in a pediatric intensive care unit. Pediatr Crit Care Med 2006:7(4): 329–334.

45. Fortenberry JD, DelToro J, Jefferson LS, et al.: Management of pediatric acute hypoxemic respiratory insufficiency with bilevel positive pressure (BiPAP) nasal mask ventilation. Chest 1995:108: 1059–1064.

46. Padman R, Lawless ST, Kettrick RG: Noninvasive ventilation via bilevel positive airway pressure support in pediatric practice. Crit Care Med 1998:26: 169–173.

47. Tobin MJ: Advances in mechanical ventilation. N Engl J Med 2001:344: 1986–1996.

48. Benjamin PK, Thompson JE, O'Rourke PP: Complications of mechanical ventilation in a children's hospital multidisciplinary intensive care unit. Respir Care 1990:35: 873–878.

49. Chadda K, Annane D, Hart N, et al.: Cardiac and respiratory effects of continuous positive airway pressure and noninvasive ventilation in acute cardiac pulmonary edema. Crit Care Med 2002:30(11): 2457–2461.

50. Simonson DA, Adams AB, Wright LA, et al.: Effects of ventilatory pattern on experimental lung injury caused by high airway pressures. Crit Care Med 2004:32(3): 781–786.

51. Fuhrman BP: Cardiopulmonary Interactions. In Fuhrman BP, Zimmerman J (eds.). Pediatric Critical Care, 3rd ed. Philadelphia, Mosby Elsevier, 2006, Chapter 24, pp. 332–345.

52. Alexander AB, Simonson DA, Dries DJ: Ventilator-induced lung injury. Respir Care Clin 2003: 343–362.

53. Stockwell JA: Nosocomial infections in the pediatric intensive care unit: Affecting the impact on safety and outcome. Crit Care Med 2007:8(suppl): 521–537.

54. Kissoon N, Rimensberger PC, Bohm D: Ventilation strategies and adjunctive therapy in severe lung disease. Pediatr Clin N Am 2008:55: 709–733.

55. Girard TD, Bernard GR: Mechanical ventilation in ARDS: A-State-of-the-Art-Review. Chest 2007:131(3): 921–929.

56. The Acute Respiratory Distress Syndrome Network. Ventilation with lower tidal volumes as compared with traditional tidal volumes for acute lung injury and the acute respiratory distress syndrome. N Engl J Med 2000:342: 1301–1308.

57. Hikling KG: Permissive hypercapnia. Respir Care Clin 2002:8: 155–169.

58. Rotta AT, Steinhorn DM: Is permissive hypercapnia a beneficial strategy for pediatric acute lung injury? Respir Care Clin 2006:12: 371–387.

59. Arnold J, Anas N, Luckett P, et al.: High-frequency oscillatory ventilation in pediatric respiratory failure: a multicenter experience. Crit Care Med 2000:28(12): 3913–3919.

60. Moriette G, Paris-Llado J, Walti H, et al.: Prospective randomized multicenter comparison of high-frequency oscillatory ventilation and conventional ventilation in preterm infants of less than 30 weeks with respiratory distress syndrome. Pediatrics 2001:107(2): 363–372.

61. Mehta S, Lapinsky SE, Hallett DC, et al.: Prospective trial of high-frequency oscillation in adults with acute respiratory distress syndrome. Crit Care Med 2001:29(7): 1360–1369.

62. Imai Y, Slutsky AS: High-frequency oscillatory ventilation and ventilator-induced lung injury. Crit Care Med 2005:33(3 Suppl): S129–S134.

63. Froese AB, Kinsella JP: High-frequency oscillatory ventilation: Lessons from the neonatal/pediatric experience. Crit Care Med 2005:33(3 Suppl): S115–S121.

64. Hill JD, O'Brien TG, Murray JJ, et al.: Prolonged extracorporeal oxygenation for acute post-traumatic respiratory failure (shock-lung syndrome). Use of the Branson Membrane lung. N Engl J Med 1972:286(12): 629–634.

65. Green TP, Timmons OD, Facler JC, et al.: The impact of extracorporeal membrane oxygenation on survival in pediatric patients with acute respiratory failure. Pediatric Critical Care Study Group. Crit Care Med 1996:24(2): 323–329.

66. Lequier L: Extracorporeal Life Support in Pediatric and Neonatal Critical Care: A Review. J Intensive Care Med 2004:19(5): 243–258.

67. Cengiz P, Seidel K, Rycus PT, et al.: Central nervous system complications during pediatric extracorporeal life support: incidence and risk factors. Crit Care Med 2005:33(12): 2817–2824.

68. Phillipson EA, Duffin J: Hypoventilation and hyperventilation syndromes. In Murray JE, Nadel JA (eds.). Textbook of Respiratory Medicine, 4th ed. Philadelphia, Elsevier 2005, Chapter 73, p. 2077.
69. Dubose TD: Acid–Base Disorders. In Brenner BM, Rector FC (eds.). The Kidney, 7th ed. Philadelphia, Elsevier 2005, Chapter 20, p. 938.
70. West JB: Gas Exchange Pulmonary Pathophysiology The Essentials, 6th ed. Baltimore, Lippincott Williams and Wilkins, 2003, Chapter 2, p. 20.

11 Diagnosis and Treatment of Respiratory Alkalosis

Otwell Timmons

Key Points

1. Respiratory alkalosis is defined as a pH above 7.45 due to an arterial carbon dioxide tension less than 35 mmHg.
2. Respiratory alkalosis accompanies pregnancy and the hyperventilation anxiety syndrome, making it the most common acid–base imbalance.
3. Carbon dioxide production and elimination are usually matched, but illness, medication, or injury can decrease production or increase elimination and effect respiratory alkalosis.
4. Among the determinants of carbon dioxide elimination are the cerebral cortex, the brainstem respiratory centers, and the peripheral receptors that sense chemical and physical phenomena.
5. The most common cause of respiratory alkalosis, the hyperventilation anxiety syndrome, arises in the cerebral cortex. It often masquerades as an organic pulmonary or cardiovascular disorder.
6. Hyperventilation constricts the coronary and cerebral circulations and dilates the pulmonary circulation.
7. Metabolic compensation for respiratory alkalosis reaches steady state in about 3 days. Over a longer time, metabolic compensation can return pH to normal despite ongoing hypocarbia.

Key Words: Respiratory alkalosis; respiratory drive; anxiety hyperventilation syndrome; respiratory stimulants; vascular tone

1. DEFINITION

Respiratory alkalosis is the elevation of body pH above 7.45 due to hypocapnia, generally accepted as an arterial partial pressure ($PaCO_2$) less than 35 torr. Respiratory alkalosis may be a primary disturbance, or it may be compensatory to metabolic acidosis. It may be acute or chronic. In chronic cases, metabolic compensation may partially correct the arterial pH or it may normalize the pH.

From: *Nutrition and Health: Fluid and Electrolytes in Pediatrics*
Edited by: L. G. Feld, F. J. Kaskel, DOI 10.1007/978-1-60327-225-4_11,
© Humana Press, a part of Springer Science+Business Media, LLC 2010

2. ETIOLOGY/CAUSATION

All body cells generate carbon dioxide (CO_2) in the course of energy metabolism. All cellular fuels, whether consumed aerobically or anaerobically, generate CO_2. The amount of CO_2 generated varies among fuels. This amount is reflected in the respiratory quotient (RQ), the ratio of moles of CO_2 produced per mole of oxygen consumed. Carbohydrate has the highest RQ, 1. The RQ for protein is about 0.8, and for fat it is 0.7.

From cells, CO_2 diffuses to the capillary blood. There, it initially dissolves in plasma. The solubility of CO_2 in plasma is relatively high, but only a small portion of CO_2 retains the form of a dissolved gas. Gaseous CO_2 is in equilibrium with its hydration product, carbonic acid (H_2CO_3), and the bicarbonate ion (HCO_3^-) in plasma (Fig. 1). H_2CO_3 and HCO_3^- interact to affect pH, as the Henderson–Hasselbalch equation describes:

$$pH = pK + \log \frac{HCO_3^-}{H_2CO_3} \text{ (when } pK = 6.1)$$

pK is the dissociation constant of carbonic acid in blood, which is 6.1. pH reflects the hydrogen ion (H^+) concentration in plasma, and it is easily measured. However, clinical utility of the Henderson–Hasselbalch equation is limited by its reliance on logarithms and by the general lack of clinical measures of H_2CO_3 *(1)*. Practical insight into the

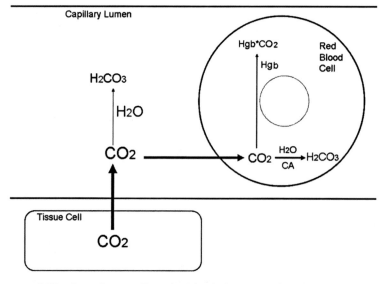

Fig. 1. Transport of CO_2 from tissue cells to the blood. CA, carbonic anhydrase; Hgb, hemoglobin; Hgb*CO_2, carbaminohemoglobin.

interrelationship of gaseous CO_2 and its metabolic congeners comes from the Henderson equation:

$$H^+ = 24 \times \frac{PCO_2}{HCO_3^-}$$

The Henderson equation points out the relationship of plasma acidity to the ratio of PCO_2 and HCO_3^-.

Larger than the plasma CO_2 stores are intracellular ones. Hydration of CO_2 occurs more rapidly in red blood cells (RBCs) due to the availability of carbonic anhydrase, and most of the CO_2 transported in blood is intracellular (Fig. 1). In RBCs, three storage forms exist. In order of importance from greatest to least, these are hydrated CO_2, hemoglobin-bound CO_2, and dissolved gaseous CO_2 *(2)*.

Maintenance of acid–base homeostasis requires excretion of CO_2 and metabolic acids. The lungs exhale CO_2, and the kidneys secrete most metabolic acids. The kidneys also regulate the concentration of plasma buffers, of which HCO_3^- is the most important. Bases are molecules that can combine with H^+. When the combination produces a weak acid, the base and its corresponding acid are termed a buffer system. Buffers blunt the degree of change in pH when the concentrations of CO_2, other acids, and bases are altered.

Changes in general physiology can rapidly alter CO_2 production (Table 1). Fever, exercise, drug intoxication, and sepsis increase CO_2 production and alter acid–base status. A simple change in the source of non-protein calories from carbohydrate to fat can decrease CO_2 production 43%. Acid–base homeostasis requires, among other actions, that the body match the decrease in CO_2 production with decreased CO_2 excretion.

The circulation delivers CO_2, carbonic acid, and bicarbonate to the lungs. In perfused lung units, CO_2 diffuses from the plasma to the alveolus. Hydrolysis of carbonic acid to gaseous CO_2 maintains the concentration gradient necessary to drive diffusion. From the alveoli, CO_2 is excreted by ventilation (Fig. 2). The amount of CO_2 exhaled per minute is proportional to the minute volume, which is the product of respiratory rate per minute and the effective tidal volume. The arterial partial pressure of CO_2 ($PaCO_2$) is proportional to CO_2 production (VCO_2) and is inversely proportional to alveolar ventilation per unit of time (VA):

$$PaCO_2 \propto \frac{VCO_2}{VA}$$

The lungs excrete the great majority of moles of acid the body produces. Healthy adult lungs exhale 13,000 mEq of carbonic acid daily, where the kidneys excrete 40 to 80 mEq of metabolic acid daily *(2)*. The alveolar ventilation is the most important instantaneous determinant of the body's acid–base status.

Regulation of alveolar ventilation is performed in the brain. The primary drivers of respiratory drive and respiratory pattern are the medullary respiratory centers of the brainstem. These centers take inputs from brain chemoreceptors, from peripheral

Table 1
Causes of Respiratory Alkalosis

Central nervous system
    Hyperventilation–anxiety syndrome
    Volitional hyperventilation
    Pain
    Increased intracranial pressure
    Brain hypoxia or ischemia
    Tumor
    Trauma
    Stroke

Pharmacologic
    Aspirin and other salicylates
    Progestational hormones
    Methylxanthines
    Adrenergic agents
    Doxapram
    Nikethamide
    Ethamivan
    Nicotine
    Dinitrophenol
    Metformin

Pulmonary
    Restrictive chest wall disease
    Pulmonary edema
    Pneumonia
    Interstitial pneumonitis
    Asthma
    Pneumothorax
    Hemothorax
    Pulmonary embolism
    Pulmonary fibrosis
    Pulmonary hypertension
    Mechanical hyperventilation

General state of the patient
    Sepsis
    Hypoxemia
    Anemia
    Exercise
    Fever
    Carbon monoxide poisoning
    Methemoglobinemia

Altitude
Asphyxia
Pregnancy
Liver failure
Inborn errors of metabolism
Heat illness
Cold shock
Change in diet
Thyroid dysfunction

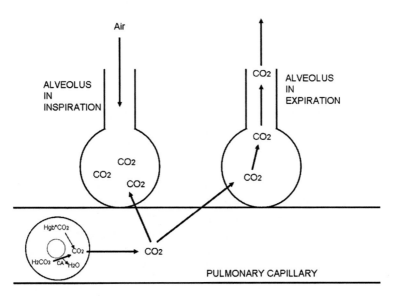

Fig. 2. Transport of CO_2 from blood to expired gas. Hgb∗CO2, carbaminohemoglobin; CA, carbonic anhydrase.

chemoreceptors, from receptors that respond to physical inputs in the lungs, and from other sites in the central nervous system (CNS) (Fig. 3). The interaction of the medullary respiratory centers with their sensors allows feedback control of alveolar ventilation. This control makes extremes of pH unusual in most cases of respiratory alkalosis.

The most active sources of stimuli to the medullary respiratory centers are the central chemoreceptors. These are chemically sensitive areas that are also located in the medulla. These chemoreceptors sense the pH of the cerebrospinal fluid (CSF). As CSF pH varies from physiologic, these receptors signal the medullary respiratory centers to alter alveolar ventilation and restore normal CSF pH.

The pH of CSF does not change instantly after a change in systemic pH. The blood–brain barrier allows equilibration of ions, such as bicarbonate, by relatively slow means. Equilibration of bicarbonate takes hours to days *(3)*. Respiratory compensation for metabolic acidosis or alkalosis will not be at equilibrium in the interim. By contrast, dissolved gases, such as CO_2, cross from the systemic circulation to the CSF and back more rapidly because they can diffuse. Their diffusion, though rapid, is not instantaneous.

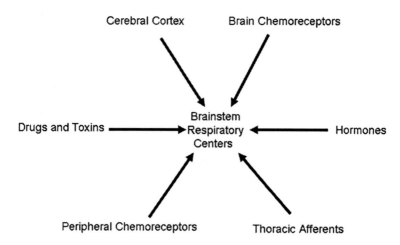

Fig. 3. Inputs to the brainstem respiratory centers.

The response of the chemoreceptors is delayed in congestive heart failure and shock states where arterialized blood may take longer to reach the cerebral circulation.

Augmenting the central chemoreceptors are the peripheral chemoreceptors, which consist of the carotid bodies and the aortic bodies. These receptors sense a wider variety of stimuli, including pH, $PaCO_2$, PaO_2, and oxygen delivery, directly from the blood stream *(4)*. Their contribution to respiratory drive is relatively weak when compared to that of the central chemoreceptors. The ability to sense PaO_2 and stimulate alveolar ventilation in response to hypoxemia is the basis for the hypoxic respiratory drive. Significant respiratory drive in response to hypoxemia is weak until frank hypoxemia, a PaO_2 less than 60 torr, exists.

The central and peripheral chemoreceptors may work together, or they may oppose each other. The receptivity of peripheral receptors to hypoxia and their potential faster response than the central chemoreceptors increase their influence in rapidly changing conditions or when the patient is hypoxemic. At any point, the interaction of chemoreceptors, the cerebral cortex, and neural sensors within the lungs determines the respiratory centers' output.

Lung reflexes are sensed locally and transmitted by vagal afferent fibers to the brain. Together, the inflation and deflation reflexes are considered the Hering–Breuer reflex *(4)*. The inflation reflex ceases inspiration in the presence of lung over distension. It has a protective function, and it helps regulate tidal volume and respiratory rate to minimize breathing work. The deflation reflex stimulates alveolar ventilation when low lung volume is sensed. Individually or together, the inflation and deflation reflexes may promote rapid shallow breathing or, if stimulation of the deflation reflex predominates, deep breathing. Either pattern may produce respiratory alkalosis. Separate from the stretch receptors are pulmonary juxtacapillary (J) receptors. These sense increased thickness of the alveolar–capillary membrane during pulmonary vascular congestion, as in pulmonary edema. Their stimulation increases alveolar ventilation.

As may be expected from the presence of these receptors, lung disease can manifest as hyperventilation. Asthma, emphysema, fibrosing alveolitis, pneumonia, pulmonary hypertension, and pulmonary embolism have all been associated with hypocapnia. No one pathway explains the resulting hyperventilation in most of these conditions. Hypocapnia likely results from hypoxemia and from stimulation of vagal and chest wall afferents. The breathing pattern may be rapid shallow breathing, or tidal volume may increase in isolation. That these patterns also manifest during changes in lung elasticity implicates the J receptors and the Hering–Breuer reflex *(5–15)*. Air hunger and chest pain may also increase respiratory drive due to volitional or other integrated cortical inputs.

Higher CNS centers also affect respiratory drive. The anxiety–hyperventilation syndrome reflects cerebral cortical inputs that override the usual inhibitory mechanisms. Body pH can rise substantially, and the resulting clinical signs can feed the initial anxiety. Neurological diseases and trauma can produce hyperventilation by disrupting the regularity of breathing or by damaging inhibitory pathways. Damage to the upper midbrain and pons can produce unabated, regular hyperventilation. Lower pontine lesions mediate apneustic breathing: very prolonged inspiration that is sometimes associated with other irregularities of the breathing pattern *(4)*.

Alteration in hormone levels can cause respiratory alkalosis directly or indirectly. The most familiar cause of hormonal hyperventilation occurs in pregnancy. Progesterone, which is necessary to support embryonic implantation and subsequent development of the placenta, is a direct stimulant of the medullary respiratory centers *(16)*. The $PaCO_2$ falls throughout pregnancy, paralleling the rise in progesterone *(17)*. Hypocapnia is also seen in the luteal phase of the menstrual cycle *(17)*, also a response to progesterone levels that are higher than baseline. In menopausal women, hypocapnia has been found to associate with hormone replacement therapy that includes medroxyprogesterone acetate *(18)*. Severe hypothyroidism has caused hypocapnia, probably due to an extremely low basal metabolic rate with relative preservation of minute volume *(19)*.

Numerous drugs directly or indirectly cause respiratory alkalosis. The most commonly used drug with this effect is aspirin. Aspirin at doses of several grams per day in adults directly stimulates the medullary respiratory centers. This primary respiratory alkalosis is distinct from any compensation for the metabolic acidosis aspirin may also cause. Blood gases in aspirin-intoxicated patients may be consistent with respiratory alkalosis, with metabolic acidosis, or with a picture of mixed primary disturbances.

Several drugs have received use as respiratory stimulants in hypoventilatory states. Ingestion of these drugs may cause modest respiratory alkalosis. Among these agents are nikethamide, ethamivan, doxapram, almitrine, progesterone, medroxyprogesterone, and methylxanthines *(20–22)*. Drugs that primarily impact other organ targets but which also can stimulate alveolar ventilation include epinephrine, norepinephrine, angiotensin II, nicotine, dinitrophenol, and metformin *(23–28)*.

Hepatic insufficiency may allow accumulation of toxic products of metabolism. Ammonia is a product of normal protein metabolism that can accumulate in hepatic disease. In pediatric patients, a common cause of chronic, recurrent hyperammonemia is ornithine transcarbamylase deficiency, of which hyperventilation is a clinical sign. The hypocapnia that is characteristic of liver disease correlates well with blood ammonia concentration *(29)*. The mechanism by which ammonia may stimulate respiration has not been elucidated.

Shock due to sepsis, extreme anemia, or cardiogenic failure can cause hyperventilation *(30, 31)*. Theoretically, the spontaneously breathing patient delivers a reduced volume of oxygen to the oxygen-responsive peripheral chemoreceptors. These receptors fire sufficiently to induce hypocapnia. A metabolic acidosis severe enough to offset the respiratory alkalosis is typically present, so a mixed acid–base disturbance or frank acidosis is the usual case. In the particular case of gram-negative sepsis, bacterial lipopolysaccharides may stimulate central chemoreceptors directly, accounting for part of the hypocapnia *(32)*.

Thermal insults, both hypothermia and hyperthermia, can cause respiratory alkalosis. Heat exhaustion and heat stroke both cause hyperventilation through an unknown mechanism. Cold shock occurs after immersion in ice-cold water for more than a few minutes. It elicits a gasp followed by involuntary hyperventilation, cutaneous vasoconstriction, and tachycardia. The hyperventilation is sufficiently severe that it reduces cerebral blood flow by vasoconstricting cerebral arterioles, and disorientation results *(33)*.

Numerous patients receive mechanical ventilation in a variety of settings. Hundreds of thousands of patients receive ventilator support in intensive care units in the United States each year. Patients are also ventilated in step-down units, rehabilitation hospitals, long-term custodial care facilities, and at home. The number of such patients whom are hyperventilated at any time is unknown, but it is likely high. Hyperventilation may be inadvertent. Patients may have normoventilation until a change in physical activity, physiologic dead space, lung compliance, or diet occurs. If such a change reduces the VCO_2 or increases the minute volume, respiratory alkalosis will occur. Intensivists and pulmonologists may favor mild hyperventilation over hypoventilation in routine care because the former offers a "cushion" of stability in case the ventilator ceases to operate.

Therapeutic hyperventilation is offered for a variety of clinical conditions. In each, an attempt is made to capitalize on the pH raising effect of hyperventilation, as in metabolic acidosis states, or to use the influence of pH and PCO_2 on vascular tone.

When metabolic acidosis threatens disability or increases a patient's mortality risk, maintenance of pH is important. Extremes of acidosis may reduce cardiac contractility and alter the kinetics of vital enzyme systems. A very common cause of metabolic acidosis is ketoacidosis in diabetes mellitus (DKA). While DKA itself rarely indicates mechanical ventilation, patients with DKA may have diminished neurological responsiveness or coma that would indicate mechanical ventilation to maintain a patent airway. If ventilation is offered for this reason, particular care must be taken to simulate the minute volume and, thus, the $PaCO_2$ the patient had maintained spontaneously. Whether spontaneous or mechanical, hyperventilation may be the only means to maintain a pH adequate for myocardial contractility and enzyme function. Allowing the $PaCO_2$ to normalize (increase) may also result in increased cerebral blood flow in the setting of existing brain hyperemia, which is known to occur in DKA. Such increased cerebral blood flow may provoke a harmful increase in intracranial pressure *(34, 35)*.

The brain benefits from a complex system to maintain vascular tone. In health and in many disease states, the brain autoregulates its blood flow. The end point of this autoregulation is a matching of cerebral oxygen supply to cerebral oxygen demand. Autoregulation is affected by correlates of oxygen delivery, such as cardiac output, hemoglobin concentration, and arterial oxygen saturation. It can also be affected by changes in the cerebral oxygen demand. Cerebral perfusion depends on sufficient systemic blood pressure, though blood pressure is not a direct determinant of oxygen delivery. Another determinant of cerebral vascular tone is CO_2. Cerebral blood flow is linearly related to $PaCO_2$ in the normal range of $PaCO_2$. For $PaCO_2$ values between 22 and 60 torr, cerebral blood flow decreases 2% for each 1 torr decline in $PaCO_2$ (36). In short, hypocarbia equals a cerebral vasoconstrictor.

Clinicians have used hyperventilation for several decades to reduce the cerebral blood volume and lower intracranial pressure (ICP). At one time, a low ICP was felt to be a surrogate for successful resuscitation of the brain in a variety of illnesses and injuries, including trauma, stroke, hypoxia-ischemia, and space-occupying lesions of the brain. Recently, instrumentation has been developed to measure brain tissue PO_2. Hemphill et al. showed reduced brain tissue PO_2 as end-tidal CO_2 was lowered between 20 and 60 torr (37). Of concern is that the tissue PO_2 may fall into the ischemic range as therapeutic hyperventilation reduces brain blood volume and brain blood flow. One clinical trial has addressed the potential impact on clinical outcome from hyperventilation of patients with head trauma (38). Those patients hyperventilated to a $PaCO_2$ of 25 torr for 5 days had worse outcome at 3 and 6 months than patients who had $PaCO_2$ tensions above 30 torr. In adult and pediatric guidelines for the initial treatment of traumatic brain injury, hyperventilation is reserved for patients who have neurological instability refractory to less toxic care or for neurologically deteriorating patients (39, 40).

Pulmonary vascular tone also varies with blood gas and pH values. Alveolar gas tensions and pH appear to be the usual determinants of pulmonary vascular tone. In general, oxygen is a pulmonary vasodilator while hydrogen ion and CO_2 are pulmonary vasoconstrictors. The vasodilation seen in oxygenated and ventilated lung units assures good blood flow to the portions of the lung that are aerated well. The vasoconstriction seen with local hypoxia or hypercarbia reduces blood flow to poorly ventilated lung units. These relationships assure good ventilation–perfusion matching in health and mild lung disease. Pulmonary hypertension includes a failure of lung vasculature to appropriately vasodilate in response to ventilation and oxygenation. In forms of pulmonary hypertension that reflect short-term abnormalities in pulmonary vasomotor response, such as persistent pulmonary hypertension of the newborn, hyperventilation, and hyperoxygenation have been used to vasodilate the pulmonary vasculature. Hyperventilation has not been proven effective in controlled trials, however, and concern exists that it may cause ventilator-associated lung injury. A modern approach is to use selective pulmonary vasodilators, such as inhaled nitric oxide, and sufficient minute ventilation to maintain normocarbia (41).

3. EVALUATION

Respiratory alkalosis itself may be mild and symptomless or it may be sufficiently severe to provoke secondary organ failure. Often, the most prominent findings are those of the inciting condition. Signs of increased alveolar ventilation may predominate. These may include increased respiratory rate, increased depth of respiration, rapid shallow breathing, and increased work of breathing. As a general rule, minute ventilation must increase 10% for significant hypocapnia to result.

By far, the most common cause of respiratory alkalosis is the hyperventilation syndrome, in which hyperventilation and anxiety are associated. In voluntary hyperventilation, patients experience breathlessness as well as the effects of hypocarbia on neuronal excitability and on blood flow to various tissues. Among symptoms of neuronal excitability are paresthesias and tetany in the hands, face, and trunk. Symptoms referable to reduced cerebral blood flow include giddiness, paresthesias, visual disturbance, headache, ataxia, tremor, tinnitus, hallucination, unilateral somatic symptoms that predominate on the left side, and loss of consciousness. Systemic vascular resistance falls during the first several minutes of hyperventilation. Blood pressure falls, and heart rate and cardiac output both increase. Cutaneous vascular resistance increases, accounting for cold extremities and some tingling *(42)*. Coronary blood flow parallels $PaCO_2$, so it falls during respiratory alkalosis. Myocardial oxygen supply falls, but not to a level that would limit myocardial oxygen consumption *(43, 44)*. Atypical chest pain is commonly seen, and it may worsen anxiety by mimicking coronary disease. Coronary spasm and cardiac arrhythmias may occur in patients who have pre-existing artery disease *(42)*. Air hunger is out of proportion to other clinical signs of pulmonary disease. An effective screening tool for hyperventilation syndrome in adults is the Nijmegen questionnaire (Table 2) *(45)*.

Physical examination may show the increased work of breathing that is associated with the increase in minute ventilation. A patient may sigh frequently. His abdomen may be distended from aerophagia. The breath-hold time may be short, though patient

Table 2

The Nijmegen Questionnaire for Evaluation of the Hyperventilation Syndrome in Adults

Symptom	Never	Seldom	Sometimes	Often	Very often
Chest pain	0	1	2	3	4
Feeling tense	0	1	2	3	4
Blurred vision	0	1	2	3	4
Dizziness	0	1	2	3	4
Confusion or loss of touch with reality	0	1	2	3	4
Fast or deep breathing	0	1	2	3	4
Shortness of breath	0	1	2	3	4
Tightness across chest	0	1	2	3	4
Bloated sensation in stomach	0	1	2	3	4
Tingling in fingers and hands	0	1	2	3	4
Difficulty in breathing or taking a deep breath	0	1	2	3	4
Stiffness or cramps in fingers and hands	0	1	2	3	4
Tightness around the mouth	0	1	2	3	4
Cold hands or feet	0	1	2	3	4
Palpitations in the chest	0	1	2	3	4
Anxiety	0	1	2	3	4

Patients circle the frequency with which they experience each symptom. Points are added, and a score equal or greater than 23 indicates hyperventilation with 91% sensitivity and 95% specificity *(45)*. From van Doorn P, Colla P, Folgering H *(56)*.

and operator variability widen the reference range of this test. Anxiety and air hunger may be prominent, and they prompt concern that significant organic respiratory disease exists.

Blood gas criteria for simple respiratory alkalosis are arterial pH above 7.45, $PaCO_2$ less than 35 torr, and no evidence to implicate hypoxia as a drive to breathe, e.g., PaO_2 below 60 torr or arterial blood oxygen saturation less than 0.9. Blood gas sampling may itself be anxiety provoking and may yield data that are not representative of the patient's condition. This might be particularly true in the crying infant. Non-invasive tests in centers experienced with their use may prove more valuable for individual patients. Non-invasive measures include end-tidal CO_2, transcutaneous CO_2, and pulse oximetry.

Acute hypocarbia reduces the ratio of CO_2 to HCO_3^- in the plasma. As per the Henderson equation, H^+ concentration will fall and pH will rise. The degree of pH rise has inherent variability. Plasma and intracellular buffers will blunt some of the rise. Among these buffers, HCO_3^- acutely falls about 0.2 mEq/L for each one torr decrease in $PaCO_2$ *(46)*. This change is a function of equilibria among the elements of the Henderson equation and is not dependent on HCO_3^- excretion by the kidneys. Organic acids, especially lactic acid, may accumulate. The activity of proton and HCO_3^- transporters in the cell membrane changes in the direction necessary to maintain pH *(47)*. Thus, the 95% confidence limits for pH and HCO_3^- after acute onset of hypocarbia are broad bands (Fig. 4) *(46)*.

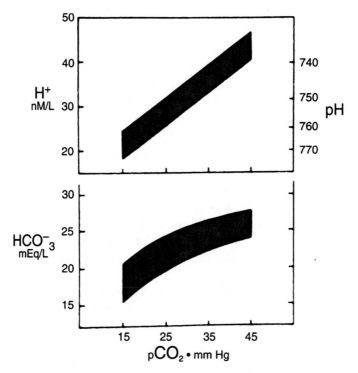

Fig. 4. Ninety-five percent confidence bands for pH and HCO_3^- across varying levels of $PaCO_2$ in patients undergoing acute hyperventilation. From Madias and Adrogue *(57)*. Modified from Arbus et al. *(46)*.

Within hours of the onset of hypocarbia, the kidneys reduce acid excretion and increase HCO_3^- excretion to begin renal compensation for respiratory alkalosis. In about 3 days, a new steady state occurs during which pH has returned about half-way to normal. Plasma HCO_3^- declines approximately 0.4 mEq/L and H^+ increases about 0.4 nEq/L for each 1 torr decrement in $PaCO_2$ (47, 48). Chronic hypocarbia can elicit sufficient metabolic compensation that pH returns to normal in the absence of an obvious source of metabolic acidosis. Chronic respiratory alkalosis is the only simple acid–base disturbance known to be compatible with a normal pH (1).

In the setting of cardiopulmonary resuscitation, arterial blood gases may falsely show respiratory alkalosis despite an increased total body burden of CO_2. The low pulmonary blood flow inherent in cardiac arrest diminishes the delivered volume of CO_2 from the venous blood to the alveoli. If ventilation is supported, ordinary minute volume provides more than sufficient ventilation to eliminate this small volume of CO_2 and the end-tidal CO_2 and the pulmonary capillary CO_2 plummet. Blood from the pulmonary capillaries determines the makeup of arterial blood, and arterial blood gases may appear very alkalotic. At the same time, venous blood may show a significant respiratory acidosis. This venous acidosis more accurately reflects the total body acid–base balance. It normalizes after the return of spontaneous circulation. The discrepancy between arterial and venous CO_2 tension limits the value of arterial blood gas sampling during cardiopulmonary resuscitation. Venous blood gases may be needed to show the patient's true acid–base status (49, 50).

4. TREATMENT

The most common cause of respiratory alkalosis is the hyperventilation syndrome. Treatment must focus on reassurance, reducing the minute volume, and relieving the symptoms of hypocarbia. When a single source for the anxiety can be found, counseling can be structured to improve the patient's response to the provocation. There are cases, however, when such counseling focuses such thought on the breathing process that the patient may worsen (42). Rebreathing from a paper sack may normalize the $PaCO_2$, but it has no demonstrated benefit to control the anxiety. Its value may mostly be educational in those patients who can accept their diagnosis.

Drugs are of limited usefulness in hyperventilation syndrome. Anxiolytics include benzodiazepines, beta-adrenergic blockers, and anti-depressants. Benzodiazepines may only be given within a limited time because of dependence and withdrawal potential. Beta blockers may exacerbate mild asthma, which is among the differential diagnoses of the anxiety–hyperventilation syndrome. Anti-depressants may normalize CO_2 in panicked patients (51).

Relief of mechanical hyperventilation is usually straightforward. The approach differs based on the nature of the hyperventilation. Inadvertent hypocarbia of patients receiving complete mechanical support should respond to reduction of minute ventilation, through use of either a lower tidal volume or a lower respiratory rate. Notably, high-frequency oscillatory ventilation differs from conventional ventilation in that lower minute volume occurs at higher, rather than lower, respiratory rates. If an anomaly of ventilator triggering causes numerous controlled or assisted breaths, the use of intermittent mandatory ventilation without assisted spontaneous breaths may resolve the problem *(52)*. Such anomalies include air-leak syndromes of the airway or the lungs, pressure waves generated by splashes of condensate within the ventilator circuit, and excessive sensitivity of the demand valve. Patients in controlled ventilatory modes receive full volume breaths whenever they breathe spontaneously. They may benefit from intermittent mandatory ventilation or from measures to reduce the spontaneous respiratory rate. Effective measures may include optimizing inspiratory flow to match patient demand, sedating patients, or pharmacologically paralyzing patients. Finally, adding dead space to the ventilator circuit may reduce the effective tidal volume.

5. MIXED ACID–BASE DISORDERS INVOLVING RESPIRATORY ALKALOSIS

Mixed acid–base disturbances occur when a metabolic disorder coexists with a respiratory disorder, when two metabolic disorders coexist, or when three disorders occur together. Most diagnoses are made by taking a history, and this should be true in the diagnosis of mixed acid–base disorders. When laboratory methods must be called on to establish the diagnosis, the following discussion may be helpful.

Simple acid–base disorders have predictable biochemical effects. Most of these involve pH, blood gas tensions, and total CO_2, which is the sum of HCO_3^- and H_2CO_3. Others include the anion gap and the serum potassium concentration. The anion gap is the difference between the concentration of sodium, the major extracellular cation, and the sum of the concentrations of the major measured anions, chloride and HCO_3^-. The anion gap measures the influence of minor, usually unmeasured anions on body chemistry. The anion gap is elevated after intake of exogenous acids, generation of unmeasured endogenous acids, and by several acid–base disturbances. Potassium is a predominantly intracellular cation. Its extracellular (plasma) concentration varies with pH, increasing with acidosis and decreasing with alkalosis. In simple acid–base disorders, the pH is defended by compensatory mechanisms. These include renal actions on the balance of electrolytes in the plasma to compensate for primary respiratory disturbances. They also include changes in the respiratory drive, usually in response to a change in cerebrospinal fluid pH that has occurred due to a primary metabolic disturbance. Respiratory compensation can occur quickly because of the large capacity of the lungs to excrete acid as CO_2. Metabolic compensation, controlled in the kidneys, occurs more slowly and may take days to weeks to complete.

A simple way to assess for complex acid–base disturbances is to inspect an acid–base nomogram. Acid–base nomograms vary, but they commonly relate $PaCO_2$, pH, and either HCO_3^- or measured base excess. Use of a nomogram allows interpretation of the acid–base status without the need for mathematical calculations *(53)*. An interactive acid–base map is available on the World Wide Web at http://www.acid–base.com/diagram.php *(54)*. Its usual ranges were established by meta-analysis of 35 years of human case reports. A simple paper-based acid–base map is also available (Fig. 5) *(55)*.

Mixed acid–base disorders may include one or two metabolic disturbances with or without a single respiratory disturbance. Multiple respiratory disturbances are not

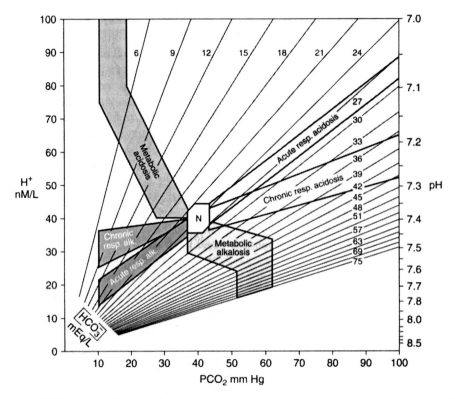

Fig. 5. An acid–base map. This graph relates pH, PCO_2, and H^+ across concentrations of HCO_3 to suggest proper assessment of acid–base status. The user plots a patient's blood gas data to find the point where pH, PCO_2, and HCO_3^- intersect. The central area, N, denotes normal acid–base status. Labeled bands reflect single acid–base derangements. Patients whose points of intersection lay outside the labeled areas likely have a mixed acid–base disturbance. From Malley *(55)*.

possible because a patient cannot have hypocarbia and hypercarbia at the same time. Diagnosis of the acid–base state relies on history, physical examination, and interpretation of electrolytes and blood gases. Use of an acid–base nomogram may simplify diagnosis.

CASE SCENARIOS

Case Scenario 1. A 20-year-old patient is ventilated for a pulmonary contusion. His lung compliance improved markedly 4 days ago, and for 3 days his pH has been above 7.5 with $PaCO_2$ 30–34 torr. When you reduce his mandatory breath rate, he is apneic. You should expect this patient's respiratory drive to improve

1. in 12 min
2. in 12 h
3. in 72 h

This patient has an uncompensated acute respiratory alkalosis of 3 days duration. Though his $PaCO_2$ may normalize within minutes, the pH of the cerebrospinal fluid and brain extracellular fluid will take hours to normalize. In the absence of active treatment with systemic acid or other measures, the respiratory drive will likely stay depressed for 12–24 h.

Case Scenario 2. A 13-year-old girl is found unresponsive with an open bottle of aspirin. Perhaps 200 tablets, each containing 325 mg aspirin, are missing. After initial stabilization, an arterial blood gas shows pH 7.3, PCO_2 20 torr, PO_2 350 torr, and base deficit 16 mEq/L. Based on the acid–base derangement, the next steps in medically managing this girl should include the following:

1. Decrease the minute volume to prevent cerebral vasoconstriction
2. Increase minute volume to normalize the pH
3. Hemodialyze to remove aspirin
4. Treat metabolic acidosis with intravenous fluid containing bicarbonate

The high base deficit and low PCO_2 indicate this patient's acid–base derangement is acute metabolic acidosis with acute respiratory alkalosis. The respiratory alkalosis is a direct effect of aspirin on the respiratory centers. The metabolic acidosis is due to aspirin's block of the electron transport chain in mitochondria. Aerobic metabolism cannot occur, and the body becomes anaerobic despite elevated oxygen tension. This results in excessive generation of heat and lactic acid. Though the first choice may prevent cerebral vasoconstriction and the second choice may raise the pH, neither will prevent death or disability from this potentially lethal aspirin overdose. The patient will likely die unless timely hemodialysis can remove the aspirin and restore aerobic cellular metabolism. Because the acidosis is not due to hypovolemia or bicarbonate loss, fluid repletion with bicarbonate solutions will help only transiently.

REFERENCES

1. Narins RG and Emmett M. Simple and mixed acid–base disorders: a practical approach. Medicine 1980; 59:161–187.
2. Malley WJ. Acid–base homeostasis. In Malley WJ (ed.), Clinical Blood Gases, 2nd ed., St. Louis: Elsevier Saunders, 2005:196–218.
3. Hlastala MP and Berger AJ. Acid–base regulation. In Physiology of Respiration, 2nd ed., New York: Oxford University Press, Inc., 2001:222–239.
4. Malley WJ. Regulation of acids, bases, and electrolytes. In Malley WJ (ed.), Clinical Blood Gases, 2nd ed., St. Louis: Elsevier Saunders, 2005:307–331.
5. Sietsema KE, Simon JI, Wasserman K. Pulmonary hypertension presenting as a panic disorder. Chest 1987; 91:910–912.
6. McFadden ER, Lyons HA. Arterial blood gas tension in asthma. N Engl J Med 1968; 278:1027–1032.
7. Kassabian J, Miller KD, Lavietes MH. Respiratory center output and ventilatory timing in patients with acute airway (asthma) and alveolar (pneumonia) disease. Chest 1982; 81:536–543.
8. Bleecker ER, Cotton DJ, Fischer SP, et al. The mechanism of rapid, shallow breathing after inhaling histamine aerosol in exercising dogs. Am Rev Respir Dis 1976; 144:909–916.
9. Cotton DJ, Bleecker ER, Fischer SP, et al. Rapid, shallow breathing after *Ascaris suum* antigen inhalation: role of vagus nerves. J Appl Physiol 1977; 42:101–106.
10. Shea SA, Winning AJ, McKenzie E, et al. Does the abnormal pattern of breathing in patients with interstitial lung disease persist in deep, non-rapid eye movement sleep? Am Rev Respir Dis 1989; 139:653–658.
11. Turino GM, Lourenco RV, Davidson LAG. The control of ventilation in patients with reduced pulmonary distensibility. Ann NY Acad Sci 1963; 109:932–940.

12. Stockley RA, Lee KD. Estimation of the resting reflex hypoxic drive to respiration in patients with diffuse pulmonary infiltration. Clin Sci 1976; 50:109–114.

13. Trenchard D, Gardner D, Guz A. Pulmonary vagal afferent nerve fibres in the development of rapid shallow breathing in lung inflammation. Clin Sci 1972; 42:251–263.

14. Phillipson EA, Murphy E, Kozar LF, et al. Role of vagal stimuli in exercise ventilation in dogs with experimental pneumonitis. J Appl Physiol 1975; 39:76–85.

15. Gardner WN. The pathophysiology of hyperventilation disorders. Chest 1996; 109:516–534.

16. Lim VS, Katz AI, Lindheimer MD. Acid–base regulation in pregnancy. Am J Physiol 1976; 231:1764.

17. Machida H. Influence of progesterone on arterial blood and CSF acid–base balance in women. J Appl Physiol 1981; 51:1433.

18. Orr-Walker BJ, Horne AM, Evans MC, Grey AB, Murray MA, McNeil AR, Reid IR. Hormone replacement therapy causes a respiratory alkalosis in normal menopausal women. J Endocrin Metab 1999; 84(6):1997–2001.

19. Lee HT, Levine M. Acute respiratory alkalosis associated with low minute volume in a patient with severe hypothyroidism. Can J Anesth 1999; 46: 185–189.

20. Hunt C, Inwood R, Shannon D. Respiratory and nonrespiratory effects of doxapram in congenital central hypoventilation syndrome. Am Rev Respir Dis 1979; 119:263–269.

21. Shannon D, Sullivan K, Perret L, Kelly D. Use of almitrine bismesylate to stimulate ventilation in congenital central hypoventilation. Eur J Respir Dis 1983; 64 (Suppl 126):295–301.

22. Sanders JS, Berman TM, Bartlett MM, et al. Increased hypoxic ventilatory drive due to administration of aminophylline in normal men. Chest 1980; 78:279.

23. Barcroft H, Basnayake V, Celander O, et al. The effect of carbon dioxide on the respiratory response to noradrenaline in man. Am J Physiol 1957; 137:365.

24. Miller LC, Schilling AF, Logan DL, et al. Potential hazards of rapid smoking as a technic for the modification of smoking behavior. N Engl J Med 1977; 297:590.

25. Mitchell RA, Loeschcke HH, Severinghaus JW, et al. Regions of respiratory chemosensitivity on the surface of the medulla. Ann NY Acad Sci 1963; 109:661.

26. Potter EK, McCloskey DI. Respiratory stimulation by angiotensin II. Respir Physiol 1979; 36:367.

27. Whelan RF, Young IM. The effect of adrenaline and noradrenaline infusions on respiration in man. Br J Pharmacol 1953; 8:98.

28. Bryant SM, Cumpston K, Lipsky MS, Patel N, Leikin JB. Metformin-associated respiratory alkalosis. Am J Therapeut 2004; 11:236–237.

29. Karetzky MS, Mithoefer JC. The cause of hyperventilation and arterial hypoxia in patients with cirrhosis of the liver. Am J Med Sci 1967; 254:797.

30. Mazzara JT, Ayres SM, Grace WJ. Extreme hypocapnia in the critically ill patient. Am J Med 1974; 56:450.

31. Winslow EJ, Loeb HS, Rahimtoola SH, et al. Hemodynamic studies and results of therapy in 50 patients with bacteremic shock. Am J Med 1973; 54:421.

32. Simmons DH, Nicoloff J, Guze LB. Hyperventilation and respiratory alkalosis as signs of gram-negative bacteremia. JAMA 1960; 174:2196.

33. Butcher J. Profile: Lewis Gordon-Pugh—polar swimmer. Lancet 2005; 366:523–524.

34. Roberts JS, Vavilala MS, Schenkman KA, et al. Cerebral hyperemia and impaired cerebral autoregulation associated with diabetic ketoacidosis in critically ill children. Crit Care Med 2006; 34:2217–2223.

35. Tasker RC, Lutman D, Peters MJ. Hyperventilation in severe diabetic ketoacidosis. Pediatr Crit Care Med 2005; 6:405–411.

36. Raichle ME, Plum F. Hyperventilation and cerebral blood flow. Stroke 1972; 3:566–575.

37. Hemphill JC 3rd, Knudson MM, Derugin N, et al. Carbon dioxide reactivity and pressure autoregulation of brain tissue oxygen. Neurosurgery 2001; 48:377–383.

38. Muizelaar JP, Marmarou A, Ward JD, et al. Adverse effects of prolonged hyperventilation in patients with severe head injury: a randomized clinical trial. J Neurosurg 1991;75:731–739.

39. The Brain Trauma Foundation, the American Association of Neurological Surgeons, and the Joint Section on Neurotrauma and Critical Care. Initial management. J Neurotrauma 2000; 17: 463–469.

40. Adelson PD, Bratton SL, Carney NA, et al. Guidelines for the acute medical management of severe traumatic brain injury in infants, children, and adolescents. Pediatr Crit Care Med 2003; 4:S45–S48.
41. Suchomski S, Morin III FC. Diseases of pulmonary circulation. In Fuhrman BP, Zimmerman JZ (eds.), Pediatric Critical Care, 2nd ed., St. Louis: Mosby-Year Book, Inc., 1998, pp. 512–528.
42. Gardner WN. The pathophysiology of hyperventilation disorders. Chest 1996; 109:516–534.
43. Rowe CG, Castillo CA, Crumpton CW. Effects of hyperventilation on systemic and coronary hemo-dynamics. Am Heart J 1962; 63:67–77.
44. Neill WA, Hattenhauer M. Impairment of myocardial O_2 supply due to hyperventilation. Circulation 1975; 52:854–856.
45. van Dixhoorn J, Duivenvoorden HJ. Efficacy of Nijmegen questionnaire in recognition of the hyper-ventilation syndrome. J Psychosom Res 1985; 29:199–206.
46. Arbus GS, Hebert LA, Levesque PR, et al. Characterization and clinical application of the "significance band" for acute respiratory alkalosis. N Engl J Med 1969; 280:117.
47. Krapf R, Beeler I, Hertner D, et al. Chronic respiratory alkalosis: the effect of sustained hyperventila-tion on renal regulation of acid–base equilibrium. N Engl J Med 1991; 324:1394.
48. Gennari FJ, Kaehny WD, Levesque PR, et al. Acid–base response to chronic hypocapnia in man. Clin Res 1980; 28:533A.
49. Weil MH, Grundler W, Yamaguchi M, et al. Arterial blood gases fail to reflect acid–base status during cardiopulmonary resuscitation: a preliminary report. Crit Care Med 1985; 13:884–885.
50. Weil MH, Rackow EC, Trevino R, et al. Difference in acid–base state between venous and arterial blood during cardiopulmonary resuscitation. N Engl J Med 1986; 315:153–156.
51. Hoes MJ, Colla P, Folgering H. Clomipramine treatment of hyperventilation syndrome. Pharmacopsy-chiatry 1980; 13:25–28.
52. Pruitt RF, Messick WJ, Thomason MH. Respiratory alkalosis caused by assist control mechanical ventilation in a patient with a bronchopleural fistula. J Trauma 1996; 40:481–482.
53. Siggaard –Anderson O. The Siggaard-Anderson curve nomogram. Scand J Clin Lab Invest 1962; 14:598.
54. Schlichtig R, Grogono, AW, Severinghaus, JW. Human $PaCO_2$ and standard base excess compensation for acid–base imbalance. Crit Care Med 1998; 26:1173-1179. Interactive acid–base map available at http://www.acid–base.com/diagram.php., accessed December 14, 2008.
55. Malley WJ. Mixed acid–base disturbances and treatment. In Malley WJ (ed.), Clinical Blood Gases, 2nd ed., St. Louis: Elsevier Saunders, 2005: pp. 365–367.
56. van Doorn P, Colla P, Folgering H. Control of end-tidal CO_2 in the hyperventilation syndrome: effects of biofeedback and breathing instructions compared. Bull Eur Physiopathol Respir 1982; 18:829–836.
57. Madias NE, Adrogue HJ. Respiratory alkalosis. In Dubose TD, Hamm LL, eds. Acid–base and Elec-trolyte Disorders: a Companion to Brenner & Rector's the Kidney. Philadelphia: Elsevier Science, 2002: 151

IV

Special Situations of Fluid and Electrolyte Disorders

12 Liver Disorders

Vani Gopalareddy and Joel Rosh

Key Points

1. Always obtain an ultrasound marking of the site prior to abdominal paracentesis to increase the yield.
2. In the setting of cholestasis and coagulopathy always administer vitamin K IM daily for 3 days and recheck INR to evaluate for liver failure.
3. Hepatorenal syndrome can occur in the setting of portal hypertension without ascites.

Key Words: Ascites; fluid; electrolytes; sodium; cirrhosis; liver failure; hepatorenal syndrome

1. ASCITES

The term "ascites" refers to the pathologic accumulation of excess fluid within the peritoneal cavity. With reference to the liver, ascites can result from pre-hepatic, intra-hepatic, or post-hepatic processes. When ascites occurs secondary to intrinsic disease of the liver, it is usually in the setting of advanced cirrhosis and hepatic decompensation (1).

1.1. Pathophysiology of Ascites

There are two proposed theories for the formation of ascites that can be referred to as the "overfill" and the "underfill" theories (Fig. 1). The overfill theory postulates that there is a primary renal tubular retention of sodium that serves to increase the plasma volume and a subsequent extravasation of fluid into the peritoneal cavity. In the underfill theory, a primary decrease in effective arterial blood volume results in renal retention of sodium and the cascade outlined above. Impaired hepatocellular functioning and portal hypertension trigger the release of the endogenous vasodilators such as nitric oxide, glucagon, and prostaglandins. The resulting peripheral vasodilatation leads to a decrease in central blood volume. Decreased plasma volume stimulates the neurohormonal system consisting of the renin–angiotensin–aldosterone (RAAS) pathway, sympathetic nervous system (SNS), and arginine vasopressin (AVP) (antidiuretic hormone). The combined effect leads to renal retention of sodium and water. Cirrhosis is also

From: *Nutrition and Health: Fluid and Electrolytes in Pediatrics*
Edited by: L. G. Feld, F. J. Kaskel, DOI 10.1007/978-1-60327-225-4_12,
© Humana Press, a part of Springer Science+Business Media, LLC 2010

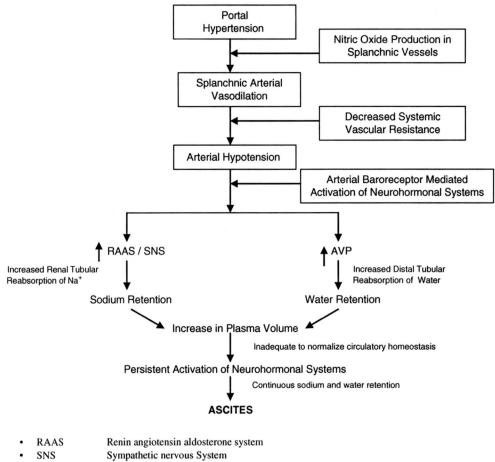

Fig. 1. Pathogenesis of ascites and hyponatremia.

associated with an increase in both atrial and ventricular atrial natriuretic peptide (ANP) release. Currently, support for the underfill theory seems most common *(2)*.

In addition to the above theories, there are several other physiologic factors that contribute to the development of ascites. Individuals with late-stage liver disease often have hypoalbuminemia secondary to poor nutrition and synthetic liver dysfunction. The hypoalbuminemia leads to a significant decrease in vascular oncotic pressure and subsequent sodium and water retentive state through RAAS and AVP as reviewed above. Additionally, portal hypertension serves to facilitate localization of this excessive amount of fluid to the peritoneal space.

1.2. Diagnosis and Treatment

Ascites may be graded as grades 1–3 or as mild, moderate, or severe (Table 1). When patients no longer respond to maximum doses of spironolactone (400 mg/day) and

Table 1
Grading of Ascites

Grade	Definition
Grade I (mild)	Normally detectable only by ultrasound examination
Grade II (moderate)	Manifest clinically by symmetric distension of the abdomen
Grade III (severe)	Gross tense ascites with marked abdominal distension

furosemide (160 mg/day) or they develop serious side effects that prohibit continued use of diuretic therapy, they are said to have untreatable (refractory) ascites.

Clinical findings of massive ascites include abdominal distension with shifting dullness and/or fluid thrill with associated lower-extremity edema and can accompany other clinical findings of chronic liver disease. Dietary restriction of sodium to about 2 g/day in adult patients (90 mEq/day), diuretic therapy with spironolactone alone or in combination with furosemide is standard practice (Figs. 2, 3, 4)

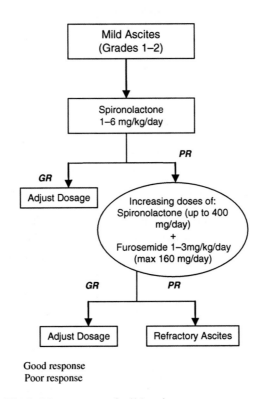

- GR   Good response
- PR   Poor response

Fig. 2. Management of mild ascites.

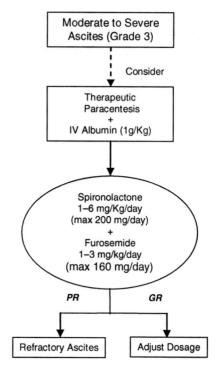

- IV   Intravenous
- GR   Good response
- PR   Poor response

Fig. 3. Management of moderate ascites.

2. HEPATORENAL SYNDROME

Hepatorenal syndrome (HRS) is a state of functional renal failure in a patient with end-stage liver disease and occurs despite structurally normal kidneys. While relatively rare in pediatric patients, it can occur in 18–39% of adult cirrhotics over a 1–5 year interval without liver transplantation *(2)*.

The syndrome is characterized by persistent oliguria (<500 ml/day), urine osmolality greater than plasma osmolality, urine–plasma creatinine ratio greater than 30:1, an elevated serum creatinine level, and urinary sodium excretion of <10 mEq/L, with a fractional excretion of sodium (FENa) < 1%. The oliguria does not respond to plasma volume expansion alone.

2.1. Pathophysiology

HRS is a severe complication of cirrhosis occurring as a consequence of an intense vasoconstriction of the renal circulation, resulting from a loss of renal autoregulation. This leads to reduced renal perfusion and a reduced glomerular filtration rate.

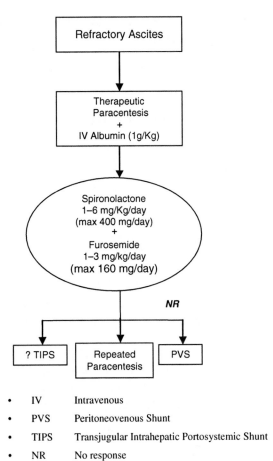

Fig. 4. Management of refractory ascites.

2.2. Management

Patients with HRS are usually candidates for liver transplantation if no other contraindications are present. Volume expansion and large volume paracentesis have been used for acute control of HRS. Volume expansion increases mean arterial pressure and paracentesis increases cardiac output and decreases renal venous pressure. The net effect of this is an increase in renal perfusion pressure and the renal flow. This leads to temporary improvement in renal function in patients with HRS. Vasodilators such as dopamine, or shunt procedures such as LeVeen (peritoneovenous), TIPS (transjugular intrahepatic portosystemic stent shunt), or orthotopic liver transplantation may be required for long-term improvement.

3. ACUTE LIVER FAILURE

The broadest definition of fulminant hepatic failure (FHF) is the development of hepatic necrosis leading to loss of liver function occurring within weeks of onset of liver disease *(3)*.

Ascites in acute liver failure is the result of acute portal hypertension, vasodilatation, poor vascular integrity, and reduced oncotic pressure. Possible fluid and electrolyte imbalances that should be anticipated include

- Hypo/hyperkalemia.
- Hypo/hypernatremia.
- Hypophosphatemia: It should be noted that there is a risk for hypophosphatemia with hepatic regeneration and ATP synthesis.
- Hypoglycemia due to decreased production and increased utilization: Defective gluconeogenesis and inadequate hepatic uptake of insulin.

3.1. Management

1. Maintain hydration without inducing fluid overload. Often 2/3 routine maintenance fluids are used to maintain urine output >0.5 cc/kg/h.
2. Restrict sodium <0.5 mEq/kg/day.
3. Diuretics spironolactone (1–6 mg/kg/day) with or without furosemide.
4. Hypoglycemia: Addition of 10% dextrose to intravenous fluids may be necessary. Frequent monitoring of blood glucose levels. Maintain blood glucose >70 mg/dL.
5. Sodium: 0.5–1 mmol/kg/day.
6. Potassium: 3–6 mmol/kg/day.
7. Phosphorus: Give IV potassium phosphate if hypophosphatemic.
8. Decreased renal perfusion (hepatorenal syndrome): State of intravascular hypovolemia hence at risk for oliguria; may need to maintain renal perfusion with

   - High-dose loop diuretics: furosemide 1–3 mg/kg q 6 h.
   - Dopamine: 2–5 μg/kg/min and FFP.
   - Hemofiltration or dialysis for severe oliguria.

CASE SCENERIO: 1

A 16-year-old male with a known diagnosis of cryptogenic cirrhosis and awaiting liver transplantation is brought to the hospital in a confused state with decreased urine output over the last 2 days. His medical condition was also complicated by marked ascites and fatigue for the last few weeks. His oral maintenance medications include lactulose given as 30 ml three times a day, spironolactone 50 mg three times a day, and ursodeoxycholic acid 300 mg twice a day.

On examination, he was afebrile with icteric sclera. His laboratory results revealed sodium of 120 mEq/L, BUN of 80 mg/dL, creatinine of 2.0 mg/dL. His serum albumin was 2.5 g/dL and conjugated bilirubin was 6.0 mg/dL.

What Is the Assessment of This Patient?

It is important to establish a diagnosis. With no history of recent medications causing nephrotoxicity, this represents acute renal deterioration in a patient with end-stage liver disease. Make sure the patient does not have excessive diarrhea and dehydration related to lactulose or diuretic therapy. The diagnosis of true hepatorenal syndrome (HRS) is

made by having an appropriate level of suspicion while excluding other potential pre-
cipitating factors.

What Is the Next Step in Management?

Obtain urinary electrolytes and creatinine to determine fractional excretion of sodium
(FE_{Na}). Central vascular pressure monitoring can be considered to help assess intravascular volume status although, in this compromised host, the risk of infection from
this intervention must be carefully considered. An $FE_{Na} < 1\%$ is consistent with the
diagnosis of HRS.

How Will You Treat This Patient?

1. *Hyponatremia*: Fluid restriction to 75% maintenance fluid with normal saline to correct
   hyponatremia. Dialysis may be required in this patient. Rapid correction with hypertonic
   saline is contraindicated as it may lead to pulmonary edema, worsening ascites, and central pontine myelinolysis. In asymptomatic patients, the target rate of rise of the serum
   sodium should not exceed 2–4 mEq/L every 4 h or about 20 mEq/L in 24 h.
2. *Hypoalbuminemia and Oliguria*: Large volume paracentesis with concomitant albumin
   infusion can be considered. Alternative to this may be a trial of albumin infusion followed
   by a high dose of a loop diuretic like furosemide. A low-dose infusion of dopamine may
   be helpful as well by stimulating renal dopaminergic receptors leading to renal vasodilatation. If these measures fail to induce an adequate diuresis, then dialysis should be
   considered pending procurement of a suitable liver donor and transplantation.

CASE SCENERIO: 2

A 15-year-old boy with end-stage liver disease due to primary sclerosing cholangitis
has just undergone orthotopic liver transplantation. The patient's intra-operative course
was remarkable for a significant transfusion requirement of 15 units of packed red cells,
10 L of crystalloid, and 4 L of coagulation products. Postoperatively, he demonstrates
good liver graft function; however, he has had a 15 kg weight gain and a decreased urine
output to 10 cc/h for last few hours.

What Is the Assessment of This Patient?

The patient is in acute renal failure in the postoperative period (Fig. 5). The origin
of renal failure in this patient may be due to a variety of factors such as post-operative
acute tubular necrosis (ATN), intravascular volume depletion with pre-renal azotemia,
and less likely, post-renal causes such as obstructive uropathy. A component of acute
nephrotoxicity from immunosuppressive medications should be considered especially if
calcineurin inhibitors are being administered. Since ATN is a salt-wasting entity, patients
with ATN usually have granular casts present in the urine, high urinary sodium, and an
$FE_{Na} > 1\%$. A normal renal ultrasound will usually exclude any obstructive uropathy.
Central vascular monitoring may be necessary to exclude pre-renal causes such as volume depletion.

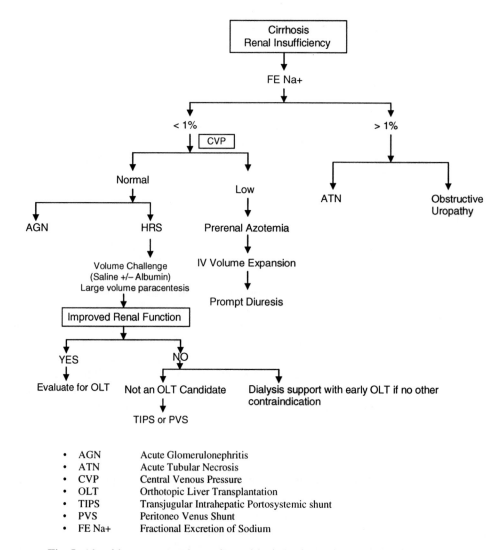

Fig. 5. Algorithm to approach a patient with cirrhosis and impaired renal function.

- AGN   Acute Glomerulonephritis
- ATN   Acute Tubular Necrosis
- CVP   Central Venous Pressure
- OLT   Orthotopic Liver Transplantation
- TIPS   Transjugular Intrahepatic Portosystemic shunt
- PVS   Peritoneo Venus Shunt
- FE Na+   Fractional Excretion of Sodium

How Will You Treat This Patient?

Carefully evaluate the patient to assess possible etiology for renal failure as in Fig. 5. Reassess intravascular volume and total body fluid status. Once this is determined, volume expansion or slow diuresis with careful monitoring of calcineurin inhibitor levels can be instituted.

REFERENCES

1. Runyon B: Care of patients with ascites. N Engl J Med 1994; 330:337–342
2. Roberts LR, Kamath PS. Ascites and hepatorenal syndrome: pathophysiology and management. Mayo Clin proc 1996 Sep; 71(9):874–881
3. Whitington PW, Alonso EM. Fulminant hepatitis and acute liver failure. In: Kelly DA, ed. Diseases of the Liver and Biliary System in Children, 2nd ed., Oxford: Blackwell publishing, 2004; 107–126

13 Special Consideration on Fluid and Electrolytes in Acute Kidney Injury and Kidney Transplantation

Oluwatoyin Fatai Bamgbola

Key Words: Acute kidney injury; Pre-renal azotemia; pRIFLE; post-transplant kidney injury; children

A normal kidney regulatory function is essential in order to maintain optimal body fluid dynamics and preserve electrolyte homeostasis. Similarly, a good kidney function is dependent on adequacy of its perfusion. The initial phase of this review will highlight the progress made so far in a consensus definition of acute kidney injury (AKI). Emphasis on the prospect of a future application of tissue biomarkers as a more accurate diagnostic tool will follow. Second, the pathogenesis and clinical outcome of pre-renal azotemia and intrinsic AKI will be differentiated. The mechanisms of renal injury in the course of fluid and electrolyte disorders are then discussed. Finally, clinical management of AKI and the challenges of fluid and electrolyte status in surgical kidney transplantation are delineated.

1. DEFINITION

Acute kidney injury is an abrupt and sustained decline in renal function that occurs over a period of few hours or days, resulting in a buildup of nitrogenous toxins, and loss of fluid, electrolyte, and acid–base homeostasis. The impairment of glomerular filtration causes fluid and salt retention leading to oliguria while excessive urine output is the likely outcome in a predominant tubular injury.

Partly because of a wide variation in operational definition, epidemiological data on AKI are often inaccurate. Indeed it is estimated that there are more than 30 definitions of AKI in the literatures *(1)*. In an effort to standardize clinical evaluation and promote comparison of research studies, AKI Network proposed a consensus definition by modifying the previously recommended RIFLE criteria. The pediatric version of RIFLE criteria is shown in the Table 1. Loss of kidney function is graded by severity into three categories on the basis of creatinine clearance [derived from Schwartz formula] and per-

From: *Nutrition and Health: Fluid and Electrolytes in Pediatrics*
Edited by: L. G. Feld, F. J. Kaskel, DOI 10.1007/978-1-60327-225-4_13,
© Humana Press, a part of Springer Science+Business Media, LLC 2010

Table 1
Pediatric RIFLE Criteria

pRIFLE criteria		Estimated creatinine clearance	Urine output
Early	R (risk)	↓ 25%	<0.5 ml/kg/h × 8 h
	I (injury)	↓ 50%	<0.5 ml/kg/h × 12 h
	F (failure)	↓ 75%	<0.5 ml/kg/h × 24 h or anuria
Late	L (loss)	Renal failure > 4 weeks	
	E (end stage)	Renal failure > 3 months	

sistence of oliguria *(2, 3)*. The late manifestations of kidney dysfunction, namely acute renal loss and acute renal failure, are recommended as outcome variables *(2, 4)*.

Furthermore, AKI qualitatively describes a spectrum of renal dysfunction that includes an asymptomatic elevation in serum creatinine concentration on one end and acute kidney failure (AKF) at the other end of the spectrum. Because of its severity, AKF has the highest probability of evolving into a permanent structural renal damage. In support of its validity, subjects with AKI as defined are hospitalized for longer duration (14 vs. 7 days, $p < 0.01$) and sustain a higher mortality rate (45.8 vs. 16.4%, $p < 0.01$) compared to the control *(4)*.

2. DIAGNOSTIC CHALLENGES

Kidney is a highly adaptive organ, with an efficient auto-regulatory mechanism and is therefore able to withstand an extreme variation in hemodynamic changes. In addition, because of a substantial renal reserve, there may be no immediate increase in serum creatinine with impairment in kidney function. Furthermore, tubular secretion of creatinine increases with severe reduction in glomerular filtration leading to an over-estimation of its clearance *(5)*. In view of these, serial evaluation of trend rather than absolute values of serum creatinine may lead to early detection of AKI *(6)*. Unfortunately, baseline information on serum creatinine value is seldom available in clinical practice. Nevertheless, highlighting its limitation as a diagnostic tool for an early kidney injury, even a marginal increase in serum creatinine value is associated with a high mortality rate in critical illness *(7)*.

Unlike creatinine, serum cystatin C does not vary with skeletal muscle mass or is it secreted by the renal tubules and may serve as a better index of glomerular filtration *(8)*. However, a multidimensional diagnostic approach that takes into account different phases of kidney injury may be more accurate than a single index. Such candidate biomarkers are cystatin C for glomerular filtration, kidney injury molecule-1 (KIM-1) for tubular function, cysteine-rich protein (CYP 61) and neutrophil gelatinase-associated lipocalin (UNGAL) for ischemia, and interlukin-18 for inflammation *(9–12)*. This novel technique may facilitate early diagnosis of AKI giving a hope for a timely therapeutic intervention and an improved mortality outcome (that had otherwise remained stagnant in the last two to three decades).

3. PRE-RENAL AZOTEMIA: PATHOPHYSIOLOGY

Pre-renal azotemia is an adaptive physiological response to an inadequate perfusion pressure that may result from either extracellular (EC) fluid depletion (e.g., acute gastroenteritis) or an ineffective circulatory volume (e.g., congestive heart failure). Normally, systemic blood flow is protected by the vascular activity of baroreceptors, which respond to hypovolemia by amplifying signal transmission to the vasomotor centers. This results in an activated sympathetic outflow, which increases the systemic arteriolar resistance and stimulates intra-renal β-adrenoreceptors for plasma renin release. In addition, release of vasopressin and aldosterone with a reduction of atrial natriuretic peptides causes salt and water retention in an effort to restore the blood volume *(13, 14)*.

Similarly, low tubular sodium delivery from impaired renal perfusion induces plasma renin release by the stimulation of macula densa (within the juxtaglomerular apparatus). In turn, plasma renin stimulates an increased synthesis of angiotensin II, a potent vasoconstrictor. With the dilatation of afferent arteriole by prostaglandin E and I_2, and an efferent vasoconstriction by angiotensin II, greater fraction of the (otherwise poor) glomerular capillary flow is filtered. This auto-regulatory process is sometimes called tubulo-glomerular feedback *(14, 15)*.

4. INTRINSIC AKI: PATHOGENESIS

Etiology of AKI includes renal vascular obstruction [e.g., hemolytic–uremic syndrome], acute nephritis, acute tubular necrosis (ATN), toxic nephropathy, interstitial nephritis, and post-renal obstruction. Acute tubular necrosis is a term that is broadly applied to all instances of kidney injury outside of arterial, glomerular, or obstructive nephropathy. Common causes of ATN are severe hypovolemia, endotoxemia, and exposure to toxins. Acute kidney injury, arising from drug toxicity, irradiation injury, sepsis, and dehydration, is a potential complication of bone marrow transplantation *(16)*. Similarly, pathogenesis of ATN in critical illness is multi-factorial and may include drugs, hypovolemia, sepsis, coagulopathy, and major organ failure. Furthermore, association of AKI with a major organ failure (or sepsis) increases the attributed mortality rate by a factor of 7–10 *(7, 13–17)*.

Failure of auto-regulatory mechanism with inadequate restoration of hemodynamic status ultimately results in loss of tubular function and structural integrity. The blood flow to the medullary kidney falls short of its intense metabolic demand, making the distal third of proximal tubules and the loop of Henle most susceptible to ischemic injury. Nephrotoxic and ischemic injuries, by increasing the local synthesis of endothelin, induce vasoconstriction by binding to ETa receptor. In addition, pro-inflammatory cytokine up-regulates endothelial wall adhesion molecules and increases activity of migratory leucocytes. Finally, the tubular injury causes a disruption of the epithelial cytoskeleton and promotes cell apoptosis and necrosis. Debris from the desquamated epithelial cells causes obstruction of the tubular lumen resulting in a backleak of its filtrate contents. The recovery phase is heralded by histological de-differentiation and regeneration of the tubular cells, which may be clinically associated with an increased urine output *(13, 14, 18)*.

5. NORMAL FLUID AND ELECTROLYTE DYNAMICS

Water constitutes close to 80% of the body weight of a newborn infant. With the growth of skeletal muscle and fat mass, water content is reduced to 50–60% of the body weight by the end of puberty. Greater amount of total body water (TBW) is situated in the intracellular (IC) space (30–40%) while EC fluid shares 20–25% of the volume. Extracellular fluid consists of plasma water (5% of TBW) and interstitial space is derived from 15% of the body fluids. To maintain adequate plasma flow, sufficient hydrostatic force must be generated by cardiac output to counteract the opposing effect of the interstitial (oncotic) pressure. Although EC and IC fluid spaces are separated by cellular membrane, osmotic equilibrium is maintained by free water permeability across the two compartments. Sodium and chloride ions are the major solutes in the EC fluid while potassium and phosphate anions are predominant in the IC unit *(19)*.

6. EXTRACELLULAR FLUID LOSS AND ACUTE KIDNEY INJURY IN CHILDREN

Children are more prone to dehydration than adults because of their unique physiological characteristics. Thus there is a greater insensible water loss in young children due to a high body surface area to weight ratio. In addition, children have a higher incidence of gastroenteritis while they depend on caregivers for an adequate access to water. Common sources of EC fluid loss are gastrointestinal tract (diarrhea, emesis), skin (fever, deep burns), and urine (forced diuresis) *(18, 19)*.

Hyper-oncotic kidney injury: Hyperglycemia, as in diabetic ketoacidosis, causes osmotic induced diuresis and severe dehydration. Poor renal perfusion is followed by azotemia in the short term while a prolonged course may lead to ischemic injury *(20)*. ATN may be prevented by an early and aggressive fluid resuscitation *(19)*. Particularly at high risk for permanent kidney injury are diabetic patients with poorly controlled hyperglycemia and a pre-existing nephropathy.

Similarly, the use of hyper-osmolar substances for forced diuresis such as mannitol in cerebral edema and 25% albumin in severe nephrotic syndrome is a potential source of AKI. Osmotic-induced renal toxicity was a common complication of sucrose-based intravenous gamma globulin (IVIG) therapy. Over the years, incidence of IVIG-mediated nephrotoxicity has been minimized with the avoidance of the sucrose medium *(21)*.

Ineffective circulatory volume: Renal perfusion may be compromised because of poor circulatory volume in spite of a positive gain in total body water. Accumulation of body fluid at the expense of plasma water deficit occurs in congestive heart failure due to reduction in cardiac output, diminished hydrostatic pressure, and expansion of venous capacitance. Similarly, low plasma oncotic pressure from severe hypoalbuminemia in nephrotic syndrome invariably results in excessive fluid retention. Cumulative gain in total body water is facilitated by pituitary vasopressin (VP) release, thirst stimulation, activated sympathetic nervous system, and induction of renin–angiotensin mechanism. Indeed there is correlation between mortality attributable to the predisposing disease and dilutional hyponatremia *(18)*.

Surgery and AKI: The incidence of an AKI after cardiac surgery in children ranges from 5 to 20%. Mortality associated with post-cardiac renal injury has remained essentially unchanged in the last two decades *(22)*. Extracorporeal diversion of blood (or cardiopulmonary bypass) during cardiac surgery may potentiate low tissue oxygen delivery and causes acute ischemic kidney injury *(23)*. To avoid life-threatening post-operative complications, a pre-emptive placement of peritoneal dialysis catheter during surgical repair of complex cardiac anomaly is desirable *(24)*. Furthermore, strategies to prevent hypovolemia are necessary in order to minimize sources of kidney injury, including rhabdomyolysis, in critically ill surgical patients. In addition to surgical hemorrhage, poor circulatory volume from capillary leaks may result from ischemic-reperfusion phenomenon, elaboration of free oxygen radicals, and cytokine-mediated endothelial injury *(22, 25)*.

7. LABORATORY EVALUATION

Serum analysis: Serial analysis showing the trend of hematocrit, hemoglobin, and serum albumin may be a useful adjunct in the evaluation of severe dehydration and adequacy of the following rehydration therapy. Metabolic acidosis may result from stool bicarbonate loss in diarrhea, and lactic acid may be generated from poor tissue perfusion in hypovolemia, sepsis, and multi-organ failure. Serum biochemistry is seldom necessary in assessing most cases of dehydration. If serum analysis is obtained, a bicarbonate concentration less than 16 mEq/L may discriminate moderate and severe dehydration from the milder form *(26)*.

Blood urea nitrogen (BUN)/serum creatinine (Cr) ratio: Extracellular fluid depletion with poor renal blood flow causes an increase re-absorption of urea by the proximal tubules. Compared with the elevation in serum creatinine, renal retention of urea is an earlier manifestation of poor kidney perfusion. Hence, BUN/Cr ratio is often greater than 20 in pre-renal azotemia. Unfortunately, blood urea nitrogen is not a reliable index of glomerular filtration as it may vary with skeletal muscle catabolism, gastrointestinal bleeding, and dietary protein intake. Similarly, serum uric acid is a sensitive but poorly specific index of renal perfusion, its concentration increases with arterial volume contraction and decreases with its expansion *(27)*.

Urine analysis and biochemistry: Urine sample is not only easy to collect; its random analysis often indicates the degree of volume deficit. In the absence of poor concentrating capacity or osmotic diuresis, a specific gravity in excess of 1015 may signify dehydration while values that are less than 1010 may suggest adequate hydration.

Urine microscopy in acute tubular necrosis may demonstrate a non-specific finding of hyaline and granular casts, few white and red blood cells, and mild proteinuria. These urinary sediments of tubular injury are reversible, subsiding few days after a successful restoration of fluid status.

In severe dehydration, poor renal perfusion with impaired glomerular filtration causes an adaptive increase in tubular sodium and water absorption, leading to a fall in urine sodium concentration (UNa) to a value less than 20 mEq/L (Table 2). The fractional excretion of urinary sodium (FENa) is less than 1% (or <2.5% in neonates), tubular concentration capacity (U/Osmol > 500 mOsm/kg) is preserved while urinary creatinine

Table 2

Diagnostic Urinary Indices to Differentiate Pre-renal Azotemia and Intrinsic Kidney Injury

Urine test	Pre-renal AKI	Intrinsic AKI	SIADH
UNa (mEq/L)	<20	>40	>40
U/SG	>1020	<1010	Generally >1020
U/Osmol (mOsm/kg)	>500	<350	Generally >500
U/P Osmol	>1.3	<1.3	Generally >2
U/Cr (mg/dL)	>40	<20	>30
FENa	<1%	>1%	~1%

UNa = urine sodium, U/SG = urine specific gravity, U/Osmol = urine osmolality, U/P Osmol = urine: plasma osmolality ratio, U/Cr = urine creatinine, FENa = fractional excretion of sodium, AKI = acute kidney injury, SIADH = syndrome of inappropriate anti-diuretic hormone secretion.
FENa = [Urine Na/Plasma Na] × [Plasma Cr/ Urine Cr] × 100

(U/Cr) is greater than 40 mg/dL. On the other hand, the loss of tubular function in intrinsic AKI results in salt wasting (FENa > 3% or > 5–10% in neonates) and poor renal concentration (U/Osmol < 350 mOsm/kg) while impaired glomerular filtration causes a reduction in urine creatinine to a value below 20 mg/dL *(18, 27)*.

Because of its correction for creatinine clearance, FENa is more sensitive (96% vs. 90%) and specific (95% vs. 82%) than urinary Na in differentiating pre-renal azotemia from intrinsic AKI. Unfortunately, accuracy of urine indices is confounded by excessive Na excretion in forced diuresis (e.g., furosemide and saline infusion). Therefore, these tests are only reliable when performed prior to institution of fluid challenge. However, given the limited diagnostic yield, therapeutic intervention should not be delayed on the account of these urinary indices *(18, 27)*.

8. CLINICAL MANAGEMENT

Pre-renal AKI: To prevent irreversible kidney injury prompt correction of EC fluid depletion is mandatory. Clinical approach is a function of the underlying cause of renal hypoperfusion. While volume restoration is critical in hypovolemia, forced diuresis and ionotropic supports (e.g., milrinone) are needed in cardiac failure. Because kidney injury in sepsis syndrome is multi-factorial, therapeutic intervention must include correction of volume deficit, hypotension (e.g., dopamine and dobutamine), coagulopathy, and endo-toxemia. In addition to the repair of fluid deficit in diabetic ketoacidosis, normoglycemia must be restored with insulin therapy. Immediate restoration of plasma oncotic pressure with slow infusion of 25% albumin and furosemide therapy will improve renal perfusion in severe nephrotic syndrome complicated by fluid overload. Exposure to therapeutic and diagnostic agents with a potential for renal insult such as hypotensive substances, renal vasoconstrictors (e.g., nonsteroidal anti-inflammatory drugs), radiopharmaceutical agents, and antibiotics (e.g., gentamicin) must be avoided or minimized. If toxic thera-peutic agent (e.g., vancomycin) must be used, serum trough levels must be monitored to avoid renal injury *(18, 27)*. At high risk of a permanent kidney injury are patients with a pre-existing glomerular impairment and a limited renal reserve, e.g., solitary kidney, renal transplant, hypoplastic–dysplastic kidney, renal artery stenosis, and use of angiotensin receptor inhibitor.

Normal saline bolus with 10–20 ml/kg over 30 min to correct peripheral circulatory failure is of utmost priority *(28)*. Assessment of mental alertness, pulse rate, blood pressure, central venous pressure (CVP), and urine output (UOP) may signify adequacy of fluid resuscitation. Lack of urine output within 2 h of fluid resuscitation should warrant examination of bladder for distension. If unsure of bladder findings, urethral catheterization is performed to determine if there is urinary retention. For patients with central vascular access, in the absence of cardiac insufficiency CVP (5–10 cm H_2O) may indicate if there is adequate volume status. If there is no urine output in spite of adequate resuscitation, diuretic challenge may be attempted with an intravenous administration of 2–4 mg/kg furosemide. If oliguria persists (UOP < 0.5 ml/kg/h) furosemide dose may be repeated either as a bolus or as a continuous infusion. Failure of diuretic fluid challenge may indicate there is an intrinsic rather than pre-renal AKI *(18, 27)*.

After a successful fluid resuscitation, volume deficit in severe dehydration is replaced as 10–15% of the body weight, moderate dehydration as 6–10%, and mild dehydration as 3–5%. Many cases of dehydration are treated with oral rehydration therapy (see Chapter 7).

Oliguric intrinsic AKI: Once there is an established kidney injury, modality of treatment will depend on the severity of glomerular filtration loss. To avoid fluid overload, intake is restricted to replace ongoing output (ml-for-ml) and the insensible water loss (400 ml/m^2/24 h) in oliguric kidney injury. To avoid sodium retention and fluid overload, metabolic acidosis is corrected only if severe (arterial pH < 7.15; serum bicarbonate <12 mEq/L). In addition, rapid correction of acidosis may decrease ionization of calcium and therefore precipitate hypocalcemic tetany. In the event of a concomitant metabolic acidosis and hyperkalemia, infusion of 1–2 mEq/kg of sodium bicarbonate over 5–10 min may normalize the serum potassium. Acidosis promotes hyperkalemia by supplying hydrogen ions for an exchange with intracellular potassium. Although furosemide diuresis does not increase renal survival in oliguric AKI, it may improve fluid control and increases renal clearance of potassium and hydrogen ions. Nebulization with albuterol solutions produces beta-agonist effect to stimulate intracellular uptake of potassium. Additional means of correcting hyperkalemia (>6 mEq/L) is the infusion of 0.1 units of regular insulin and 1 ml/kg 50% glucose over 1 h (drives potassium into the cells). Furthermore, oral or rectal administration of sodium polystyrene sulfonate resin (1 g/kg kayexalate) causes an exchange of Na for a fecal elimination of potassium *(18, 27, 29)*.

The risk of aggressive use of furosemide for volume control may outweigh its potential benefit, as it does not decrease the need for dialysis use and may in fact increase the risk of death because of delayed onset of dialysis therapy *(29)*.

Non-oliguric intrinsic AKI: In general, AKI without oliguria has a more favorable renal survival. Non-oliguric kidney injury requires a liberal fluid supply to replace the loss from the associated water diuresis. Furthermore, fluid requirement may vary with the phase of renal injury; thus the initial oliguria in ATN may give way to polyuria during the recovery phase. Hence frequent but scheduled evaluation of urine output and body weight is necessary to guide the amount of fluid requirement *(18, 27)*.

Hyperhydration and reno-protection: Generous hydration may be required to enhance renal excretion of potentially toxic endogenous or exogenous substances. Thus there is a lower incidence of contrast nephropathy with the infusion of normal saline prior to cardiac catheterization than the control. Additionally, renal sparing benefit is observed with intravenous saline support (for volume expansion) and the use of non-ionic contrast agents (290–850 mOsm/kg) in radio-imaging studies *(29)*. Adequate hydration is also a necessity to minimize possible kidney injury from acute tumor lysis during chemotherapy. The same precaution is needed to protect kidney from oncologic irradiation injury. Furthermore, renal survival is increased with an early and aggressive fluid support in traumatic rhabdomyolysis *(27)*.

Renal replacement modality: Development of fluid overload, severe hyperkalemia (>6.5 mEq/L), intractable metabolic acidosis, and inability to maintain basic nutritional needs may necessitate a renal replacement therapy. The options available in AKI are acute peritoneal dialysis (PD), acute hemodialysis (HD), and continuous renal replacement therapy (CRRT). Acute PD is a practical choice for infants because of the limited option for vascular access. Although not as technologically advanced as CRRT, it may be used in an unstable patient with hypotension. Because solute clearance is remarkably slow, PD is of no use in rapid removal of poisons or toxic metabolites (inborn errors of metabolism). Hemodialysis is the treatment of choice in systemic intoxication (e.g., acetyl salicylate poisoning) or in a sudden fluid overload. Dialysis is not an appropriate modality in the removal of any toxic substance with a wide body tissue distribution. Patients with unstable hemodynamic status (e.g., sepsis) are preferably managed with CRRT rather than a conventional dialysis. Because of improved technology, modern conventional hemodialysis may be run slowly and for longer hours to achieve a bio-equivalent outcome with the CRRT in selected patients. Although quite efficient for ultrafiltration and dialysis, use of CRRT in AKI does not improve renal outcome or mortality rate *(18, 27, 30)*.

9. KIDNEY TRANSPLANTATION: FLUID AND ELECTROLYTES

During the immediate pre-operative care of renal transplant recipients efforts should be made to avoid dehydration in order to minimize the risk of allograft hypoperfusion. Similarly, the potential recipients on chronic dialysis are prone to peri-operative pulmonary edema because of a cumulative fluid retention. The need for a pre-transplant dialysis must be individualized depending on the fluid status, time of the last dialysis, presence of residual renal function, and type of electrolyte disorders. Immediate dialysis should be instituted to correct pre-operative hyperkalemia [serum K > 5.5] or metabolic acidosis [serum HCO_3 < 18]. Fluid removal is minimized during pre-operative dialysis to protect the transplanted kidney from poor perfusion and a delayed graft function *(31, 32)*.

A pre-requisite for successful kidney transplantation is an optimal cooperation between nephrology and transplant surgical teams. An adequate knowledge of the peculiar clinical characteristics of both the allograft recipient and donor is invaluable. For an example, the nature of the primary renal disease may influence the fluid status of the recipient. Thus a poor tubular concentrating capacity in children with a previous

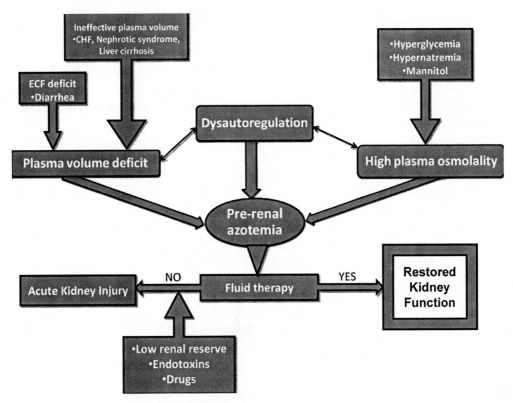

Fig. 1. Schematic illustration of the relationship between fluid and electrolyte dysregulation and acute kidney injury.

obstructive uropathy may result in a negative fluid balance. On the other hand, increased total body water is likely in hypoalbuminemia from a pre-existing nephrotic syndrome. Furthermore, patients with long-standing kidney disease may have a limited cardiac reserve due to uremic-induced diastolic dysfunction, dysautonomia, and chronic hypertension *(32)*.

Small-sized pediatric patients (<10 kg) are particularly at risk of allograft vein thrombosis because of the disparity between body mass, kidney volume, and size of the renal vessels. Adequate perfusion of the donor kidney is readily undermined by the diminutive systemic pressure and low blood volume that are typical of pediatric recipients. Consequently, the transplanted kidney is prone to vascular thrombosis from poor plasma perfusion, ischemic endothelial injury, and surgery-related mechanical stress. To minimize the occurrence of vascular thrombosis, enough fluid is administered during surgery to maintain CVP at 16–20 cm H_2O prior to allograft vascular anastomosis. Use of 5% albumin may be preferred if serum albumin is <2.5 g/dL. Sometimes, the volume of intra-operative fluid required to sustain an adequate perfusion may lead to the development of post-operative pulmonary edema (29%) and a need for assisted ventilation (8.3%) *(33, 34)*.

Intra-operative administration of (hypertonic) mannitol solution has the potential not only to enhance allograft perfusion but it also minimizes oxidative stress (as a free oxygen radical scavenger) from ischemic reperfusion injury. Pulse steroid therapy, though primarily used for immuno-suppression, may increase vasoactivity and improve renal blood flow. Immediate UOP after allograft vascular anastomosis is a good indicator of an adequate renal perfusion. In the absence of prolonged ischemia, brisk diuresis occurs within few minutes of surgical anastomosis. Initial urine output is massive because of osmotic effect of urea nitrogen load, intra-operative fluid challenge, and mobilization of retained body water from chronic kidney disease *(32, 35)*.

Prolonged cold ischemia, inadequate renal perfusion, and loss of autoregulation in a denervated graft are predisposing factors for a delayed function. Post-operatively, adequate fluid input must be maintained by keeping CVP between 8 and 10 cm H_2O. Estimated from the average daily urinary Na excretion (>40 mEq/L) and gastric Na secretion (20–80 mEq/L), post-transplant loss of urine or nasogastric secretions is replaced ml-for-ml with half-normal saline (77 mEq/L). The insensible water loss is replaced with 5% dextrose water as 45–50 ml/100 kcal of daily energy expenditure. Insensible water loss may also be crudely estimated as 40–50% of the maintenance fluid requirements *(31, 32)*.

Frequent evaluation of fluid status is essential to allow for adjustment in intake if necessary. Normal saline fluid boluses (10–20 ml/kg body weight) is given if there is a fall in CVP below 7 cm H_2O and/or reduction in UOP below 1–2 ml/kg/h and/or progressive fall in BP below the baseline. If there is no increase in UOP after 2–3 boluses of NS, forced diuresis with furosemide may be attempted. Absence of urine output in spite of an elevated CVP is another reason for a furosemide diuresis. It should be noted that forced diuresis does not necessarily improve graft outcome; its major advantage is to forestall fluid overload and postpone an immediate need for dialysis *(31, 32)*.

The rate of intravenous fluid infusion is reduced by 25% every 1 h if urine output exceeds 5 ml/kg/h. Urine volume should be maintained at 2–5 ml/kg/h. Post-ischemic diuresis may follow the recovery of renal allograft from ATN. Therefore, inadequate fluid support may compromise long-term allograft function *(31)*.

CASE SCENARIO

AR is an 11-year-old African American female who was previously healthy until few months prior to the presentation at a local emergency room (ER). She had anorexia, sleepiness, body weakness, and close to 15 kg weight loss in the last five months. She had an increased frequency of emesis in the last few weeks, and an associated diarrhea for 3 days. Her current medications included "apple cider vinegar" and an unidentified "enzyme supplement;" both of which were obtained from a health food store for symptomatic relief. Her perinatal history was uneventful and immunization was up to date.

What in the history suggests a possible diagnosis of kidney injury?
The history highlights a common clinical scenario in the presentation of chronic kidney disease. This girl had been sick for a minimum of 5 months. She presented with protracted uremic symptoms but apparently because of an adequate renal reserve visit to the ER was avoided until the later phase of the illness. Uremia alters the control of

hunger–satiety cycle by increasing brain secretion of anorectic serotonin, and causing a decreased synthesis of (appetite stimulant) neuropeptide Y. In addition to low caloric intake, catabolism with weight loss is promoted by pro-inflammatory cytokines (IL-1), elaboration of leptin, and metabolic acidosis. Anemia and metabolic acidosis are contributory to body weakness and somnolence. The protracted symptoms, in the setting of a poor accessibility to health care services, may promote risky behavior such as seeking homeopathic medicine or over-the-counter therapy. Often, these non-FDA approved alternative agents (largely untested for nephrotoxicity) may cause further kidney injury. Medication such as nonsteroidal anti-inflammatory drug may also cause a rapid loss in renal function leading to deterioration in a compensated kidney disease. Her symptoms progressively worsen over the months, and in the last 1 week an acute deterioration necessitates urgent medical services.

What are the common chronic kidney diseases in which family history could be helpful in making diagnosis?

Common kidney diseases with strong family history are Alport nephritis (X-linked or autosomal inheritance), polycystic kidney disease (autosomal recessive or dominant), and nephrogenic diabetes insipidus (X-linked or autosomal). Focal segmental glomerulosclerosis (FSGS) is a common cause of nephrotic syndrome particularly in African American population. FSGS is heterogeneous kidney disease, some of which have clearly defined genetic mutation that involves functional integrity of podocytes (a component of foot process in the glomerulus; important for ultrafiltration).

The family history in this patient is highly suspicious of a possible diagnosis of FSGS. Both parents and a maternal aunt were on dialysis for end-stage kidney disease. Except for the maternal aunt who had a preceding nephrotic syndrome the etiology of end-stage kidney disease was unknown in both parents. Her paternal grandmother died of chronic kidney disease. Her 20-year-old brother and 14-year-old sister were healthy, and both had tested negative for proteinuria. Review of the system was unremarkable.

If this is an acute on chronic kidney injury, what are the expected physical findings?

Protracted fluid loss might have resulted in dehydration. On the other hand, long standing oliguria may predispose to fluid retention including body edema, congestive heart failure (CHF), and pulmonary edema. Severe hypertension with or without encephalopathy is a likely complication. Advanced kidney disease may present with anemia because of erythropoietin deficiency or dilutional effect of fluid retention. Deficient 1-alpha hydroxylation of 25-vitamin D and secondary hyperparathyroidism may result in hypocalcemia. Impaired glomerular filtration reduces renal phosphate clearance. Metabolic acidosis may lead to lethargy and acidotic hyperventilation. Hyperkalemia is a possible complication due to impaired potassium clearance and an extracellular shift of potassium in exchange for hydrogen ions. On the other hand, she may also have hypokalemia because of the protracted emesis and total body potassium depletion from skeletal muscle wasting.

Her clinical and laboratory findings reflect a number of the projected possibilities: she had a normal mental status, good nutritional status, moderate pallor, mild–moderate dehydration, but there was no jaundice, body edema, or peripheral adenopathy. Her axillary temperature was 99°F, pulse rate 75/min, RR 20/ min, BP 162–177/100–115 mmHg, and pulse oximetry was 99% in room air. Her height was 153 cm and weight was 48.7 kg. Other physical findings were not clinically significant.

Laboratory analysis: WBC was 5.1, hemoglobin 8.1 gm/dL, hematocrit 22.6%, and platelet count was 145,000. Serum Na was 137 mEq/L, K 2.6 mEq/L, Cl 97 mEq/L, HCO_3 19 mEq/L, glucose 77 mg/dL, BUN 93 mg/dL, Cr 18.7 mg/dL, Ca 4.3 mg/dL, P 9.6 mg/dL, and albumin 4.1 gm/L. Urine had a pH of 6.5, protein was >300 mg/dL, was positive for ketones, but glucose was negative. EKG showed a prolonged QTc interval with no arrhythmia. Echocardiogram showed a mild decrease in ventricular contractility.

Her calculated GFR (cGFR) by Schwartz formula is

$$cGFR = k \times Ht\,(cm)/Serum\,Cr\,(mg/dL) = 0.55 \times 153/18.7 = 4.7\,ml/min/1.73m^2$$

(k; proportionality constant for age and sex = 0.55)

$$\%\,loss\,in\,GFR = eGFR - cGFR/eGFR \times 100 = 127 - 4.7/127 \times 100 = 96.3\%$$

(where eGFR = estimated normal GFR for age)

Using the pRIFLE criteria (see Table 1), she has a stage 3 AKI or acute kidney failure (AKF). Thus, most likely she has an acute loss in GFR on a pre-existing kidney injury. Because there is hardly any chance for renal recovery, a chronic maintenance dialysis will be ultimately required.

Note that she presented with a weight of 48.7 kg which is >90th percentile for height. With the loss of 15 kg in the course of the illness her real weight exceeds 64 kg (>99th, percentile for height). Using the baseline weight to calculate her body mass index (BMI), the value equals 28.4 kg/m^2 (which is >95th percentile = 26 kg/m^2). Thus obesity is a contributing factor to the kidney failure. The ensuing weight-loss in the course of her illness is an adaptive mechanism by the kidney to minimize the metabolic load of obesity. This is one of the reasons why kidney may be so resilient, and why kidney injury may last long before obvious clinical manifestation.

What are the immediate and long-term therapeutic concerns?

Life-threatening complications must be addressed immediately including cardiac toxicity (prolonged QTc) from hypocalcemia and/or hypokalemia and correction of fluid deficiency. Infusion of bicarbonate was not a priority because of its less severe deficit and due to the danger of hypocalcemic tetany. Blood transfusion may be avoided if there are no symptoms attributed to anemia. Otherwise, it may be given during dialysis to avoid fluid overload in the presence of oliguric kidney injury. Severe hypertension should be reduced slowly (50–75% over 24 h) with oral antihypertensive agents in the absence of symptoms. If there is hypertensive encephalopathy, immediate intravenous therapy with nicardipine, labetalol, diazoxide, or sodium nitroprusside is administered. After the initial hemodynamic stability, central dialysis catheter is inserted and acute hemodialysis is provided. To maintain fluid and electrolyte homeostasis, and restore important renal function deficit, chronic dialysis is offered while supportive care is instituted for anemia, Vitamin D deficiency, hyperphosphatemia, hypertension, and nutritional deficit. Dialysis modality is not an end in itself but a transitional procedure that will allow for eventual renal allograft transplantation.

Acute therapy for the patient included infusion of 5% dextrose and half saline with 20 mEq/L per liter of potassium chloride to correct dehydration and hypokalemia, intravenous Ca gluconate for severe hypocalcemia (restoring EKG changes back to normal), and thereafter acute hemodialysis. Chronic supportive care included home peritoneal dialysis, sevelamer hydrochloride as phosphate binder, erythropoietin for anemia, nifedipine for hypertension, and 1, 25 Vitamin D as maintenance therapy for Ca deficiency.

After an extensive pre-transplant work up, she was placed on a waiting list for cadaveric transplantation. Ten months after the initial diagnosis, she was offered the kidney of a 31-year-old head injury victim of a motor vehicle accident. Cold ischemic time for the allograft was 10 h. She had oliguria in the first 3 h of surgery with urine output of 15–20 ml/h. Although BP was 150/95 mmHg, CVP was low, 2–5 cm H_2O. She received three boluses of normal saline, which was followed by a prompt increase in rate of UOP to 100–150 ml/h. Blood urea nitrogen was 48 mg/dL, while serum Cr was 18.8 mg/dL shortly after the graft surgery. By post-operative day 3, serum creatinine had decreased to 7.4 mg/dL while by the 7th day the Cr was 1.6 mg/dL.

REFERENCES

1. Bellomo R, Ronco C, Kellum JA, Mehta RL, Palevsky P and the ADQI workgroup. Acute renal failure – definition, outcome measures, animal models, fluid therapy and information technology needs: the Second International Consensus Conference on the Acute Dialysis Quality Initiative (ADQI) Group. Crit Care 2004, 8 (4): R204–R212

2. Mehta RL, Kellum JA, Shah SV, Mollitoris BA, Ronco C, Warnock DG, Levin A. Acute kidney injury network: report of an initiative to improve outcomes in acute kidney injury. Crit Care 2007, 11(2): R31

3. Akcan-Arikan A, Zappitelli M, Loftis LL, Washburn KK, Jefferson LS, Goldstein SL. Modified RIFLE criteria in critically ill children with acute kidney injury. Kidney Int 2007, 71(10): 1028–1035

4. Barrantes F, Tian J, Vazquez R, Amoateng-Adjepong Y, Manthous CA. Acute kidney injury criteria predict outcomes of critically ill patients. Crit Care Med 2008, 36(5): 1397–1403

5. Doolan PD, Alpen EL, Theil GB. A clinical appraisal of the plasma concentration and endogenous clearance of creatinine. Am J Med 1962, 32: 65–72

6. Lassnigg A, Schmid ER, Hiesmayr M, Falk C, Druml W, Baeuer P, Schmidlin D. Impact of minimal increase in serum creatinine on outcome in patients after cardiothoracic surgery: do we have to revise current definitions of acute renal failure? Crit Care Med 2008, 36(4): 1129–1137

7. Chertow GM, Burdick E, Honour M, Bonventre JV, Bates DW. Acute kidney injury, mortality, length of stay, and costs in hospitalized patients. J Am Soc Nephrol 2005, 16:3365–3370

8. Herrero-Morin JD, Malaga S, Fernandez N, Rey C, Dieguez MA, Solis G, Concha A, Medina A.. Cystatin C and beta2-microglobulin: markers of glomerular filtration in critically ill children. Crit Care 2007, 11: R59

9. Bennett M. Urine NGAL predicts severity of acute kidney injury after cardiac surgery: a prospective study. Clin J Am Soc Nephrol 2008, 3(3): 665–673

10. Parikh CR, Devarajan P. New bio-markers of acute kidney injury. Crit Care Med 2008, 36: S159–S165

11. Mehta RL, Chertow GM. Acute renal failure definitions and classification: Time for change? J Am Soc Nephrol 2003, 14: 2178–2187

12. Zappitelli M, Washburn KK, Arikan AA, Loftis LL, Ma Q, Devarajan P, Parikh CR, Goldstein SL. Urine neutrophil gelatinase-associated lipocalin is an early marker of acute kidney injury in critically ill children: A prospective cohort study. Crit Care 2007, 11(4): R84

13. Galloway E, Doughty L. Electrolyte emergencies and acute renal failure in pediatric critical care. Clin Pediatr Emerg Med 2007, 8(3): 176–189

14. Bailey D, Phan V, Litalien C et al. Risk factors of acute renal failure in critically ill children: A prospective descriptive epidemiological study. Pediatr Crit Care Med 2007, 8: 29–35
15. Iglesias J, Lieberthal W. Clinical evaluation of acute renal failure. In: Johnson RJ, Feehaly J, eds. Comprehensive clinical nephrology, 1st edn. London: Mosby, 2000, (4): 15.1–15.16
16. Detaille T, Anslot C, de Clety SC. Acute kidney injury in pediatric bone marrow patients. Acta Clin Belg Suppl 2007, 2:401–404
17. Wolfson RG, Hillman K. Causes of acute renal failure. In: Johnson RJ, Feehaly J, eds. Comprehensive clinical nephrology, 1st edn. London: Mosby, 2000, (4): 16.1–16.15
18. Khalil P, Murty P, Palevsky PM. The patient with acute kidney injury. Primary Care: Clinics in Office Practice 2008, (35): 239–264
19. Greenbaum LA. The pathophysiology of body fluids and fluid therapy. In: Kliegman RM, Behrman RE, eds. Nelson textbook of pediatrics, 18th edn. Philadelphia, PA: Saunders Elsevier, 2007, (52): 300–319
20. Moritz ML, Ayus JC. Preventing neurological complications from dysnatremias in children. Pediatr Nephrol 2005, 20(12): 1687–1700
21. Orbach H, Katz U, Sherer Y, Shoenfeld Y. Intravenous immunoglobulin: adverse effects and safe administration. Clin Rev Allergy Immunol 2005, 29(3): 173–184
22. Thakar CV, Worley S, Arrigain S, Yared JP, Paganini EP. Improved survival in acute kidney injury after cardiac surgery. Am J Kidney Dis 2007, 50(5): 703–711
23. Ranucci M. Perioperative renal failure: hypoperfusion during cardiopulmonary bypass? Semin Cardiothorac Vasc Anesth 2007, 11(4): 265–268
24. Alkan T, Akcevin A, Turkoglu H, Paker T, Sasmazel A, Bayer V, Ersoy C, Askn D, Aytac A. Preoperative prophylactic peritoneal dialysis in neonates and infants after complex congenital cardiac surgery. ASAIO J 2006, 52(6): 693–697
25. Sharp LS, Rozycki GS, Feliciano DV. Rhabdomyolysis and secondary renal failure in critically ill surgical patients. Am J Surg 2004, 188(6): 801–806
26. Wathen JE, MacKenzie T, Bothner JP. Usefulness of the serum electrolyte panel in the management of pediatric dehydration treated wit intravenously administered fluids. Pediatrics 2004, 114(5): 1227–1234
27. Vogt BA, Avner ED. Acute renal failure. In: Kliegman RM, Behrman RE, eds. Nelson Textbook of Pediatrics, 18th edn. Philadelphia, PA: Saunders Elsevier, 2007, (535): 2206–2209
28. Neville KA, Verge CF, Rosenberg AR, O'Meara MW, Walker JL. Isotonic is better than hypotonic saline for intravenous rehydration of children with gastroenteritis: a prospective randomized study. Arch Dis Child 2006, 91(3): 226–232
29. Venkataraman R. Can we prevent acute kidney injury? Crit Care Med 2008, 36(4): S166–S171
30. Ricci Z, Ronco C. Dose and efficiency of renal replacement therapy: Continuous renal replacement therapy versus intermittent hemodialysis versus slow extended daily dialysis. Crit Care Med 2008, 36(4): 229–237
31. Brenan DC. Immediate postoperative management of the kidney transplant recipient. In: Norman DJ, Turka LA eds. Primer on Transplantation 2nd edn. New Jersey: American Transplantation Society, 2001, (54): 440–451.
32. Urizar RE.. Renal Transplantation. In: Kliegman RM, Behrman RE, eds. Nelson Textbook of Pediatrics, 18th edn. Philadelphia, PA: Saunders Elsevier, 2007, (536): 2214–2219
33. Chavers B, Najarian JS, Humar A. Kidney transplantation in infants and small children. Pediatr Transplant 2007, 11(7): 702–708
34. Sprung J, Kapural L, Bourke DL, O'Hara JF Jr. Anesthesia for kidney transplant surgery. Anesthesiol Clin North Am 2000, 18(4): 919–951
35. Markmann JF, Yeh H, Naji A, Olthoff KM, Shaked A, Barker CF. Transplantation of abdominal organs. In: Townsend CM Jr. ed., Sabiston Textbook of Surgery, 18th ed. Philadelphia, PA: Saunders Elsevier 2008, (28): 692–707

14 Adrenal Causes of Electrolyte Abnormalities: Hyponatremia/Hyperkalemia

Lawrence A. Silverman

Key Points

1. Sodium and potassium homeostasis is tightly controlled by adrenal mineralocorticoid production.
2. Disorders of sexual differentiation are frequently associated with electrolyte disorders.
3. Inborn errors of aldosterone biosynthesis and bioactivity leading to lead hyponatremia and hyperkalemia.

Key Words: Congenital adrenal hyperplasia; Aldosterone deficiency; 17-OHP; aldosterone; plasma renin activity

1. CONGENITAL ADRENAL HYPERPLASIA

An 8-day-old baby boy presents to the emergency department. He is ill appearing, lethargic, and hypotensive. Initial laboratory assessment reveals a serum sodium of 131 mEq/L and potassium of 6.3 mEq/L.

The diseases of the adrenal glands that result in disorders of salt and water metabolism can be classified as diseases of either aldosterone deficiency or aldosterone excess. Further classification of diseases of aldosterone deficiency includes disorders of decreased aldosterone production or decreased activity.

Case Scenario 1: The most common cause of decreased aldosterone production lies within the group of disorders commonly referred to as congenital adrenal hyperplasia (CAH). CAH is a group on inherited disorders of adrenal steroid biosynthesis (Fig. 1). While this group of diseases is commonly thought of only as a disorder of sexual differentiation at birth, the associated disorders in production of aldosterone and its precursors frequently lead to abnormalities in sodium and potassium homeostasis. Eventually, these disorders can lead to issues of severe dehydration, sodium and potassium imbalance, and, ultimately, life-threatening shock (Table 1) *(1)*.

From: *Nutrition and Health: Fluid and Electrolytes in Pediatrics*
Edited by: L. G. Feld, F. J. Kaskel, DOI 10.1007/978-1-60327-225-4_14,
© Humana Press, a part of Springer Science+Business Media, LLC 2010

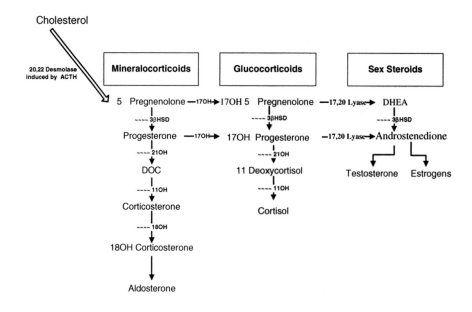

DHEA – Dehydroepiandrosterone, OH – Hydroxylase, HSD – Hydroxysteroid dehyrogenase

Fig. 1. Pathway of adrenal steroid synthesis.

As noted in earlier chapters, aldosterone is produced by the cells of the zona glomeru-losa of the adrenal gland. Its production is regulated by angiotensin II, which in turn is regulated by renin levels. Renin production reflects intravascular volume, as detected by renal perfusion through the juxtaglomerular apparatus. Both potassium and to a lesser degree adrenocorticotropic hormone (ACTH) levels are also important in the regulation of aldosterone levels. Aldosterone in turn acts at the distal tubule, via the mineralocor-ticoid receptor, resulting in activation of sodium channels and the sodium–potassium pump. This results in resorption of sodium and water and excretion of potassium. This ultimately controls electrolyte and fluid regulation *(2)*.

Table 1
Forms of CAH with Electrolyte Disturbances

Lipoid adrenal hyperplasia (StAR or 20,22 desmolase deficiency)
3β-Hydroxysteroid dehydrogenase deficiency
21-Hydroxylase deficiency
Aldosterone synthetase deficiency

Of the six forms of CAH, 21-hydroylase deficiency is the most common, accounting for 90% of all CAH *(3)*. With an incidence of approximately 1 in 15,000, up to 75% of cases are noted to be "salt wasters." As noted in the adrenal steroidogenic pathway, this disease state is not a primary defect in aldosterone biosynthesis, but rather the inability to synthesize aldosterone precursors leading to aldosterone deficiency and a consequent inability to resorb sodium and excrete potassium in the tubules. Hence hyponatremic hyperkalemic metabolic acidosis is observed in untreated patients.

The presentation of infants with 21-hydroxylse deficiency may be dependent upon the sex of the newborn. An overvirilized female will frequently be noted to have a disorder of sexual differentiation and generally be observed in the nursery for signs of salt wasting, once the diagnosis of CAH is entertained. However, a newborn male with salt losing 21-hydroxylase deficiency may only have the subtle stigmata of mild hyperpigmentation. Thus, an infant boy may present ill appearing with hyperkalemic, hyponatremic acidosis. This presentation is usually after the first week of life, as the control of fetal electrolytes relies on the placenta and the mother's kidneys. With the institution of newborn screening programs for 21-hydroxylase deficiency throughout the United States, this presentation will hopefully become less common. However, normal newborn screening results do not rule out the possibility of disease.

The other, less common causes of CAH may similarly present with ambiguous genitalia and abnormalities related to salt wasting and hypertension. These include 3β-hydroxysteroid dehydrogenase deficiency as well as StAR (congenital lipoid hyperplasia) deficiency (4, 5). As noted from Table 1, both of these forms of CAH also lead to decrease production of aldosterone with subsequent salt wasting crisis in the newborn period. Both of these enzyme deficiencies may lead to disorders of sexual differentiation, as males with StAR deficiency and males with 3β-hydroxysteroid dehydrogenase deficiency will be undervirilized while females will be overvirilized.

2. ALDOSTERONE BIOSYNTHETIC DEFICIENCIES

Specific disorders in aldosterone biosynthesis have also been described that are not usually associated with either disorders of sexual differentiation or cortisol production (2). Aldosterone synthetase deficiency, also known as corticosterone methyl oxidase (CMO) I and II, deficiency are among this subgroup. These patients will present with failure to thrive and mild salt-wasting crisis, hyponatremic, hyperkalemic, metabolic acidosis in the first few months of life. The secretory rate of deoxycorticosterone (DOC) is insufficient to meet the mineralocorticoid requirement of a newborn. As they also have normal cortisol production, hypotension and shock are less likely.

3. DEFECTS IN ALDOSTERONE ACTION

With less than 100 cases reported in the literature, a rare resistance to aldosterone has been reported. These patients with pseudohypoaldosteronism type I would present in a fashion similar to those with aldosterone deficiency, but laboratory findings would note elevated aldosterone levels and elevated plasma rennin activity (PRA). As noted in earlier chapters, patients with primary renal disease, including obstructive and infective process, may also present with aldosterone resistant picture, sometimes referred to as type 4 RTA.

4. CONGENITAL SYNDROMES

There are rare syndromes associated with lack of development of the adrenal gland (Table 2). These are not specifically related to enzyme deficiency in the gland, but a lack of development of a normally functioning gland from an anatomic/physiologic perspective. Among these disorders are syndromic disorders, including Smith–Lemli–Opitz and deficiencies of two genes important to adrenal gland development, DAX and SF-1. This specific X-linked adrenal hypoplasia may also be associated with muscular dystrophy and glycerol kinase deficiency.

Table 2
Syndromes Associated with Adrenal Insufficiency

Smith–Lemli–Opitz
X-linked muscular dystrophy/glycerol kinase deficiency/adrenal hypoplasia
Zellweger syndrome
Wolman disease
Adrenal leukodystrophy
Allgrove syndrome

Other congenital syndromes may affect lipid production, and hence an inability to provide the cholesterol precursors necessary for adrenal steroid biosynthesis. These include Zellweger and Wolman syndromes. The adrenal leukodystrophies and the AAA syndrome of achalasia–addisonianism–alacrima often present later in childhood and have variable mineralocorticoid deficiency.

5. ACQUIRED ADRENAL INSUFFICIENCY

Case Scenario 2: A 13-year-old girl with a history of Hashimoto's thyroiditis presents with fatigue and weight loss.

While less common, there are a number of acquired forms of adrenal insufficiency. Included among these are insufficiency secondary to adrenal hemorrhage, either in the newborn period, or secondary to infection, i.e., Waterhouse–Friderichsen syndrome. Viral, fungal, and tuberculin infections leading to adrenal insufficiency have been described, as has infiltrative disorders, including sarcoidosis, amyloidosis, and histiocytosis X *(6)*.

Perhaps more relevant to pediatric practice are those disorders that fall into the autoimmune classification. While frequently isolated, acquired adrenal insufficiency may be associated with other endocrine hypofunction, as well as vitiligo and mucocutaneous candidiasis. Certainly in the setting of other autoimmune disease, as well as a positive family history, an increased index of suspicion will help in making the diagnosis.

It is important to note that those diseases that lead to ACTH deficiency rarely cause disturbances in electrolyte balance, as this system is under the control of the renin–angiotensin–aldosterone system, which is independent of ACTH production.

6. HYPOKALEMIA

While rare, 17α-hydroxylase deficiency presents later in life, usually around the time of puberty, with hypokalemia and hypertension and delayed puberty. Increased substrate, specifically deoxycorticosterone (DOC), which has aldosterone-like effects in the mineralocorticoid pathway, leads to increased production of precursors, hence leading to hypokalemia (7).

7. ACUTE ADRENAL INSUFFICIENCY WITH MINERALOCORTICOID DEFICIENCY

7.1. Evaluation and Treatment

Most commonly acute adrenal insufficiency with electrolyte disturbances presents in the neonatal period.

Referring to the vignette (Case Scenario 1) at the beginning of this chapter, an 8-day-old baby boy presents to the emergency department. He is ill appearing, lethargic, and hypotensive. Initial laboratory assessment reveals a serum sodium of 131 mEq/L and a potassium of 6.3 mEq/L. Serum glucose is 35 mg/dL. Further history reveals persistent vomiting and poor feeding as well as decreased wet diapers. A family history reveals a previous male child died at 3 weeks of age of reported diarrhea, dehydration, and shock. On physical exam, the infant is ill appearing and markedly dehydrated. He is in shock. His weight is 15% below birth weight. He has a generous sized phallus, with hyperpigmented nipples, and scrotum.

The patient's history, physical, and laboratory exam are consistent with the diagnosis of salt losing congenital adrenal hyperplasia (Table 3). The most likely disease in the CAH spectrum is 21-hydroxylase deficiency.

Table 3
Signs of Mineralocorticoid Deficiency

Weakness
Weight loss
Anorexia
Fatigue
Salt craving
Hypotension
Hyperpigmentation
Hyponatremic, hyperkalemic acidosis

As with any patient, the first goal is acute resuscitation. In this case, fluid in the form of normal saline, with or without dextrose, to correct shock is of primary importance. In addition, a stress dose of hydrocortisone should be given, 25 mg/m^2 IV; this may be life saving. During the initial workup, a "red top tube" can be set aside for serum analysis of adrenal steroid precursors, the most important of which is 17-hydroxyprogesterone. Additional laboratory evaluation that may be obtained to help diagnose mineralocorticoid deficiency include urine electrolytes and a plasma renin activity (obtained in a "purple top" EDTA tube and placed on ice).

Once the patient has been stabilized and is no longer in extremis, the diagnosis is confirmed by elevation of adrenal precursors, either random or after ACTH testing, and DNA analysis, replacement therapy can begin. The goal of therapy in CAH is to decrease adrenal androgen production by replacing cortisol and to insure electrolyte homeostasis by replacing aldosterone. To achieve this goal, hydrocortisone replacement requirements are generally higher than the normal cortisol secretory rate of 7.5–12.5 mg/m^2 divided into every 8-h oral dosing In addition mineralocorticoid replacement is given as 9-alpha-fluorocortisol acetate (fludrocortisone). This dose is titrated to blood pressure, electrolytes and plasma renin activity levels. Infants generally need larger doses than older children. As infants generally receive very little sodium though either breast milk (7.7 mEq/l) or infant formula (18.5 mEq/l), sodium replacement, frequently as 2 g of table salt daily, is needed until enough dietary sodium is ingested daily. The sodium requirement of an infant is 2–3 mEq/kg/day.

CASE SCENARIO 2

A 13-year-old girl with a history of Hashimoto's thyroiditis presents with fatigue and weight loss. History reveals intermittent abdominal pain and occasional vomiting in the afternoon. Upon further questioning there is increased intake of salty foods. Family history is positive for a relative with type 1 diabetes and premature ovarian failure. Upon exam, the girl is cachectic, with a 10-pound weight loss. There is mild hyperpigmentation on the palms, soles, and gums, and no tan lines are noticed. Laboratory evaluation reveals a serum sodium concentration of 131 mEq/L, potassium 5.4 mEq/L. A morning cortisol level is low, 3.2 mcg/dL (3–21), with an inappropriately elevated ACTH of 824 pg/ml (6–48).

This patient appears to have acquired adrenal insufficiency. In the setting of another autoimmune endocrinopathy in the patient, and the family history of a relative with autoimmune endocrinopathy, the history and findings are consistent with polyglandular autoimmune syndrome (8). The autoimmune etiology can be confirmed by measuring anti-21-hydroxylase antibodies. Treatment in this situation is related to long-term replacement of glucocorticoids and mineralocorticoid; as the patient is not in extremis, stress coverage may not be necessary (Table 4). In general, older patients will have their

Table 4
Maintenance and Stress Glucocorticoid and Mineralocorticoid Replacement

Medication	Maintenance dosage range	Stress dosage
Glucocorticoid replacement (mg/m^2/24 hours)	7.5–12.5 /every 8 hours	25–50
Mineralocorticoid (mg/day)	0.05–1.5	0.05–1.5

Note: no additional mineralocorticoid stress dosage is required, as the increased glucocorticoids will provide enough mineralocorticoid effect.

own "salt seeking" behavior and supplemental sodium is rarely necessary to maintain sodium and potassium in the normal range.

REFERENCES

1. New, M. Diagnosis and management of congenital adrenal hyperplasia. Ann Rev Med 1998;49: 311–328.
2. White PC. Disorders of Aldosterone Biosynthesis and Action, NEJM 1994;331: 250–258.
3. White PC, Speiser PW. Congenital adrenal hyperplasia due to 21-hydroxylase deficiency. Endocr Rev 2000;21: 245–291
4. Pang S, Congenital adrenal hyperplasia owing to 3 beta-hydroxysteroid dehydrogenase deficiency. Endocrinol Metab Clin North Am 2001 Mar;30(1): 81–99
5. Bose H, Sugawara T, Strauss Jr, Miller W, The pathophysiology and genetics of congenital lipoid adrenal hyperplasia. International Congenital Lipoid Adrenal Hyperplasia Consortium. N Engl J Med 1996;335: 1870–1878
6. Shulman DI, Palmert MR, Kemp SF, Adrenal insufficiency: Still cause of morbidity and death in childhood. Pediatrics 2007;119: e484–494.
7. Yanase T, Simpson E, Waterman M, 17 alpha-hydroxylase/17,20-lyase deficiency: from clinical investigation to molecular definition. Endocr Rev 1991;12: 91–108
8. Ten S, New M, Maclaren N, Clinical Review 130: Addison's disease 2001. J Clin Endocrinol Metab 2001;86: 2909–2922

15 A Physiologic Approach to Hereditary Tubulopathies

Marva Moxey-Mims and Paul Goodyer

Key Points

1. The primary function of the proximal tubule is the bulk reabsorption of inorganic and organic solutes.
2. Fanconi syndrome is a generalized term applied to a large number of disorders characterized by defective proximal tubular reabsorption of numerous solutes. The most common inherited cause is cystinosis.
3. Normally, 99% of filtered sodium is actively reabsorbed by the renal tubules, with sequential fine-tuning as the glomerular filtrate moves along the nephron.
4. Isolated salt-losing syndromes result from luminal transporter disorders along the thick ascending limb of Henle, the distal convoluted tubule, or the cortical collecting tubule.

Key Words: Fanconi syndrome; cystinosis; salt-losing syndromes; aminoaciduria; bicarbonaturia; proximal tubule; phosphaturia; pseudohypoaldosteronism; nephrogenic diabetes insipidus; Bartter syndrome

1. CASE SCENARIO

A 4-month-old boy presents to his pediatrician with failure to thrive (birth weight was 2800 g but body weight is now <3rd percentile). He was born 1 month prematurely and the mother reports polyhydramnios during pregnancy. She is bottle-feeding her child and reports that he drinks vigorously, going through more diapers than his older sister used to. The boy has been circumcised and has an excellent urinary stream. He is afebrile and there are no dysmorphic features but the baby seems irritable and occasionally vomits in the morning. Serum creatinine is at the high end of the normal range.

Although the investigation of failure to thrive in infancy requires us to consider a broad differential diagnosis, the history of polyhydramnios and polyuria in this case suggest the possibility of an inborn renal tubulopathy. One approach is to consider specific investigations for a fairly long list of rare inherited diseases that might affect renal tubular transport, but a more efficient diagnostic strategy is to begin with simple screening

From: *Nutrition and Health: Fluid and Electrolytes in Pediatrics*
Edited by: L. G. Feld, F. J. Kaskel, DOI 10.1007/978-1-60327-225-4_15,
© Humana Press, a part of Springer Science+Business Media, LLC 2010

tests of tubular function to define the dysfunctional nephron segment causing polyuria. This narrows the differential diagnosis and helps to define the therapeutic plan that might correct growth failure.

Here, we take a physiologic approach to diagnosis of inherited forms of infantile polyuria and divide the causes into those arising from salt wasting in the proximal tubule, loop of Henle, or collecting duct and polyuria arising from defective water reabsorption in the collecting duct. We focus on functional tests of specific nephron segments, which can be obtained with single blood and urine samples at the time of a clinic visit.

2. DYSFUNCTION OF THE RENAL PROXIMAL TUBULE (FANCONI SYNDROME)

2.1. Renal Fanconi Syndrome

Fanconi syndrome is the term used to describe a generalized dysregulation of proximal tubular function. This disorder may be inherited, acquired or idiopathic (Tables 1 and 2). Since the proximal tubule is where most solute and water reabsorption normally occur, impaired reabsorption results in excessive urinary excretion of many solutes, specifically glucose, bicarbonate, phosphate, amino acids, low molecular weight proteins, and uric acid.

Table 1
Inherited Causes of Fanconi Syndrome

Cystinosis
Tyrosinemia
Lowe's syndrome
Galactosemia
Fructosemia
Fanconi–Bickel syndrome
Dent's disease
Mitochondrial disorders
Wilson's disease

Cystinosis is the most common cause of the Fanconi syndrome in children. It is an autosomal recessive disorder characterized by intracellular deposits of cystine. The genetic mutation here is in the CTNS gene that encodes cystinosin, a lysosomal membrane cystine transport protein (1). As a result, cystine cannot be transported to the cytosol after protein degradation, causing progressive lysosomal cystine accumulation. Cystinosis is a systemic disease, but the initial clinical presentation is dominated by the signs and symptoms of the proximal tubular dysfunction. In contrast, the clinical presentations of the other inherited causes of Fanconi syndrome (Table 1) tend to be dominated by their systemic findings.

Table 2
Drugs that Can Induce Fanconi Syndrome

Anticancer Drugs
    Ifosfamide
    Cisplatin and carboplatin
    Streptozocin
    Azacitidine
    Mercaptopurine
Antiviral Agents
    Didanosine
    Adefovir
    Cidofovir
    Tenofovir
Antibacterial drugs
    Tetracyclines
    Aminoglycosides
Other drugs/toxins
    Suranim
    Valproate
    Fumaric acid
    Ranitidine
    Salicylates
    Methyl-3-chromone
Glue sniffing

2.1.1. CLINICAL PRESENTATION

Many inherited tubulopathies can lead to renal Fanconi syndrome. Laboratory findings include glucosuria (in the face of normoglycemia), aminoaciduria, low molecular weight proteinuria, renal tubular acidosis due to loss of bicarbonate, hypokalemia, uricosuria, and phosphaturia. Children with genetic causes for tubular dysfunction often present in infancy. For example, the most severe form of cystinosis (infantile) presents between 6 and 12 months with the biochemical abnormalities described above, along with rickets.

2.1.2. PATHOPHYSIOLOGY/PATHOGENESIS

There is now evidence for a single common pathogenetic mechanism for all Fanconi syndrome etiologies, rather than multiple defective transporters causing excess solute loss. The unifying defect appears to be the reduced availability of ATP for the enzyme Na,K-ATPase. This is caused by various metabolic disorders, which reduce sodium extrusion from the tubular cell, reducing the gradient for transport of solutes coupled to sodium reabsorption (2, 3) (Fig. 1).

In 1935, Fanconi described several children with a broad pattern of proximal tubular dysfunction; subsequent autopsy studies indicated that his patients probably had nephro-

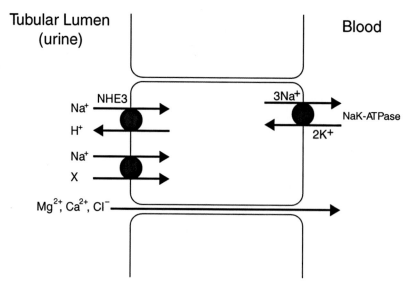

Fig. 1. Proximal tubule. X = solutes coupled to sodium reabsorption, e.g., amino acids, glucose, phosphate. If sodium absorption is impaired, the gradient for transport of these solutes is reduced.

pathic cystinosis. In this disease, homozygous null mutations of the cystinosin gene preclude normal efflux of cystine from the lysosome. Lysosomal cystine accumulation causes progressive tissue injury, beginning with renal proximal tubular dysfunction in the first year of life. The renal proximal tubule is damaged earlier than many other tissues, presumably because of the high burden of protein delivered to lysosomes during endocytosis of low molecular weight (LMW) proteins from the proximal tubular fluid. Thus, the polyuria and failure to thrive described in the index case above could easily be caused by cystinosis or some other cause of congenital renal Fanconi syndrome. Evidence of proximal tubule function based on the tests below allows one to focus differential diagnosis on the causes of hereditary renal Fanconi syndrome.

2.1.3. PROXIMAL TUBULE PHYSIOLOGY

A 5-month-old infant with normal glomerular filtration rate ultrafilters about 40 L of isotonic fluid into Bowman's space each day. More than two-thirds of the filtered load is reabsorbed during its passage along the convoluted and straight portions of the proximal tubule. Proximal tubular cells are endowed with elaborate microvilli to expand the luminal reabsorptive surface and are richly supplied with mitochondria to generate energy for active transport. Luminal reabsorption of sodium chloride is coupled to the uptake of both inorganic (bicarbonate, phosphate, sulfate) and organic (glucose, amino and carboxylic acids) solutes; transfer across the basolateral membrane into the peritubular space is driven largely by Na–K-ATPase and $3HCO_3$-Na co-transport. Active transport generates a small but powerful osmotic gradient (4 mOsm/L) across the proximal tubule, which drives the flow of water through aquaporin-1 water channels in the cell membrane and via the leaky paracellular pathway between cells. Flow through the paracellular pathway causes additional reabsorption of NaCl through passive solvent drag. Together, these mechanisms remove about 65% of the filtered NaCl and water and nearly 100% of the filtered bicarbonate, phosphate, and organic solutes.

The renal glomerulus effectively restricts the flux of large proteins into the urine, but LMW proteins such as beta-2 microglobulin (12 kDa), alpha-1 microglobulin (33 kDa), retinol binding protein (21 kDa), or peptide hormones easily enter the tubular fluid along with other small solutes and water. Proteins in the tubular fluid are efficiently adsorbed to non-specific cationic sites in the luminal membrane the proximal tubular cell and are taken up through endocytosis. Endocytotic vesicles traffic to lysosomes where the protein is cleaved into its constituent amino acids and recycled by exiting the compartment through selective channels in the lysosomal membrane. Once the protein cargo has been delivered, endocytotic vesicles are recycled to the luminal membrane.

2.1.4. CLINICAL TESTS TO IDENTIFY PROXIMAL TUBULAR DYSFUNCTION

As mentioned above, dysfunction of the renal proximal tubule may cause profound polyuria when bulk reabsorption of salt and water is compromised. However, the unique features of proximal tubule dysfunction are best identified by clinical tests, which measure reabsorption of organic solutes and protein or specific inorganic solutes primarily absorbed in the proximal tubule such as phosphate, bicarbonate, and potassium. Because proximal tubular bicarbonate transport is quantitatively important, polyuria may be expected in infants with isolated proximal renal tubular acidosis. However, this is an extremely rare condition. Isolated transport defects affecting phosphate (e.g., X-linked hypophosphatemic rickets) or specific groups of amino acids (e.g., cystinuria) do not produce significant polyuria. Practically speaking, therefore, infants presenting with the syndrome above should be investigated for evidence of a broad dysfunction of the proximal tubule, i.e., renal Fanconi syndrome.

2.1.5. AMINO ACIDURIA

Since approximately 99% of the filtered load of amino acids are reabsorbed in the proximal tubules, quantification of urine amino acids (factored for urine creatinine) in a random aliquot of urine provides a robust indicator of broad proximal tubule dysfunction. The widespread transport defect of renal Fanconi syndrome should, however, be distinguished from selective patterns of aminoaciduria (e.g., cystinuria), which affect only one of the many amino acid transport mechanisms. Cystinuria carriers (affecting only cystine, ornithine, arginine, and lysine) are not uncommon (1:75 live births) and might be present by chance in children without a broad Fanconi syndrome. Urine amino acids are usually measured on automated amino acid analyzers, however, with an inherent cost and delay in obtaining the result.

2.1.6. LOW MOLECULAR WEIGHT ("TUBULAR") PROTEINURIA

Healthy infants excrete about 40–50 μg of protein per day in the urine (109 μg/m^2/day); urine protein/creatinine ratio is normally <0.49 mg protein/mg creatinine in infants or <0.18 mg protein/mg creatinine in children over 1 year of age. About half of this is albumin and half is constituted by other proteins such as the LMW proteins (molecular weight <40 kDa), which are more freely filtered through the glomerular slit pore diaphragm. In renal Fanconi syndrome, urinary excretion of both albumin and LMW proteins increases. Dipsticks (embedded with tetrabromophenol blue) commonly used to detect proteinuria may detect the increased albuminuria, but are relatively insensitive to most LMW proteins. A simple "bedside" test, which detects both albumin and LMW protein, involves addition of 3 drops of 20% sulfosalicylic acid to 5 ml of urine; proteinuria is evident if the urine becomes turbid (due to protein denaturation at low pH). For convincing evidence of proximal tubular dysfunction, however, quantification of a specific LMW is usually required. In normal children, urinary beta-2 microglobulin concentration is less than 0.36 mg/L (less than 0.4% of the filtered load), whereas it typically ranges from 10 to 30 mg/L in children with renal Fanconi syndrome *(4)*. Beta-2 microglobulin, normalized for urine creatinine, should be <40 mg/mmol creatinine *(5)*.

2.1.7. PHOSPHATURIA

The renal proximal tubule normally reabsorbs between 85 and 95% of the filtered load of phosphate during infancy. Excessive phosphaturia is common in Fanconi syndrome, often depleting the body pool of phosphate and causing hypophosphatemic rickets. In the setting of low serum levels of phosphate, failure to reabsorb at least 85% of the filtered load is abnormal. The tubular reabsorption of phosphate (TRP) is easily calculated from simultaneous blood and urine samples:

$$1 - \frac{[\text{Urine PO}_4 \times \text{serum creatinine}]}{[\text{Serum PO}_4 \times \text{urine creatinine}]} \times 100\%$$

Two important caveats must be considered, however, in the interpretation of TRP values. In the setting of hyperparathyroidism (e.g., vitamin D-deficient rickets or renal failure) phosphaturia is physiologic and represents the normal effect of parathyroid hormone rather than proximal tubular dysfunction. Conversely, TRP may be close to normal when serum phosphate (and thus the phosphate load presented to the proximal tubule) is markedly decreased; in this case, TRP should be re-evaluated after partial correction of phosphate depletion. Alternatively, nomograms estimating the renal threshold for phosphate (TmP/GFR) from the parameters above have been published; TmP/GFR should be >2.8 mg/dL *(6)*.

2.1.8. BICARBONATURIA (PROXIMAL RTA)

In infants with renal Fanconi syndrome, variable degrees of proximal tubular transport dysfunction may cause urinary bicarbonate wasting, systemic acidosis, and low serum bicarbonate levels. The challenge is to distinguish proximal from distal renal tubular acidosis. At the time of presentation, physicians have the opportunity (often missed) to determine whether distal nephron acid secretion is intact. This may be accomplished by assessing urine pH in a urine sample obtained prior to any bicarbonate therapy. In the face of acidosis caused by proximal RTA, the distal tubule can acidify the urine to a pH below 5.3. Insertion of a urinary catheter allows serial measures of urine pH during slow intravenous bicarbonate infusion to repair acidosis; simultaneous measures of serum bicarbonate allow an estimate of the renal bicarbonate threshold – the point at which the bicarbonate filtered load exceeds proximal tubule reabsorptive capacity, spilling into the distal nephron to increase urinary pH to >6.0. The renal bicarbonate threshold measured in this fashion should be above 18 mEq/L.

2.1.9. PROXIMAL POTASSIUM REABSORPTION

The interpretation of urinary potassium excretion is complex, since bulk reabsorption (normally greater than 90% of the filtered load) occurs in the proximal tubule, but also in the loop of Henle and (in states of potassium depletion) in the collecting duct. Furthermore, the daily intake of potassium is secreted by principal cells of the renal collecting duct. Thus, urinary potassium excretion is not a simple measure of proximal tubule function. Nevertheless, infants with renal Fanconi syndrome exhibit potassium excretion in excess of the usual amount secreted by the collecting duct.

Fractional excretion of potassium (FE_K) is calculated as

$$FE_{K+} = \frac{[\text{Urine potassium} \times \text{serum creatinine}]}{[\text{Serum potassium} \times \text{urine creatinine}]} \times 100\%$$

Potassium excretion by normal infants is slightly higher than in older children and adults; among normal infants, mean $FE_K = 12.2\%$ (range $= 5$–27%); values above 27% indicate potassium wasting (7).

2.1.10. WORKUP

The laboratory workup includes serum electrolytes, urea, creatinine, calcium, phosphate, and magnesium to document metabolic acidosis and hypophosphatemia and rule out evidence of kidney failure. The urinary pH should be documented when the patient is acidotic. Urinary phosphate and glucose excretion, as well as aminoaciduria need to be evaluated. A check of urinary low molecular weight proteins (retinol binding protein, beta-2 microglobulin, or N-acetylglucosaminidase) should also be considered for diagnostic confirmation. If cystinosis is suspected, a slit lamp examination by an ophthalmologist to look for corneal cystine crystals is a must, as well as a check for elevated leukocyte cystine levels. In cases of a family history of the disease, the diagnosis can actually be made prenatally via amniocentesis or chorionic villus sampling (8).

2.1.11. TREATMENT

Once the diagnosis of cystinosis is made, it is very important to start definitive treatment with cysteamine (β-mercaptoethylamine), as early treatment has been shown to substantially delay the progression of renal failure (9–11). The recommended dose is 1.3–1.9 g/1.73 m^2/day. Without treatment, these patients progress to end-stage kidney disease during the first decade of life in the majority of cases. Despite its efficacy, the odor and taste of cysteamine are impediments to long-term medication compliance. In addition, patients require correction of the metabolic acidosis with sodium or potassium citrate at a dose of 10–20 mEq/kg/day. The hypophosphatemia and rickets are treated with oral phosphate at 25–75 mg/kg and calcitriol 10–30 ng/kg/day. Sodium supplements are often necessary as well to address the mild hyponatremia and improve growth. Many children with cystinosis also develop hypothyroidism, so appropriate supplementation with thyroxine should be initiated.

2.2. Salt-Wasting Syndromes

Salt wasting can occur because of a central stimulus to increase renal excretion (cerebral salt wasting – see Chapter 1), or because of mutations in sodium transporters that result in decreased distal reabsorption (renal salt wasting).

2.2.1. RENAL SALT-WASTING SYNDROMES

The two major proximal tubular salt and water transporter mechanisms involve the water channel aquaporin (AQP1) and the sodium proton exchanger, NHE3. Despite the fact that 60–70% of total renal salt and water absorption occurs in the proximal tubule, defects in this region are unlikely to lead to clinically significant sodium losses. Knockout mice with mutations of genes encoding AQP1 or NHE3 exhibit efficient hemodynamic compensatory mechanisms that result in a decreased glomerular filtration rate and consequently minimal impact on sodium excretion (37). Severe syndromes of salt wasting are caused by transport deficiencies downstream from the proximal tubule, in the thick ascending limb of Henle (TALH), the distal convoluted tubule (DCT), or the cortical collecting tubule (CCT).

3. DYSFUNCTION OF THE LOOP OF HENLE (BARTTER SYNDROME)

3.1. Loop of Henle Physiology

Nearly 30% of filtered NaCl is reabsorbed in the TALH, but the segment is largely impermeable to water (Table 3). At the luminal surface, uptake of sodium, potassium, and chloride are accomplished by the furosemide-sensitive cotransporter, NKCC2. At the basolateral surface, sodium is pumped into the peritubular space by Na–K-ATPase, while chloride exits passively down its electrochemical gradient through two chloride

Table 3
Tubular Transporter Defects of Primary Renal Salt Wasting

Syndrome	Affected nephron segment	Defective transporter
Bartter syndrome	TALH	NKCC2
		ROMK
		ClC-Kb
		Barrtin
Gitelman's syndrome	DCT	NCCT
PHA1	CCT	NCCT

channels (ClC-Ka and ClC-Kb), which both utilize the same subunit protein, Barttin. Potassium is recycled into the lumen through an outwardly directed potassium channel, allowing the next round of $Na/K/Cl_2$ uptake. By transferring salt in the absence of water, the TALH generates a hypertonic medullary interstitium, which allows water reabsorption from the collecting duct in the presence of vasopressin. Thus mutation of any of the above proteins interferes with the overall function of the transport mechanism in the TALH, causing profound loss of salt and water resembling the effects of furosemide.

3.2. Bartter Syndrome

Infants presenting with polyuria and failure to thrive may have Bartter syndrome, a hereditary dysfunction of the TALH. Bartter first described this autosomal recessive syndrome in adults with a milder defect of $Na/K/Cl_2$ co-transport in the TALH (12). The most striking features of the syndrome (hypokalemia, alkalosis, increased urinary prostaglandins, and hyperplasia of the juxtaglomerular apparatus with elevation of plasma renin) are actually manifestations of the compensatory renal response to massive salt wasting. The syndrome is genetically heterogeneous and may be caused by half a dozen different mutant genes – all related to the complex transport mechanism for salt reabsorption in the TALH.

In Type 1 Bartter syndrome, TALH dysfunction is due to inactivating mutations of the $Na/K/Cl_2$ co-transporter gene (SLC2A1) (13). Neonates are profoundly affected and there is typically a history of polyhydramnios. Affected infants may become dehydrated in the first days of life and fail to thrive. Hyponatremia and hypokalemia are profound and early recognition of the syndrome may be life-saving. Plasma renin is typically elevated 10–20 times normal and elevated levels of urinary prostaglandins reflect stimulated production of PGE in the juxtaglomerular apparatus in an effort to maintain glomerular blood flow.

A second genetic type of neonatal Bartter syndrome has been identified in which mutations of the gene (KCNJ1) encoding the outwardly rectifying potassium channel (ROMK) in the thick ascending limb of Henle (13). While urinary salt wasting may be profound, ROMK is also needed for potassium excretion in the collecting duct, therefore serum potassium may be normal or even elevated. The presence of alkalosis, however, distinguishes this form of Bartter syndrome from pseudohypoaldosteronism, congenital adrenal hyperplasia, or adrenal insufficiency (Fig. 2).

Infants may also develop Type IV Bartter syndrome with deafness due to mutations of the BSND gene, encoding a protein (Barttin) expressed in the basolateral membrane of TALH cells, collecting duct intercalated cells and in cells of the cochlea and vestibular system of the ear (14). Barttin is a critical subunit of both the CLC-Ka and CLC-Kb chloride channels in the TALH, so affected patients develop severe salt wasting. Rarely, patients with digenic mutations of both chloride channels develop the same pattern of disease. Since CLC-Ka is expressed in the ear, these digenic type IV Bartter patients also develop deafness (15). Hypercalciuria and nephrocalcinosis are uncommon.

In slightly milder forms of Bartter syndrome, children may present during the first 2 years of life with polyuria, vomiting, episodes of unexplained fever, and growth retardation. Among these patients are those with mutations in only one chloride channel

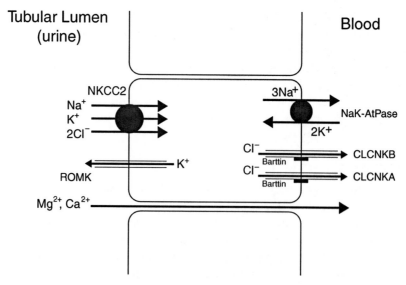

Fig. 2. Thick ascending limb of Henle. Loss of function of NKCC2 results in one form of neonatal Bartter syndrome. Loss of ROMK function causes another, and a defect in barttin causes the form of Bartter syndrome associated with deafness. "Classic" Bartter results from a defect in CLCNKB and is less severe than the neonatal form.

gene (CLCNKB) *(16)*. Since the alternative chloride channel (CLC-Ka) is intact, there is some chloride efflux and salt wasting is only moderately compromised. Patients have normal hearing and tend not to have hypercalciuria and nephrocalcinosis *(17)*.

Finally, it has been noted that patients with activating mutations of the calcium sensing receptor may exhibit modest salt wasting and hypokalemia. Since the disease is characterized by autosomal dominant hypocalcemia, it is easily distinguished from classical Bartter syndrome. However, the mechanisms for salt wasting in the two conditions are related. Increased reabsorption of calcium produces a less favorable electrical gradient for the NKCC2-mediated salt reabsorption in the TALH.

3.2.1. CLINICAL TESTS TO EXAMINE TALH FUNCTION

In the absence of Fanconi syndrome, TALH dysfunction is identified by

(1) Evidence of intravascular volume contraction (massive elevation of plasma renin and aldosterone); normal levels are slightly higher than in adults and it is difficult to distinguish recumbent from upright levels but the striking elevation in primary salt-losing states is easily distinguished from normal.

Plasma renin activity (infants): normal = 3.1 ± 3.5 ng/mL/h
Bartter syndrome = 10–30 ng/mL/h
Plasma aldosterone (infants): normal = 18.3 ± 12.2 ng/dL
Bartter syndrome = 30–300 ng/dL
(wide variation depending on hypokalemia)

(2) Evidence of inappropriate urinary excretion of NaCl; the extent of urinary sodium losses can be assessed by measuring fractional excretion of sodium after central volume restoration. If measured when the infant presents with massive renin and aldosterone elevation, $FENa^+$ excretion can be deceptively close to "normal" (1%).

$$FENa^+ = \frac{[Urine\,Na^+ \times Serum\,creatinine]}{[Serum\,Na^+ \times Urine\,creatinine]} \times 100\%$$

(3) Evidence of compensatory stimulation of sodium reabsorption in the collecting duct. In all states of severe volume contraction, elevated levels of aldosterone stimulate sodium reabsorption in the collecting duct in exchange for hydrogen ion or potassium excretion. Since restoration of central volume takes precedence over acid/base balance, infants who lose salt from the TALH exhibit an acid urine pH (<6.0) in the face of systemic alkalosis. Stimulated potassium secretion can be demonstrated by an estimate of the potassium secretory gradient from blood to the lumen of the cortical collecting tubule. A "bedside" measure of the transtubular potassium gradient (TTKG) (see below) involves an adjustment of urine potassium concentration for the amount of water reabsorbed during transit along the collecting duct. Normal infant TTKG ranges between 4 and 8; values between 10 and 13 are commonly seen in Bartter syndrome and other salt-wasting states where aldosterone levels are high and the collecting duct is intact.

(4) Evidence of hypercalciuria (salt wasting in the TALH causes unfavorable electrophysiology for distal tubular calcium reabsorption). Hypercalciuria can be identified by measuring urine calcium to creatinine ratio, but in practice, the wide range of normal values among infants greatly reduces the sensitivity of this test before the age of 1 year. Care should be taken regarding units for normal values of this ratio since the upper limit of normal for infants > 1 year is 0.6 (mmol calcium/mmol creatinine) – or 0.2 (mg calcium/mg creatinine) (18, 19).

3.2.2. TREATMENT OF BARTTER'S

Patients require sodium chloride and potassium replacement (5–10 mEq/kg/day in four divided doses). For infants, the salt content of formula can be adjusted to 40–50 mEq/L. In addition, the use of NSAIDS reduces the effect of prostaglandins on the kidney. Traditionally, indomethacin, 2–3 mg/kg/day has been used, but certain other NSAIDS have also been found to be effective, including aspirin, ibuprofen, and ketoprofen.

4. DYSFUNCTION OF SODIUM REABSORPTION IN THE CORTICAL COLLECTING DUCT (PSEUDOHYPOALDOSTERONISM)

4.1. Defective Na⁺ – H⁺/K⁺ Exchange in the Renal Collecting Duct

In pseudohypoaldosteronism (PHA), exchange of sodium for hydrogen ion or potassium is absent, despite massively elevated circulating levels of renin and aldosterone. Infants exhibit renal salt wasting accompanied by hyperkalemia and acidosis (20) and usually present in the first weeks of life with dehydration and hyponatremia. Two clinically distinct forms of this syndrome (PHA1) have been identified. The autosomal recessive form of PHA1 is caused by homozygous loss of one of either the α, β, or γ subunit of the luminal sodium channel (ENaC) in the cortical collecting tubule *(21–23)*. Dysfunction of the ENaC blocks sodium reabsorption but also eliminates the driving force for secretion of potassium and hydrogen ions. The features of this syndrome are mimicked by spironolactone because ENaC expression is normally stimulated by aldosterone. Since ENaC is expressed elsewhere, affected infants also have severe salt wasting in the colon, sweat glands and salivary glands, but are easily distinguished from cystic fibrosis patients in whom acidosis and hyperkalemia are generally absent. Children with PHA1 have recurrent episodes of salt wasting and hyperkalemia requiring therapy with oral salt supplements, sodium bicarbonate, and potassium binding resins for life.

An autosomal dominant form (PHA2) is caused by heterozygous loss of the mineralocorticoid receptor gene (Fig. 3) *(24, 25)*. While affected neonates may be extremely ill and can die from hyperkalemia, they respond well to oral salt supplementation. With volume expansion and adequate delivery of sodium to the collecting tubule, hyperkalemia is controlled. With tubular maturation, the clinical problems resolve by 1–2 years of age and heterozygous adults are asymptomatic. Aldosterone levels remain elevated (>30 ng/dL), apparently compensating for the reduced number of mineralocorticoid receptors.

Pseudohypoaldosteronism must be distinguished from adrenal insufficiency, aldosterone synthase (CYP11B2) deficiency, and salt-wasting forms of congenital adrenal hyperplasia (CAH) in which collecting duct dysfunction is caused by a defect in the adrenal pathway of cortisol and aldosterone synthesis *(26)*. Most commonly, CAH is caused by inactivating mutations of the 21-hydroxylase gene (CYP21) and is confirmed by demonstrating elevated plasma renin activity, low serum aldosterone, and

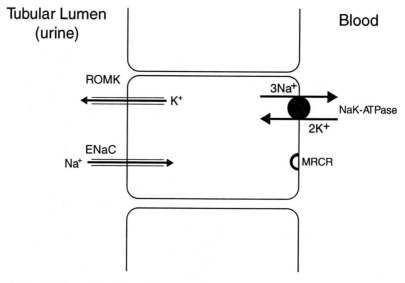

Fig. 3. Cortical collecting tubule. Pseudohypoaldosteronism is caused by a defect in ENaC or loss of the mineralocorticoid receptor (MRCR) gene.

accumulation of 17-hydroxyprogesterone and androgens in the blood. In infants with hypotension or severe electrolyte disturbances, an urgent therapeutic trial of hydrocortisone (2 mg every 8 h) may be life-saving (27). This rapidly corrects collecting duct dysfunction and directs attention toward some form of aldosterone deficiency rather than renal tubular unresponsiveness to the hormone. Ideally, blood and urine samples for physiologic tests of renal tubular function are made before and after administration of hydrocortisone.

4.1.1. PHYSIOLOGY OF SALT REABSORPTION IN THE CORTICAL COLLECTING DUCT

Only about 2–5% of the filtered load of sodium is reabsorbed in the collecting tubule. However, this site is the final arbiter of sodium excretion and is a major site of aldosterone action in states of volume contraction. Sodium reabsorption in the cortical collecting duct involves passive entry of sodium through luminal channels in the principal cells; sodium is then pumped across the basolateral membrane by aldosterone-stimulated Na–K-ATPase (28, 29) This sodium movement generates a negative potential in the lumen, which favors potassium secretion from the cell via aldosterone-stimulated potassium channels. Thus, the energy for sodium uptake is indirectly coupled to potassium secretion and can generate a substantial potassium gradient from blood to collecting duct lumen.

The negative luminal potential generated by sodium reabsorption also favors hydrogen ion secretion by alpha-intercalated cells interspersed among the principal cells. Here, H^+/K^+-ATPase pumps hydrogen in to the tubular fluid, while reabsorbing potassium. Thus, aldosterone-stimulated sodium reabsorption is indirectly coupled to acid secretion via its powerful effect on luminal electropotential.

4.1.2. TESTS OF COLLECTING DUCT SALT TRANSPORT

Collecting duct secretion of potassium can be assessed by calculating the transtubular potassium gradient (TTKG), an index first proposed by West et al. to estimate aldosterone-dependent potassium secretion in the collecting duct (30). This test assumes that urine osmolarity at the top of the collecting duct is essentially equivalent to serum osmolarity (300 mOsm/L). Measurement of final urine osmolarity then allows an approximation of the proportional increase in luminal potassium concentration due to water reabsorption en route to formation of the final urine. TTKG values for infants were reported by Rodriguez-Soriano et al. (7).

$$\text{TTKG} = \frac{[\text{Urine potassium} \times 300\,\text{mOsm/L}]}{\text{Serum potassium} \times \text{Urine osmolarity}}$$

In the setting of hypoaldosteronism or pseudohypoaldosteronism, TTKG is usually <4.1 in children and <4.9 in infants (7).

5. DYSFUNCTION OF WATER REABSORPTION IN THE COLLECTING DUCT.

5.1. Nephrogenic Diabetes Insipidus (See Chapter I Water)

While failure to thrive and polyuria in infants may be explained by one of the various salt-losing states above, it may also be caused by inability to concentrate the urine in the renal collecting duct. In 90% of infants with congenital nephrogenic diabetes insipidus (NDI), dysfunction of water reabsorption in the collecting duct is due to null mutations of the AVPR2 (vasopressin receptor) gene on the X-chromosome (Xq28) *(31)*. Thus, the disease is inherited in an X-linked pattern; males are fully affected while most women have only mild polyuria *(31)*. Some families bear mild mutations of AVPR2 and have a subtler form of NDI *(32, 33)*. Occasional females in classical X-linked kindreds may be strikingly affected (through lyonization). Thus, the physiologic tests described above should eventually be complemented by molecular genetic testing when possible. Sequence analysis detects the causative mutation in at least 95% of families; at least 180 different AVPR2 mutations have been described.

Infants with null mutations of AVPR2 typically present with a history of polyhydramnios and polyuria in infancy and exhibit striking failure to thrive in the first months of life. Periods of dehydration are associated with hypernatremia, unexplained fever, vomiting and lethargy, or irritability. Older children excrete about 8–9 L/m^2/day of urine, often associated with urinary tract dilatation and, occasionally, with bladder decompensation.

In about 10% of cases, NDI is due to mutations of the aquaporin II water channel gene (AQP2 on chromosome 12q13) and is usually inherited in autosomal recessive fashion *(31)*. The phenotype is equivalent to that in X-linked NDI. Occasional aquaporin II mutations are transmitted as a dominant trait, but produce a slightly milder form of NDI, often coming to medical attention only in late childhood.

5.1.1. Physiology of Water Reabsorption in the Collecting Duct

Tubular fluid leaving the TALH is dilute (about 50 mOsm/L). However, during its passage along the collecting tubule, between 10 and 15% of the water filtered through the glomerulus can be reabsorbed passively into the hyperosmotic medulla. Under conditions of water deprivation, circulating vasopressin binds to receptors (AVPR2) in collecting duct cells, activating the insertion of water channel proteins (aquaporin II) into the cell membrane and allowing transcellular flow of water. Final urine osmolarity may reach 1200 mOsm/L.

5.1.2. Test of Water Reabsorption in the Collecting Duct

In states of volume contraction and or hypernatremia, where the physician is certain that circulating levels of vasopressin are elevated, the urine should be concentrated; in older children with normal serum sodium it is often sufficient to screen for defective urinary concentration by measuring urine osmolarity after overnight water deprivation. However, infants in whom diabetes insipidus is suspected are at risk during water deprivation. Newborns with nephrogenic diabetes insipidus (NDI) may lose 10% of their body weight overnight. Thus, it is prudent to use a "short" dDAVP test in babies, ideally with a catheter in place to ensure quick assessment of urine output and osmolarity. Following a urine sample for baseline osmolarity, all fluids are withheld for 2 h; body weight is assessed every hour and serum sodium every 2 h to ensure that no more than 5% of the body weight is lost and serum sodium remains below 150 mEq/L. dDAVP is then administered intranasally (10 μg for infants, 20 μg for children) or intravenously (0.3 μg/kg). Urine is collected every 2 h for 6 h. Maximum urine osmolarity exceeds 500 mOsm/L in normal infants or > 800 mOsm/L in children and is less than 200 mOsm/L in infants with NDI *(32)*. If available, blood levels of vasopressin can be measured at baseline and are highly elevated in NDI.

CASE SCENARIOS

Case Scenario 1 – an 8-month-old infant is evaluated in the ER due to lethargy and fever and is found to be dehydrated on physical examination. Physical examination reveals a rachitic rosary and "popping" on palpation over the scalp. History indicates a birth weight at the 50th percentile, but the child's weight is now at the 10th percentile. Mom says she can't keep up with all the heavy, wet diapers, and the baby always seems to be thirsty.

What laboratory tests would you like?
Laboratory values show Na – 130 mEq/L, K – 2.8 mEq/L, CO_2 – 14 mmol/L, PO_4 – 2 mg/dL, Ca – 8.5 mg/dL, glucose – 70 mg/dL. As intravenous hydration progresses, polyuria becomes evident. After a renal consult, you send urine for electrolytes (Na, K, Cl, Ca, PO_4), amino acids, glucose, and creatinine.

What other evaluation is indicated?
While awaiting these results, you get an urgent ophthalmologic consult for slit-lamp examination, which reveals corneal cystine crystal deposits. Renal ultrasound reveals nephrocalcinosis, and a radiograph of the wrists shows splaying. Blood is sent for leukocyte cystine level for definitive diagnosis. The level comes back at 10 nmol half-cystine/mg protein (normal values are <0.2 nmol half-cystine/mg protein).

What is the renal prognosis?
Progression to end stage renal disease from cystinosis if untreated.

What is the appropriate treatment?
Cysteamine (beta-mercaptoethylamine), sodium or potassium citrate, oral phosphate and calcitriol.

Case Scenario 2 – a 3-month-old presents with a history of failure to thrive, vomiting, and loose stools. Physical examination shows a patient at the 5th percentile for height and weight, and he appears dehydrated. There are no other physical abnormalities. After hydration, urine output is 4–5 mL/kg/h.

What laboratory tests would you like?

Lab results – Na 127 mEq/L, K 2.0 mEq/L, Cl 85 mEq/L, HCO_3 33 mEq/L. Normal serum calcium and magnesium. Blood pH 7.49, pCO_2 40. Urine – specific gravity 1.006, Cl 45, K 40, Ca:Cr 0.38 (normal < 0.2).

What other evaluation would you like?

A renal ultrasound shows medullary hyperechogenicity. Plasma renin is reported to be 40 U/L (normal 4–8 U/L).

What is your diagnosis?

Bartter's syndrome.

What is the appropriate treatment?

After 1 week of potassium supplementation and supportive care, the patient's labs are Na 138 mEq/L, K 3.6 mEq/L, Cl 98 mEq/L, HCO_3 28 mEq/L; blood pH 7.45, pCO_2 41.

What additional therapy should be added now?

Non-steroidal anti-inflammatory drugs (NSAIDs) to reduce the effect of prostaglandins on the kidney. Traditionally, indomethacin, 2–3 mg/kg/day, but other NSAIDs have also been found to be effective, including aspirin, ibuprofen, and keto-profen.

REFERENCES

1. Town M, Jean G, Cherqui S, et al. A novel gene encoding an integral membrane protein is mutated in nephropathic cystinosis. *Nat Genet* 18:319–324, 1998.
2. Van't Hoff WG. Molecular developments in renal tubulopathies. *Arch Dis Child* 83:189–191, 2000.
3. Kalatzis V, Antignac C. New Aspects of the pathogenesis of cystinosis. *Pediatr Nephrol* 18:207–215, 2003.
4. Portman RJ, Kissane JM, Robson AM: Use of beta 2 microglobulin to diagnose tubulo-interstitial renal lesions in children. *Kidney Int* 30:91–98, 1986
5. Bergon E, Granados R, Fernandez-Segoviano P, et al.: Classification of renal proteinuria: a simple algorithm. *Clin Chem Lab Med* 40:1143–1150, 2002
6. Walton RJ, Bijvoet OL: Nomogram for derivation of renal threshold phosphate concentration. *Lancet* 2:309–310, 1975
7. Rodriguez-Soriano J, Ubetagoyena M, Vallo A: Transtubular potassium concentration gradient: a useful test to estimate renal aldosterone bio-activity in infants and children. *Pediatr Nephrol* 4:105–110, 1990
8. Jackson M, Young E. Prenatal diagnosis of cystinosis by quantitative measurement of cystine in chorionic villi and cultured cells. *Prenat Diagn* 25:1045–1047, 2005.
9. Thoene JG, Oshima RG, Crawhall JC, Olson DL, Schneider JA. Cystinosis. Intracellular cystine depletion by aminothiols in vitro and in vivo. *J Clin Invest* 58:180–189, 1976.
10. Gahl WA, Reed GF, Thoene JG, et al. Cysteamine therapy for children with nephropathic cystinosis. *N Engl J Med* 316:971–977, 1987.
11. Markello TC, Bernardini IM, Gahl WA. Improved renal function in children with cystinosis treated with cysteamine. *N Engl J Med* 328:1157–1162, 1993.
12. Bartter FC, Pronove P, Gill JR, Jr., et al.: Hyperplasia of the juxtaglomerular complex with hyperaldosteronism and hypokalemic alkalosis. A new syndrome. *Am J Med* 33:811–828, 1962.

13. Simon DB, Karet FE, Hamdan JM, et al.: Bartter's syndrome, hypokalaemic alkalosis with hypercalciuria, is caused by mutations in the Na–K–2Cl cotransporter NKCC2. *Nat Genet* 13:183–188, 1996

14. Birkenhager R, Otto E, Schurmann MJ, et al.: Mutation of BSND causes Bartter syndrome with sensorineural deafness and kidney failure. *Nat Genet* 29:310–314, 2001

15. Estevez R, Boettger T, Stein V, et al.: Barttin is a Cl⁻ channel beta-subunit crucial for renal Cl⁻ reabsorption and inner ear K⁺ secretion. *Nature* 414:558–561, 2001

16. Simon DB, Bindra RS, Mansfield TA, et al.: Mutations in the chloride channel gene, CLCNKB, cause Bartter's syndrome type III. *Nat Genet* 17:171–178, 1997

17. Rodriguez-Soriano J: Bartter and related syndromes: the puzzle is almost solved. *Pediatr Nephrol* 12:315–327, 1998

18. Alconcher LF, Castro C, Quintana D, et al.: Urinary calcium excretion in healthy school children. *Pediatr Nephrol* 11:186–188, 1997

19. Matos V, van Melle G, Boulat O, et al.: Urinary phosphate/creatinine, calcium/creatinine, and magnesium/creatinine ratios in a healthy pediatric population. *J Pediatr* 131:252–257, 1997

20. Cheek DB, Perry JW: A salt wasting syndrome in infancy. *Arch Dis Child* 33:252–256, 1958

21. Chang SS, Grunder S, Hanukoglu A, et al.: Mutations in subunits of the epithelial sodium channel cause salt wasting with hyperkalaemic acidosis, pseudohypoaldosteronism type 1. *Nat Genet* 12:248–253, 1996

22. Grunder S, Firsov D, Chang SS, et al.: A mutation causing pseudohypoaldosteronism type 1 identifies a conserved glycine that is involved in the gating of the epithelial sodium channel. *Embo J* 16:899–907, 1997

23. Strautnieks SS, Thompson RJ, Gardiner RM, et al.: A novel splice-site mutation in the gamma subunit of the epithelial sodium channel gene in three pseudohypoaldosteronism type 1 families. *Nat Genet* 13:248–250, 1996

24. Geller DS, Rodriguez-Soriano J, Vallo Boado A, et al.: Mutations in the mineralocorticoid receptor gene cause autosomal dominant pseudohypoaldosteronism type I. *Nat Genet* 19:279–281, 1998

25. Tajima T, Kitagawa H, Yokoya S, et al.: A novel missense mutation of mineralocorticoid receptor gene in one Japanese family with a renal form of pseudohypoaldosteronism type 1. *J Clin Endocrinol Metab* 85:4690–4694, 2000

26. White PC, Speiser PW: Congenital adrenal hyperplasia due to 21-hydroxylase deficiency. *Endocr Rev* 21:245–291, 2000

27. Speiser PW: Prenatal and neonatal diagnosis and treatment of congenital adrenal hyperplasia. *Horm Res* 68 Suppl 5:90–92, 2007

28. Camici M: Molecular pathogenetic mechanisms of nephrotic edema: progress in understanding. *Biomed Pharmacother* 59:215–223, 2005

29. Ecelbarger CA, Tiwari S: Sodium transporters in the distal nephron and disease implications. *Curr Hypertens Rep* 8:158–165, 2006

30. West ML, Bendz O, Chen CB, et al.: Development of a test to evaluate the transtubular potassium concentration gradient in the cortical collecting duct in vivo. *Miner Electrolyte Metab* 12:226–233, 1986

31. Fujiwara TM, Bichet DG: Molecular biology of hereditary diabetes insipidus. *J Am Soc Nephrol* 16:2836–2846, 2005

32. Sadeghi H, Robertson GL, Bichet DG, et al.: Biochemical basis of partial nephrogenic diabetes insipidus phenotypes. *Mol Endocrinol* 11:1806–1813, 1997

33. Faerch M, Christensen JH, Corydon TJ, et al.: Partial nephrogenic diabetes insipidus caused by a novel mutation in the AVPR2 gene. *Clin Endocrinol (Oxf)* 68:395–403, 2008

34. van Lieburg AF, Knoers NV, Monnens LA: Clinical presentation and follow-up of 30 patients with congenital nephrogenic diabetes insipidus. *J Am Soc Nephrol* 10:1958–1964, 1999

16 Enteral and Parenteral Nutrition

Dina Belachew and Steven J. Wassner

Key Points

1. While volume status is normally controlled by renal function and thirst, individuals maintained solely on prescribed enteral or parenteral alimentation are at increased risk for electrolyte and volume status disorders.
2. When fluid intake is limited, enteral formulas with higher osmolar concentration may lead to an osmotic diuresis and dehydration.
3. During the early phases of enteral or parenteral nutrition, fluid and electrolyte intakes should be monitored and adjusted on a regular basis.
4. The refeeding syndrome is a disorder due to metabolic abnormalities occurring in malnourished patients undergoing the initial phase of enteral or parenteral refeeding.
5. Serum potassium and phosphate concentrations may be normal prior to the initiation of eneral or parenteral regimens, only to decrease to dangerous levels early in the course of refeeding.
6. Provision of trace elements is necessary to prevent the development of trace element deficiencies associated with the rapid restoration of body mass.
7. Specific groups within pediatrics (e.g., neonates, those with renal insufficiency or eating disorders) require special attention when prescribing enteral or parenteral nutrition.

Key Words: Electrolyte abnormalities; enteral nutrition; hyperalimentation; hypokalemia; hypophosphatemia; parenteral nutrition; refeeding syndrome

1. INTRODUCTION

Enteral and parenteral nutrition are now accepted components in the care provided to vulnerable populations. While both enteral and parenteral routes can be utilized and the choice of feeding technique depends on each patient's specific requirements; unless specific contraindications exist, the enteral route is preferred *(1)*. In the almost one-half century since the introduction of total parenteral therapy (TPN) *(2, 3)* it has become part of our standard therapy for severely ill individuals, and Table 1 notes some of the indications for enteral and parenteral therapy.

Nutritional therapy has been shown to improve weight, anthropometric measures, and immune function *(4, 5)*. Unfortunately, there is no convincing evidence that improved nutrition actually decreases mortality *(6, 7)* and one meta-analysis has noted the

From: *Nutrition and Health: Fluid and Electrolytes in Pediatrics*
Edited by: L. G. Feld, F. J. Kaskel, DOI 10.1007/978-1-60327-225-4_16,
© Humana Press, a part of Springer Science+Business Media, LLC 2010

Table 1
Some Indications for the Use of Enteral and Parenteral Support

Enteral nutritional support	Parenteral nutrition
Neurologic: altered mental status, cerebral palsy	Severe illness with altered mental status
Cardiorespiratory: tracheoesophageal fistula, respiratory distress, cystic fibrosis, chronic lung disease, congenital heart disease	Premature infants with severe respiratory disease, cardiac failure, post cardiac surgery
Gastrointestinal: inflammatory bowel disease, short bowel syndrome, chronic diarrhea, malabsorption, biliary atresia	Congenital anomalies of the gastrointestinal tract, necrotizing enterocolitis, short bowel syndrome, intractable vomiting and diarrhea
Renal: chronic or acute renal failure	Renal failure
Others: prematurity, hypermetabolic states, severe trauma or head injury, oropharyngeal trauma, cancers, ulcers or burns	Extensive burns, post-chemotherapy phase, post bone marrow transplant

potential harm associated with nutritional support in the critically ill adults *(8)*. It is understandable therefore, that there is still much to learn about the proper indications, prescriptions, and complications associated with this form of therapy.

The purpose of this chapter is to delineate the alterations in fluid and electrolyte metabolism related to the use of enteral and parenteral nutrition. A full discussion of fluid and electrolyte metabolism is, however, beyond the scope of this chapter and is best found in specific chapters elsewhere in this volume. No attempt is made to discuss the nutritional aspects of this therapy and the interested reader is referred to other sources *(9)*.

2. SODIUM AND WATER

Under normal circumstances, salt intake is delicately balanced by salt excretion. However, a positive sodium balance is required for appropriate growth. It has been demonstrated that salt depletion early in life leads to diminished weight gain and linear growth associated with decreased protein synthesis rates *(10–12)*.

It is important to distinguish between the concepts of serum sodium concentration and that of total body sodium content. Serum sodium concentration is a function of total body water content so that hypo- or hypernatremia is most often related to abnormalities in water metabolism. For normal individuals, water is not limiting and both renal and posterior pituitary functions combine to maintain appropriate water balance. When enteral or parenteral diets are prescribed in patients unable to drink on their own, we substitute our calculations for the body's homeostatic controls. Table 2 lists a variety of factors that can lead to volume overload or dehydration.

Table 2
Conditions That Affect Sodium and Water Balance

Positive balance	Negative balance
Supplemental IV fluids	Vomiting, diarrhea, ostomy losses
Oral intake, tube feeds	Burns, cystic fibrosis, excessive sweating
Intravenous or enteral water "flushes"	Renal dysfunction, diuretics
Medication admixtures	Hyperosmotic states, e.g., hyperglycemia
Mist tents, respirators	Radiant warmers, phototherapy

Dehydration, either with, or without alteration of the serum sodium concentration can be induced in patients receiving enteral nutrition by a variety of dietary changes. Increasing the caloric density of formula by adding less than the standard amount of water to powdered preparations will increase the renal solute load, which may cause an osmotic diuresis and result in further dehydration. Pureed diets generally have a higher osmolality and viscosity than prepared formulas and unless monitored, may also lead to the development of hypernatremic dehydration (13). During conditions where antidiuretic hormone (ADH) secretion is increased, even the administration of "normal" quantities of water may result in hyponatremia.

Hyperglycemia is a common metabolic disturbance encountered during parenteral nutrition therapy. Severe hyperglycemia is often associated with hyponatremia due to the movement of water from the intracellular to the extracellular compartment in response to the high serum glucose concentrations (increased osmolality). Other complications associated with severe hyperglycemia include dehydration and electrolyte abnormalities due to an osmotic diuresis and hyperinsulinemia. Rarely, hyperglycemia and the resulting osmotic diuresis can result in the development of intracellular dehydration and cerebral bleeds. Glucose-induced insulin secretion may be responsible for a variety of fluid and electrolyte abnormalities including both hypokalemia and hypophosphatemia (vide infra). Insulin increases proximal tubular sodium reabsorption (14) so that rapid refeeding with the development of high insulin concentrations has been associated with the expansion of extracellular fluid volume and edema formation (15).

Since growth requires a positive sodium balance, it is understandable that anabolic states are associated with increased renal sodium retention. Under most circumstances, sodium intake is sufficient to permit growth. However, when growth is most rapid (e.g., the neonatal period) or where there are abnormal sodium losses through the skin, kidney or gastrointestinal tract, care must be taken to ensure that the formulas contain sufficient sodium for adequate growth (10). Practically, if renal function is normal and diuretics are not being administered, a urinary sodium concentration greater than 20 mEq/L suggests that sodium intake is adequate.

3. POTASSIUM

In the setting of normal renal function, hyperkalemia is uncommon during enteral feeding. In acute renal failure or in the later stages of chronic kidney disease, the ability to excrete potassium is limited and hyperkalemia may result due to a combination of decreased renal potassium excretion, inappropriately high intakes and/or the use of medications that inhibit potassium excretion (e.g., angiotensin converting enzyme inhibitors).

Hypokalemia is a common abnormality in hospitalized patients *(16)*. Severe hypokalemia, defined as a serum potassium concentration of less than 2.5 mEq/L, may be associated with significant clinical complications *(17)*. Gastrointestinal potassium loss is most often due to diarrhea or laxative abuse. Patients with chronic intravascular volume depletion (e.g., diuretics, emesis or nasogastric suction, prolonged sweating, or cystic fibrosis) develop secondary hyperaldosteronism, which predisposes them to hypokalemia. Clinical features associated with hypokalemia are numerous and consist of cardiac, gastrointestinal, neuromuscular, renal, and metabolic abnormalities *(17)*. For a full listing of possible causes and consequences of hypokalemia the reader is referred to Chapter 13.

Hypokalemia during nutritional rehabilitation is most often due to the provision of insufficient potassium along with insulin-induced transcellular potassium shifts *(18)*. Hypokalemia is a major electrolyte abnormality associated with the refeeding syndrome as discussed in the sudsequent section.

4. PHOSPHOROUS

While phosphate is best recognized for its role in bone calcification, it is important in multiple metabolic pathways and is essential for a variety of cell functions (Table 3).

Phosphate is ubiquitous in our diet and its intake is closely linked to protein intake. Since phosphate is predominantly excreted through the kidneys, hyperphosphatemia is

Table 3
The Role of Phosphate in Body Metabolism

	Function
Structural	Component of phospholipids, nucleoproteins and nucleic acids
Cellular metabolism	2,3-diphosophoglycerate regulates oxyhemoglobin dissociation and delivery of oxygen to tissues
	Production of high energy phosphates (e.g., ATP, ADP)
	Appropriate function of ion channels and maintenance of cell membrane resting potential
Enzymatic processes	Protein phosphorylation of enzymes and cellular signal compounds
Hematologic	Chemotaxis
	Phagocytosis
	Clot retraction
Cardiovascular	Myocardial contractility
Metabolic	Buffering function

most often seen in individuals with decreased kidney function. For healthy individuals with normal dietary intakes, hypophosphatemia is a rare finding *(19, 20)*. However, hypophosphatemia is frequently encountered in certain subgroups of hospitalized patients including those with sepsis, major trauma, and those in the intensive care units where it has been associated with poor clinical outcome *(21)*. Hypophosphatemia is also a major component of the refeeding syndrome.

5. CALCIUM AND MAGNESIUM

Hypercalcemia may be seen as a result of severe hypophosphatemia and will respond to increases in serum phosphate levels. Resorption hypercalcemia can also be present in individuals who are kept immobile or who have increased bone catabolism secondary to tumor infiltration. Serum calcium will also be elevated when excessive calcium is added to parenteral solutions or in individuals receiving enteral nutrition and supplemental Vitamin D or Vitamin A.

Preterm infants are a special group of patients with increased calcium requirements and minimal body calcium stores. Both enteral and parenteral solutions should contain sufficient calcium (and Vitamin D when enteral feeds are prescribed) to avoid mobilization of bone calcium stores, the development of osteopenia, and hypocalcemia *(22)*. On the other hand, neonatal hypercalcemia has also been reported as a result of excess calcium intake during nutritional support *(23)*.

While total calcium concentrations are measured routinely, it is only the ionized component of calcium that is metabolically active. Particularly in patients with malnutrition and decreased serum albumin concentrations, the concentrations of ionized calcium may be normal in spite of hypocalcemia. While there are formulas available to correct total calcium concentrations on the basis of serum albumin concentrations, the ready availability of ionized calcium determinations has made direct assessment a practical alternative.

Magnesium is found mainly in the bone and soft tissue and is mandatory for optimal cell function as well as being an essential cofactor to many enzymes *(24)*. Only about 0.3% of the total body magnesium is present in serum and exists in both the ionized and non-ionized states. Unfortunately, studies have shown that serum magnesium levels do not correlate with total body magnesium stores *(25)*. Analogous to serum calcium concentrations, it is the concentration of ionized magnesium that is active. Thus, measurements of total serum magnesium reflect only an approximation of whole body magnesium status.

The refeeding syndrome is associated with hypomagnesemia. The proposed mechanism, while not entirely clear, is thought to be due to intracellular shifts of magnesium after a period of poor intake *(26)*. Preexisting magnesium depletion appears to exacerbate the degree of hypomagnesemia *(27)*. While most cases of hypomagnesemia are not clinically significant, severe hypomagnesemia, i.e., plasma concentrations less than 1.2 mg/dL (0.5 mmol/L), can result in complications such as cardiac arrhythmia, anorexia, abdominal discomfort, tremor, paresthesia, tetany, as well as symptoms of irritability, confusion, weakness, and ataxia *(28)*.

6. BICARBONATE

Under normal circumstances, bicarbonate is reclaimed from the glomerular filtrate by the proximal renal tubule and hydrogen ion is secreted into the urine within the distal renal tubule. In adults, dietary intake of fixed bases (phosphates and sulfates) provides approximately 1–2 mmol of acid/kg/day. In children, net acid production is increased as a byproduct of bone calcification. The net result is that during periods of growth, renal acid excretion in infants and children may reach significantly high levels (up to 5 mmol/kg/day) *(29)*.

Patients receiving parenteral nutrition, particularly those with diminished renal function, may require a significant amount of bicarbonate to balance their net daily acid production. When formulating parenteral alimentation solutions, bicarbonate and chloride ions form the predominant anions required to maintain electrical neutrality. Care must also be taken to ensure that sufficient chloride is available to prevent the chloride depletion syndrome *(30)*, which is associated with the development of volume contraction and a primary metabolic alkalosis *(31)*. In individuals with metabolic alkalosis, the development of a compensatory respiratory acidosis with elevation of the pCO_2 can make it more difficult to wean patients from respiratory care.

7. THE REFEEDING SYNDROME

The refeeding syndrome is a potentially lethal condition that can be defined as severe electrolyte and fluid shifts associated with metabolic abnormalities, which occur in malnourished patients undergoing refeeding. Historically, some of the earliest reports occurred just after World War II and dealt with the refeeding of Japanese prisoners and victims of Leningrad and Netherlands famines. These reports noted that refeeding after a period of prolonged starvation was often associated with cardiac failure and death *(32)*. Although initially reported in patients undergoing enteral refeeding, this syndrome was revisited after the introduction of parenteral nutrition *(26, 33–35)*. Currently, the groups appearing to be at greatest risk include those with anorexia nervosa, oncology patients undergoing chemotherapy, malnourished elderly patients, alcoholics, and some post-operative patients. The incidence is reported to be as high as 25% in cancer patients who require nutritional support *(36)*. The same study also reported a higher incidence in those fed enterally than parenterally *(36)*. The electrolyte disturbances mainly involve the intracellular ions phosphate, magnesium, and potassium and appear similar to disturbances observed when aggressive therapy is begun in individuals with poorly controlled diabetes mellitus *(37)*.

When a malnourished patient begins nutritional support, the refeeding syndrome is most likely to occur during the first 72 h of refeeding *(38)*. While it is most commonly seen in individuals refed after prolonged periods of undernutrition, the refeeding syndrome has been reported to occur after starvation periods as short as 48 h *(34)*.

7.1. Pathophysiology of the Refeeding Syndrome

In starvation the secretion of insulin is decreased in response to a low carbohydrate intake while endogenous fat and protein stores are catabolized to produce energy.

This results in loss of intracellular electrolytes, in particular phosphate. Malnourished patients become total body phosphate depleted although they often have normal or only mildly decreased serum phosphate concentrations *(39)*. There are several mechanisms that maintain the serum phosphate during starvation *(40)*. Overall phosphate requirements are decreased and are initially maintained by mobilizing bone reserves. Poor phosphate intake suppresses parathyroid hormone (PTH) secretion, which leads to increased renal tubular phosphate reabsorption. Phosphate deficiency also leads to renal PTH resistance, further preventing phosphaturia.

When individuals resume eating, carbohydrate intake rapidly stimulates the secretion of insulin resulting in significant cellular uptake of phosphate, magnesium, and potassium. This can lead to profound hypophosphatemia, and less frequently, hypokalemia and hypomagnesemia. Since adenosine triphosphate (ATP) is required for the phosphorylation and metabolism of glucose, the administration of large carbohydrate loads to individuals with severe hypophosphatemia can lead to death due to depletion of body ATP stores *(19)*.

Hypophosphatemia can be mild (2.3–3.0 mg/dL), moderate (1.6–2.2 mg/dL), or severe (≤1.5 mg/dL). Severe hypophosphatemia can produce a plethora of clinical manifestations mostly resulting from impaired cellular energy pathways (ATP) or reduced red blood cell 2,3-diphosphoglycerate (DPG) concentrations (Table 4). Importantly, the early clinical features are often non-specific and may go unrecognized.

Table 4
Clinical Manifestations of Hypophosphatemia

Respiratory	*Musculoskeletal*
Impaired diaphragmatic contractility	Myalgia
Difficulty in weaning from mechanical ventilators *(52)*.	Weakness
	Rhabdomyolysis
Cardiac	Neurologic
Heart failure and sudden death	Change in mental status
Abnormal sarcomere contractility	Paresthesia
Direct myocardial damage *(53) (54)*	Seizures
Hematologic	Renal
Hemolysis	Renal tubular impairment
Thrombocytopenia	Acute tubular necrosis
Coagulopathy	Metabolic acidosis
Reduced leukocyte phagocytosis and chemotaxis	

Severe hypokalemia is also a concern since low serum potassium concentrations can lead to the hyperpolarization of cell membranes and the development of a flaccid paralysis. If the muscles of the diaphragm are affected this can result in death due to respiratory failure.

It is important to have a good understanding of the pathophysiology of the refeeding syndrome and have a high index of suspicion in patient populations at risk. With the increasing incidence of eating disorders, the practicing physician may encounter this problem not only in the in-patient hospital setting but also in outpatient clinics *(41)*.

To date, there are no randomized controlled studies on phosphate supplementation in children and recommendations are extrapolated from adult studies. An older regimen recommended administering 9 mmol (27.9 mg) potassium phosphate by continuous infusion over 12 hours *(42)*. More recently, a graduated dosing scheme based on the serum phosphate level has also been found to be safe and efficacious in patients receiving specialized nutrition support. In this schema, phosphate infusion is calculated based on serum level and the infusion is run at a rate of 7.5 mmol/hour or approximately 4 mmol/hour/meter^2 (Table 5). Other regimens have been utilized as well *(43)*.

Table 5
Phosphate Replacement in Hypophosphatemia (from *(55)*)

Serum Phosphate concentration	Amount of Phosphate infused
Mild (2.3–3 mg/dL)	0.033 mmol/kg
Moderate: (1.6–2.2 mg/dL)	0.066 mmol/kg
Severe: <1.5 mg/dL	1 mmol/kg

To convert mg/dL to mmol/L divide by 3 (e.g., 4.5 mg/dL = 1.5 mmol/L)

It is appropriate to begin phosphate supplementation at least 4 hours before starting feeds. Complications associated with overzealous phosphate repletion include renal failure, hyperphosphatemia, hypocalcemia, and electrocardiographic abnormalities *(44)*. Patients receiving parenteral alimentation often receive significant glucose intake but limited phosphate intake since high concentrations of calcium and phosphate will precipitate in solution. "Standard" recommendations are often inadequate and may be associated with significant hypophosphatemia. There is little information within the pediatric literature but when adults received 6.8 mmol/L (21 mg/dL) of phosphate in TPN, none became hypophosphatemic *(45)*.

8. TRACE ELEMENTS

Trace elements are components and cofactors of enzyme systems and essential to a variety of metabolic processes. They are of special concern to pediatricians as the effects of trace element deficiency are frequently most severe during periods of rapid growth. Table 6 notes the major abnormalities associated with individual trace elements as well as suggested intakes during nutritional therapy.

Copper deficiency is seen most often in premature infants and children with malnutrition secondary to chronic diarrhea, individuals receiving parenteral nutrition and after oral zinc supplementation *(46, 47)*. Preterm infants are at particular risk as copper mainly accumulates during the third trimester. Since copper metabolism can be altered by liver damage or cholestasis, serum copper levels should be measured when TPN is utilized in this group of individuals.

Table 6
Trace Elements in Enteral and Parenteral Nutrition (adapted from (56–58))

Trace element	Function	Clinical abnormality	Enteral requirements	Parenteral amount (mcg/kg/day)
Copper	Cofactor for many enzymes, connective tissue synthesis energy metabolism iron metabolism antioxidant and free radicals scavenger	Anemia Neutropenia Osteoporosis (46)	04–06 mg 0–6 m 06–07 mg 6–12 m 1–2 mg preadolescents	20
Zinc	Present in multiple metalloenzymes lymphopenia and immune dysfunction (59)	Poor growth, hypogonadism (males) decreased appetite Mental lethargy (59)	2 mg 0–6 m 5 g 6–12m 10 mg preadolescents	Preterm 400 0–3 m – 250 >3 m 100 Child 500
Manganese	Present in metalloenzymes (e.g., pyruvate kinase)	Growth retardation, impaired glucose tolerance (Abnormal bone and cartilage)	0.3–0.6 mg 0–6 m 06–1.0 mg 6–12 m	1
Selenium	Antioxidant as part of glutathione peroxides	Muscular discomfort/weakness Cardiomyopathy	5 mcg 0–6 m 15 mcg 6–12 m	2 (60)
Iodine	Thyroid hormone synthesis	Hypothyroidism, mental retardation, cretinism	50–75 mcg/day for adults. No specific levels for infants and children	1
Chromium	Cofactor for insulin	Abnormal Glucose metabolism/diabetes-like syndrome	Adult recommendations 50–200 mcg	0.2

Zinc deficiency affects rapidly dividing cells and tissues and has been implicated in growth failure. Zinc deficiency can be due to poor nutritional intake as well as steatorrhea, alcoholism, and renal disease with the development of zincuria.

Manganese is a cofactor for some enzymes but its essentiality has not been established in humans. Due to its ubiquitous presence in foods, deficiency is extremely uncommon and has not been reported in infants and children but overload is a concern. The threshold for development of toxic effects is not known but manganese toxicity can result in central nervous system dysfunction and cholestatic disease.

9. SPECIAL SITUATIONS

9.1. Renal Failure

In renal failure, care must be taken to adjust intakes to the output capability of the kidneys. In oliguric/anuric renal failure, it is generally necessary to decrease fluid intake by concentrating nutrients while limiting and monitoring electrolyte intakes. In spite of decreased excretory ability, the use of both parenteral and enteral alimentation can be associated with the development of hypokalemia and hypophosphatemia. Only general recommendations can be made and these patients require careful daily or more frequent clinical and laboratory evaluation. Often, the provision of adequate nutrition will require the institution of some form of renal replacement therapy. This should be instituted early in the course of care to prevent the development of the nutritional depletion associated with diminished intake. One additional advantage to the provision of adequate nutritional intake is the ability to limit endogenous catabolism, thus diminishing the release of endogenous acid, potassium, and phosphate associated with tissue catabolism.

In patients undergoing maintenance dialysis, studies have demonstrated that oral supplements and tube feeding do not result in significant alteration in electrolyte concentrations *(48, 49)*. When a specially prepared low-electrolyte formula was used as the main source of nutrition, it was occasionally associated with hypokalemia, hyponatremia, and hypophosphatemia; however, when used as supplementary feeding, no adverse effects on electrolyte status were reported *(50, 51)*.

9.2. Neonates

The use of parenteral and enteral nutrition in premature, frequently ill, neonates is a routine part of current practice. It should be remembered that in spite of their low serum creatinine concentrations, these infants actually have a low absolute rate of glomerular filtration and inability to concentrate their urine past 600–700 mOsm/kg water. Particular care must be paid to the use of solutions with high osmolar loads, which may result in dehydration as well as the possible development of necrotizing enterocolitis. While protein requirements are increased in this age group, the administration of excessive protein loads can be associated with the development of metabolic acidosis.

Neonates with acute renal failure present a particularly complex set of problems. They require higher calorie and protein intakes per kilogram of body weight than older individuals, and their diets are limited to liquids. Provision of adequate nutritional intake in this patient population most often requires the coordinated care of a variety of specialties within the neonatal intensive care unit.

CASE SCENARIOS

Case Scenario 1

You are covering for the weekend and receive a call from the mother of one of your patients, a 15-year-old female with anorexia nervosa. The mother was concerned that her daughter was looking more fatigued over the past 24 h and had not gotten out of bed for over a day. The patient denied any intercurrent illnesses and the rest of the family was well. Upon further questioning, you learn that the child had been binge eating for the past 3 days. You were able to access her records and learn that laboratory studies done the week prior demonstrated mild anemia, with an otherwise normal blood count as well as serum electrolytes, calcium, phosphorous, glucose, BUN, and creatinine concentrations.

The most likely explanation for this patient's condition is?

In spite of previously normal electrolyte values, individuals with anorexia nervosa are undernourished and at significant risk for metabolic/electrolyte derangements. While both intercurrent illness and refeeding can lead to the rapid development of electrolyte abnormalities, in this patient there is no evidence to support intercurrent illness. Her recent history of increased food intake (binge eating) would have led to an increase in serum insulin concentrations and likely precipitated the refeeding syndrome. The signs are often non-specific signs and can include fatigue, listlessness, decreased energy level, and muscle aches. The severity of her symptoms will be related to both her prior malnourished state and the amount/composition of her recent binge eating intake. These individuals are at significant risk and should be closely evaluated and monitored.

The most appropriate next step would be to?

Although her laboratory result from the week before had been reported to be within normal limits, it is appropriate to have her come into the emergency room to repeat her laboratory studies. While mild hypophosphatemia and hypokalemia may be treatable with oral supplementation, it is likely that she will require hospital admission for electrolyte replacement and a controlled increase in her daily calorie and fluid intake. It is recommended to start out with a calorie and fluid intake that is at about 75% of ideal daily intake and closely monitor electrolyte levels.

Case Scenario 2

A 9-year-old boy was seen for short stature. At birth he was diagnosed with aganglionosis of the large intestine and required a pull-through procedure. Postoperatively he developed hyponatremia and hypochloremia and at discharge his electrolytes were Na^+ 135 mEq/L, K^+ 5.9 mEq/L, Cl^- 97 mEq/L, and HCO_3^- 20 mmol/L. He was lost to follow-up and presented at 9 years of age with short stature and failure to thrive. History revealed that he had been having two to three large semi-liquid stools per day over the course of his lifetime. Dietary history revealed that he actively sought out salty food and salted his food liberally. He lives with his parents and sister who are all healthy and take no medications.

Physical exam revealed a pulse of 112, blood pressure 102/80 without orthostatic changes. His height was 106.7 cm (–4.5 SDS), and his weight was 17.7 kg (–2.7 SDS). He was short but well proportioned. His skin was dry but the rest of the examination was otherwise normal. Serum electrolytes revealed an Na^+ 136 mEq/L, K^+ 2.6 mEq/L, HCO_3^- of 34 mmol/L, and Cl^- of 80 mEq/L. The BUN was 24 mg/dL and the serum creatinine was 0.7 mg/dL.

What is your assessment of this patient?

This patient has evidence of volume depletion as noted by his hypokalemic hypochloremic metabolic alkalosis. In addition, the history of salt craving is highly suggestive of chronic salt depletion. Chronic salt depletion can be due to a variety of conditions including decreased intake, chronic vomiting (bulimia), as well as diarrheal, skin, or renal losses. There was no history of poor intake or vomiting but the history of previous colectomy and semi-liquid stools should strongly suggest increased intestinal salt loss. In normal individuals the large intestine reabsorbs a significant quantity of salt and water using an Na–K-ATPase mechanism, and chronic diarrhea can lead to a state of chronic salt and water depletion. It will also be necessary to rule out renal salt loss by assessing the kidneys ability to conserve sodium. In this child a random urine sample contained <10 mEq/L of sodium and of 187 mg/dL of creatinine, ruling out renal salt wasting.

How would you treat this patient?

This child required salt supplementation to counteract his ongoing intestinal sodium loss. He received sodium chloride tablets in increasing doses. The parents noted that his salt craving decreased as his sodium intake approached 10 mEq/kg/day. Treatment of this child's salt deficiency lead to a normalization of his serum electrolytes, a lowering of his BUN, and creatinine concentrations as well as a significant increase in his growth velocity. Over the next 3 years his height standard deviation score increased from –4.5 to –3.5 SDS.

It is difficult to assess salt sufficiency solely through the determination of serum electrolyte concentrations; as in this case the patient's serum sodium concentration was never lower than 135 mEq/L. When renal function is normal determination of the urinary sodium and creatinine concentrations and calculation of the fractional excretion of sodium will help assess intravascular volume status. When renal salt loss is responsible for the sodium depletion, determination of the serum renin activity can be used to assess intravascular volume.

REFERENCES

1. Seidman E, Gastrointestinal benefits of enteral feeds. In: Pediatric Enteral Nutrition, Baker SB, Baker RD, Davis A, eds., 1994, Chapman and Hall: New York, pp. 46–67.
2. Wilmore DW, The history of parenteral nutrition. In: Pediatric Parenteral Nutrition, Baker RD, Baker SS, Davis AM, eds., 1997, International Thomson Publishing, pp. 1–6.
3. Dudrick S, Wilmore D, and Vars HM, Long-term total parenteral nutrition with growth in puppies and positive nitrogen balance in patients. Surg Forum 1967, 18: 356–357.
4. Borowitz DB, Robert D, Stallings, Virginia, Consensus Report on Nutrition for Pediatric Patients with Cystic Fibrosis. J Pediatr Gastroenterol Nutr 2002, 35: 246–259.

5. Goulet O, Nutritional support in malnourished pediatric patients. Baillieres Clin Gastroenterol 1998, 12: 843–876.
6. Heyland DKM, MacDonald S, Keefe L, Drover JW, Total parenteral nutrition in the critically ill patient. A meta-analysis. J Am Med Assoc (JAMA) 1998, 280(23): 2013–2019.
7. Heyland DKM, Montalvo M, MacDonald S, Keefe L, Su XY, Drover JW, Total parenteral nutrition in the surgical patient: A meta-analysis. Can J Surg 2001. 44(2): p. 102–111.
8. Marino PLM, Finnegan, MJ, Nutrition support is not beneficial and can be harmful in critically ill patients. Crit Care Clin 1996, 12(3): 667–676.
9. Kleinman R, ed. Pediatric Nutrition Handbook. 5th ed. 2004, American Academy of Pediatrics.
10. Wassner SK, Kulin HE, Diminished linear growth associated with chronic salt depletion. Clin Pediatr 1990, 29(12): 719–721.
11. Wassner S, Altered growth and protein turnover in rats fed sodium-deficient diets. Pediatr Res 1989, 26(6): 608–613.
12. Fine BP, Ty A, Lestrange N, Maher E, Levine OR, Diuretic-induced growth failure in rats and its reversal by sodium repletion. J Pharmacol Exper Therapeut 1987, 242(1): 85–89.
13. Davis AM, Initiation, monitoring, and complications of pediatric parenteral nutrition. In: Pediatric Parenteral Nutrition, Baker RD, Baker SS, Davis AM, eds., International Thomson Publishing, pp. 212–237.
14. DeFronzo RA, Cooke CR, Andres R, Faloona GR, Davis PJ, The effect of insulin on renal handling of sodium, potassium, calcium and phosphate in man. J Clin Invest 1975, 55: 845–855.
15. Bloom WL, Carbohydrates and water balance. Am j Clin Nutr 1967, 20: 157–162.
16. Paice BJ, et al., Record linkage study of hypokalaemia in hospitalized patients. Postgrad Med J 1986 62(725): 187–191.
17. Gennari FJ, Hypokalemia. N Engl J Med 1998, 339(7): 451–458.
18. Bia MJ, DeFronzo RA, Extrarenal potassium homeostasis. Am J Physiol 1981, 240: F257–F268.
19. Knochel J, The pathophysiology and clinical characteristics of severe hypophosphatemia. Arch Intern Med 1977, 137: 203- 220.
20. Lotz M, Zisman E, Bartter F, Evidence for a phosphorus-depletion syndrome in man. New Eng J Med 1968, 278: 409–415.
21. Brunelli SM, Goldfarb S, Hypophosphatemia: Clinical consequences and management. J Am Soc Nephrol 2007, 18: 1999–2003.
22. Marks KE, Calcium and phosphorus in pediatric parenteral nutrition. J Pharm Pract 2004, 17(6): 432–446.
23. Rodd CG, Paul hypercalcemia of the newborn: etiology, evaluation, and management. Pediatr Nephrol 1999, 13: 542–547.
24. Ryan M, The role of magnesium in clinical biochemistry: An overview. Ann Clin Biochem 1991, 28: 19–26.
25. Lafrance J-P, Martine M, Metabolic, electrolytes, and nutritional concerns in critical illness. Crit Care Clin 2005, 21: 305–327.
26. Crook MB, et al., The importance of the refeeding syndrome. Nutrition 2001, 17: 632–637.
27. Solomon SM, Kirby DF, The refeeding syndrome: A review. J Parenter Enteral Nutr 1990, 14: 90.
28. Whang R, Magnesium deficiency: pathogenesis, prevalence and clinical implications. Am J Med 1987, 82: 24.
29. Wassner S, Baum M, Physiology and management. In: Pediatric Nephrology, Barratt T, Avner E, Harmon W, eds. 1999, Lippincott Williams & Wilkins: Baltimore, pp. 1155–1182.
30. Roy S3rd, The chloride depletion syndrome. Adv Pediatr 1984, 31: 235–57.
31. Kassirer JP, et al, The critical role of chloride in the correction of hypokalemic alkalosis in man. Am J Med 1965, 38: 172–189.
32. Schnitker MA, Mattman PE, Bliss TL, A clinical study of malnutrition in Japanese prisoners of war. Ann Intern Med 1951, 35: 69–96.
33. Afzal NA, Addai S, Fagbemi A, Murch S, Thomson M, Heuschkel R, Refeeding Syndrome with Enteral Nutrition in Children: A Case Report, Literature Review and Clinical Guidelines. Clin Nutr 2002, 21(6): 515–520.

34. Marik PE, Bedigian MK, Refeeding hypophosphatemia in critically ill patients in an intensive care unit. A prospective study. Arch Surg 1996, 131: 1043–1047.

35. Marinella MAM, The refeeding syndrome and hypophosphatemia. Nutr Rev 2003, 61(9): 320–323.

36. Gonzalez AG, Fajardo Rodriguez A, Gonzalex-Figueroa E, The incidence of the refeeding syndrome in cancer patients who receive artificial nutritional treatment. Nutr Hosp 1996, 11: 98.

37. Matz R, Parallels between treated uncontrolled diabetes and the refeeding syndrome with emphasis on fluid and electrolyte abnormalities. Diabetes Care 1994, 17(10): 1209–1213.

38. Hayek ME, Eisenberg PG, Severe hypophosphataemia following the institution of enteral feeding. Arch Surg 1989, 124: 1325–1328.

39. Thompson CH, Kemp GJ, Reduced muscle cell phosphate (pi) without hypophosphataemia in mild dietary pi deprivation. Clin Chem 1995, 416: 946–947.

40. Weisinger JR, Bellorin-Font E, Magnesium and phosphorous. Lancet 1998, 352: 391–396.

41. Kaysar NK, Polliack M, et al., Severe hypophosphataemia during binge eating in anorexia nervosa. Arch Dis Child 1991, 66: 138–139.

42. Vannatta JB, Andress DL, Whang R, Papper S, High-dose intravenous phosphorous therapy for severe complicated hypophosphatemia. South Med J 1983, 76: 1424–1426.

43. Terlevich A, Hearing SD, Woltersdorf WW, Smyth C, Reid D, McCullagh E, et al., Refeeding syndrome: effective and safe treatment with phosphates polyfusor. Aliment Pharmacol Ther 2003, 17: 1325–1329.

44. Chernow B, Rainey TG, Georges LP, O'Brein JT, Iatrogenic hyperphosphatemia: A metabolic consideration in critical care medicine. Crit Care Med 1981, 9: 772–774.

45. Thompson JS, Hodges RE, Preventing hypophosphatemia during total parenteral nutrition. J Parenter Enteral Nutr 1984, 8: 137–139.

46. Danks D, Copper deficiency in humans. Ann Rev Nutr 1988, 8: 235–257.

47. Fuhrman MP, Herrmann V, Masidonski P, et al., Pancytopenia after removal of copper from total parenteral nutrition. JPEN 2000, 24: 361–366.

48. Beutler K, Park GK, Wilkowski MJ, Effect of oral supplementation on nutrition indicators in hemodialysis patients. J Ren Nutr 1997, 7: 77–82.

49. Stratton RJ, et al., Multinutrient oral supplements and tube feeding in maintenance dialysis: A systematic review and meta-analysis. Am J Kidney Dis 2005, 46(3): 387–405.

50. Dare BK, Whiteside EJ, Wilson DE, An evaluation study to assess the potential use of renamil (Formerly Named Ren-O-Mil) for patients with chronic renal failure. J Hum Nutr Diet 1997, 10: 25–36.

51. Kuhlmann MK, Schmidt F, Kohler H, High protein/energy vs standard protein /energy nutritional regimen in the treatment of malnourished hemodialysis patients. Miner Electrolyte Metab 1999, 25: 306–310.

52. Newman JH, Neff TA, Ziporin P, Acute respiratory failure associated with hypophosphatemia. N Engl J Med 1977, 296: 1101.

53. O'Connor LW, Wheeler WS; Bethune JE, Effects of hypophosphatemia on myocardial performance in man. N Engl J Med 1977, 297: 901–903.

54. Weinsier RK, Krumdieck CL, Death resulting from overzealous total parenteral nutrition: the refeeding syndrome revisited. Am J Clin Nutr 1981, 34: 393–399.

55. Brown RO, Dickerson RN, et al., A new graduated dosing regimen for phosphorous replacement in patients receiving nutrition support. J Parenter Enteral Nutr 2006, 30(3): 209–214.

56. Council, NR, Recommended Dietary Allowances. 10th revised ed. 1989, Washington: National Academy of Sciences.

57. Keinman R (ed.), Parenteral nutrition. In: Pediatric Nutrition Handbook, 2004, American Academy of Pediatrics, pp. 369–389.

58. Keinman R (ed.), Trace elements. In: Pediatric Nutrition Handbook, 2004, American Academy of Pediatrics, pp. 313–337.

59. Prasad AS, Clinical manifestations of zinc deficiency. Ann Rev Nutr 1985, 5(1): 341–363.

60. Kumpulainen J, Salmenpera L, Siimes M, Koivistoinen P, Lehto J, Perheentupa J, Formula feeding results in lower selenium status than breast-feeding or selenium-supplemented formula feeding: A longitudinal study. Am J Clin Nutr 1987, 45: 49–53.

17 Understanding Uric Acid

F. Bruder Stapleton

Key Points

1. Serum uric acid concentrations vary as a function of age.
2. Certain medications may effect uric acid excretion.
3. It is important to assess extracellular volume status in the evaluation of children with hyperuricemia.

   Key Words: Hyperuricosuria; uric acid metabolism; hyperuricemia; hypouricemia; urate; serum uric acid; urinary uric acid excretion; acute uric acid nephropathy; tumor lysis syndrome; uricolysis

Physicians caring for children seldom consider measuring serum uric acid or urinary uric acid levels, most likely because gout or hyperuricemia is most often encountered in adults. Because uric acid disorders are uncommon in children, pediatricians frequently are unfamiliar with uric acid metabolism and renal handling of uric acid. At times, altered serum or urinary uric acid values can be valuable in clarifying renal and/or fluid and electrolyte disorders.

CASE SCENARIO 1: HYPERURICOSURIA WITH A NORMAL SERUM URIC ACID CONCENTRATION

Patient 1 is a 4-year-old boy with cystic fibrosis and documented pancreatic insufficiency. At 3 years and 9 months of age, he was switched from pancrelipase capsules to equivalent doses of pancrelipase powder. During the next 3 months, his mother gradually increased the daily intake of pancrelipase powder from the recommended seven packets to 15–20 packets because of persistent stool abnormalities. Shortly thereafter, the child had intermittent episodes of dysuria, with deposition of orange crystals on the penis and in the urine. Physical examination showed a well-nourished child who weighed 16 kg (25th percentile) and was 95 cm tall (<3rd percentile). Orange crystals covered the penis and inner thighs. Freshly voided urine was filled with uric acid crystals, occasional uric acid casts and had a pH of 5, with a specific gravity of 1.016 (Fig. 1). Laboratory evaluation designed to identify known renal and systemic causes of hyperuricosuria gave

From: *Nutrition and Health: Fluid and Electrolytes in Pediatrics*
Edited by: L. G. Feld, F. J. Kaskel, DOI 10.1007/978-1-60327-225-4_17,
© Humana Press, a part of Springer Science+Business Media, LLC 2010

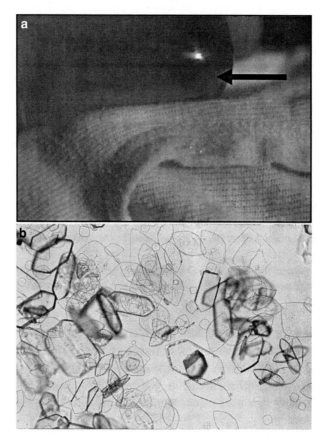

Fig. 1. (**a**) A freshly voided urine sample with a layer of uric acid crystals; (**b**) a microscopic view of uric acid crystals in this urine.

normal results. Creatinine clearance was normal. Serum electrolytes were normal and the serum bicarbonate was 23 mEq/L. The serum uric acid concentration ranged between 3 and 5.6 mg/dL, and 24-h urinary uric acid excretion ranged to 621 mg (39 mg/kg). Fractional excretion of uric acid was 40% (normal values – Table 1). Assays for red-cell hypoxanthine guanine phosphoribosyltransferase activity were comparable to those of three controls. What can explain the high urinary uric acid load with a normal serum uric acid? To answer this question, one must first consider some aspects of uric acid metabolism.

1. URIC ACID METABOLISM AND RENAL ELIMINATION

Metabolism: Uric acid is created in the body as the final oxidation product of purine catabolism. Uric acid is a weak organic acid with a pKa of 5.75. At physiologic pH, uric acid is present almost entirely as monosodium urate. The solubility of monosodium urate is nearly 15 times that of uric acid in aqueous solution. In human plasma, saturation occurs at a monosodium urate concentration of approximately 7 mg/dL. The proton

Table 1
Normal Uric Acid Values in Children

	Neonates 29–33 weeks gestation	38–40 weeks gestation	Children 3–4 years	5–9 years	10–14 years
Serum uric acid (mg/dL)	7.7 ± 2.7	5.2 ± 1.6	3.4 ± 0.8	3.65 ± 1	4.15 ± 1.2
Uric acid excretion (mg/kg/day)	n/a	n/a	13.5 ± 3.8	11.5 ± 3.8	9 ± 3.8
Fractional excretion of uric acid (%)	61 ± 12	44.5 ± 15.2	12 ± 3.75	10 ± 3	7.6 ± 3.8
Uric acid excretion (mg/dL GFR)	4.8 ± 2.2	1.7 ± 0.8	0.34 ± 0.11[1]		

Values are mean ± SD (Ref. 8–12)
[1] Value for all ages > 3 years (7)

concentration of a solution containing uric acid determines not only the relative amount of monosodium urate, but also the solubility of urate. Thus, in maximally acidified urine, uric acid predominates with minimal solubility *(1)*.

Elimination: The renal elimination of uric acid involves four components: glomerular filtration, tubular reabsorption, tubular secretion, and reabsorption beyond secretory sites. Uric acid is nearly completely filtered by the glomerular membrane; tubular reabsorption, secretion, and further reabsorption occurs along the proximal renal tubule *(2)*. Excessive excretion of uric acid may be the result of increased uric acid production or either decreased renal tubular reabsorption or increased secretion *(3)*.

1.1. Tubular Secretion and Postsecretory Reabsorption of Uric Acid

Tubular secretion of uric acid presumably occurs in the late convoluted or early proximal straight tubule *(4)*. Active cellular uptake occurs at the basolateral membrane, thereby generating a high intracellular uric acid concentration, which promotes passive diffusion across the luminal cell membrane into the tubular fluid. An active apical transporter, URAT 1, has been identified in the proximal tubule *(5)*.

The fourth component of renal uric acid transport, "postsecretory" reabsorption, was proposed from clearance studies that demonstrated an inhibition of the uricosuric effect of probenecid by pyrazinamide *(6)*. This conclusion appears justified because the simultaneous administration of these two pharmacologic agents does not affect the renal clearance of either drug. Based on calculated secretory rates, substantial reabsorption of secreted urate occurs.

Daily Uric Acid Excretion: Mean daily urinary uric acid excretion for adult men ingesting a purine-free diet is less than 600 mg/day. In adults, normal fractional excretion of uric acid is less than 10%. Daily excretion rates in women are less than men. Urinary urate excretion of greater than 800 mg/day in men eating an unrestricted diet is considered excessive *(5)*.

Clearance studies have shown that the renal handling of uric acid during early development and during childhood is significantly different from that of adults (8). Uric acid excretion is extremely high in the neonatal period with values exceeding 20 mg/kg/day in term infants. The fractional excretion of uric acid in premature and term infants is also dramatically elevated compared with adult values with mean values as high as 60% at 29–31 weeks' gestational age and 38% at term (Table 1). An inverse relationship exists between the fractional excretion of uric acid measured during the first day of life and gestational age. Fractional excretion of uric acid declines during early postnatal development at a rate comparable with intrauterine development.

Although the serum uric acid concentration in the newborn reflects maternal serum uric acid concentration and may increase with hypoxia and perinatal asphyxia, the excretion of dilute and often alkaline urine by the newborn infant helps to decrease the likelihood of uric acid precipitation and allows excretion of large amounts of uric acid without harmful effects (9). Uric acid clearance in infants is related to sodium excretion and urinary flow rate. The decline in the fractional excretion of uric acid during early life is presumed to reflect changes in renal tubular transport because the filtered uric acid load actually increases during this period of development.

The mean urate excretion is 13.5 mg/kg/day in children 3 years of age and declines during childhood (10). The high fractional excretion of uric acid in young children also progressively declines. This fall in the fractional excretion of urate with increasing age may be due to a relative increase in urate reabsorption rather than a decrease in urate secretion (Table 1).

Uric acid excretion in children has been assessed by comparing urinary uric acid to urinary creatinine concentration. This urinary uric acid to creatinine ratio is higher in young children than in adults and declines to adult levels during early childhood. Because normal values for urinary uric acid to creatinine ratio, for total urate excretion, excretion per unit body weight, and fractional excretion uric acid all vary with age, a reference table with age-related normals is required for interpretation of data.

A more reliable and constant measure of uric acid excretion (above age 2 years) is possible by measuring acid excretion per deciliter of creatinine clearance (UUA × SCr/UCr) (11). Values of random and 24-h urine samples were comparable (0.53/dL and 0.56/dL, respectively) and do not vary significantly with age in children aged 3 months to 14 years. A normal value of less than 0.56 mg uric acid per deciliter glomerular filtrate may be used after 2 years of age (Table 1). An increased value of (UUA × SCr)/UCr in a patient with normal renal function and hyperuricemia indicates an excessive production of uric acid. This rationale suggests that the patient in Case 1 had an increased production of uric acid. The high urinary uric acid excretion was due to the high-dose pancreatic extract with ingestion of large amounts or uric acid precursors (12).

CASE SCENARIO 2: HYPERURICEMIA WITH LOW URINARY URIC ACID EXCRETION

Patient 2 was a 17-year-old white male in whom an elevated serum concentration of uric acid of 11.5 mg/dL was discovered at a routine pre-school physical examination. He was entirely asymptomatic and was taking no medications. He was an above-average student and grade-appropriate. There was no family history of gout or renal disease. He had been noted to have asymptomatic proteinuria during a routine physical examination at the age of 14 years. Evaluation at that time demonstrated a normal creatinine clearance, normal excretory urogram, and orthostatic proteinuria. He had subsequently been examined at yearly intervals; his creatinine clearance, urinalyses, and 24-h protein excretion were normal. Physical examination revealed a healthy adolescent whose height was 182 cm, weight was 83.2 kg, and blood pressure was 124/82 mmHg. There were no tophi and examination of the musculoskeletal and neurological systems was normal.

Laboratory data included hemoglobin 14.8 g/dL, white blood cell count 8600 mm^3, platelet count 300,000/mm^3, reticulocyte count 1%, sodium 143, potassium 4.5, chloride 105, and bicarbonate 26 mEq/l, urea nitrogen 16, and creatinine 1.1 mg/dL.

During the evaluation of this patient, hyperuricemia was discovered in the father and four brothers. All of the members of the family with hyperuricemia were asymptomatic. A complete blood count, serum concentrations of electrolytes and urea nitrogen, and creatinine clearance were normal in all family members. Careful evaluation of renal function in this patient indicated that the patient had a selective defect in renal tubular secretion (13).

2. PHYSIOLOGICAL FACTORS AFFECTING RENAL EXCRETION OF URATE IN HUMANS

2.1. Extracellular Volume and Urine Flow Rate

The volume of the extracellular fluid compartment has an important influence on the renal handling of urate. In particular, the "effective arterial circulatory volume" is most significant in influencing renal uric acid excretion. Extracellular volume expansion with either isotonic or hypertonic (3%) saline increases uric acid excretion and promotes hypouricemia, presumably by inhibiting tubular urate reabsorption or by increasing peritubular backleak of uric acid (14). In contrast, extracellular volume depletion by diuretics diminishes uric acid excretion by 47–67% (15). Volume contraction during diarrheal dehydration in young children has been shown to increase serum uric acid concentrations, particularly in association with hypernatremia (16).

The effect of urinary flow rate on uric acid excretion can be difficult to separate from the effect of extracellular fluid volume. During antidiuresis owing to extracellular fluid volume contraction, the urinary urate concentration increases and may result in a small amount of urate back-diffusion in the distal terminal nephron tubules (17). Conversely, during diuresis, the diminished urinary urate concentration may reduce diffusion of urate.

The syndrome of inappropriate antidiuretic hormone secretion (SIADH) illustrates the important influence of extracellular fluid volume on urate clearance (18, 19). In SIADH, antidiuresis results in expansion of the extracellular fluid compartment, which then leads to increased urinary excretion of uric acid. Serum uric acid concentrations and fractional excretion of urate were studied in two groups of hyponatremic neonates, one with SIADH and the other with hyponatremic dehydration (20). The neonates with

SIADH had a mean serum urate concentration of 2.46 ± 0.54 mg/dL and an elevated fractional excretion of urate of 78 ± 0.18%, whereas volume-depleted hyponatremic infants had a serum urate concentration of 8.49 ± 2.45 mg/dL. Water restriction and subsequent correction of serum osmolality in the patients with SIADH resulted in an increase in the mean serum urate concentration to 4.95 ± 0.86 mg/dL and a significant decrease in the fractional urate excretion to 51 ± 0.08%. The site of reduced uric acid reabsorption in patients with SIADH is believed to be in the postsecretory component of urate reabsorption in the nephron.

2.2. Clinical Relevance

Extracellular volume contraction, particularly with hypernatremia, is associated with hyperuricemia. The syndrome of inappropriate ADH secretion, on the other hand, is associated with hypouricemia.

3. SYSTEMIC ACID–BASE EFFECTS AND ENDOGENOUS METABOLITES

Impaired urinary excretion of uric acid and hyperuricemia frequently accompany metabolic acidosis. Tubular secretion of uric acid is directly inhibited by both lactic acid and β-hydroxybutyrate (21). Reduced urate excretion also has been reported in severe respiratory acidosis and in diabetic ketoacidosis. During exercise, an increase in serum lactate concentration reduces urate excretion. Hyperlactic acidemia may also represent the common mechanism by which ethanol abuse, branched-chain ketoaciduria (maple syrup urine disease), type I glycogen storage disease, heat stress, and hereditary fructose intolerance affect urate excretion (1). In type I glycogen storage disease and fructose intolerance, uric acid production is increased as a result of intracellular depletion of high energy phosphates (22). Intracellular ATP depletion results in the diffusion of adenosine from the cell. Adenosine is then metabolized to uric acid and increases both the serum uric acid concentration and total uric acid excretion.

Metabolic alkalosis may promote urate retention. This effect is most likely a manifestation of extracellular volume contraction rather than a direct result of the alkalosis itself.

Hyperglycemia increases the renal excretion of urate (23). The development of glucosuria and osmotic diuresis is associated with decreased urate reabsorption in the proximal tubule. Recent studies have demonstrated that the reduced renal tubular reabsorption occurs distal to secretory sites (24).

CASE SCENARIO 3: HIGH SERUM URIC ACID WITH ELEVATED URINARY URIC ACID EXCRETION

Patient 3, a 14-year-old boy, presented to his pediatrician with fatigue. He was an honor student and was taking no medications. His physical examination was normal. Laboratory tests showed a hemoglobin 12 gm/dL, white blood cells 7000/mm³,

BUN 35 mg/dL, creatinine 8 mg/dL, sodium 137 mEq/L, potassium 5 mEq/L, chloride 107 mEq/L, bicarbonate 20 mEq/L, serum uric acid 35 mEq/L. Serum LDH concentration was normal. Urinary uric acid excretion was 1100 mg/dL (normal < 600 mg/dL) and the uric acid excretion per dL GFR was 1.2 mg/dL (normal < 0.57 mg/dL).

What caused this patient's hyperuricemia? The patient had an increased urinary excretion of uric acid secondary to increased production of uric acid. A bone marrow aspirate revealed acute T-cell leukemia *(25)*. His renal failure was due to acute urate nephropathy. This complication occurs most frequently as tumor lysis syndrome during initial chemotherapy for lymphoid malignancies.

4. HYPERURICEMIA

The serum uric acid concentration is an important physiologic regulator of uric acid excretion. Tubular secretion of urate into the urine seems to account for the major mechanisms by which urinary urate excretion increases with hyperuricemia. The capacity to increase tubular secretion in response to acute uric acid loads is greater in children than adults. This may account for the rarity of clinical gout in children and also explains why Patient 1 had a normal serum uric acid despite a high dietary load of purine precursors *(13)*. An approach to the patient with hyperuricemia is shown in Fig. 2.

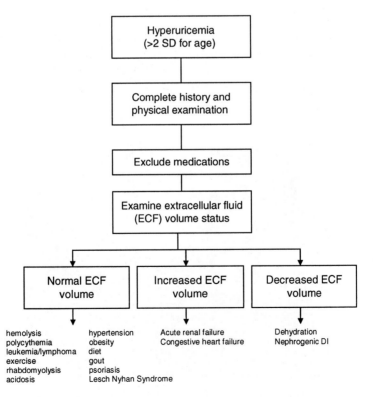

Fig. 2. Suggested approach to a child with hyperuricemia.

5. RENAL CONSEQUENCES OF HYPERURICEMIA

Acute uric acid nephropathy is an important etiology of oliguric acute renal failure among selected groups of patients in whom the serum urate concentration becomes markedly elevated or in whom a massive uricosuria develops. The most common clinical setting for acute urate nephropathy occurs with rapid turnover of nucleoproteins in patients with leukemia, lymphoma, or other neoplasms, especially during cytotoxic therapy.

Called tumor lysis syndrome, acute renal failure with hyperuricemia during therapy for leukemia or lymphomas is associated with hyperkalemia, acidosis, hypocalcemia, and hyperphosphatemia *(26, 27)*. These metabolic complications develop rapidly and may be life-threatening. Rarely, spontaneous acute urate nephropathy may precede cytotoxic therapy in patients with leukemia or lymphoma *(25)*.

Additional causes of renal failure from increased serum uric acid and uric aciduria include inherited disorders of purine metabolism (i.e., Lesch–Nyhan syndrome or hypoxanthine–guanine phosphoribosyl transferase deficiency), hemolysis, rhabdomyolysis, perinatal asphyxia, extreme exercise, and prolonged muscle contractions from status epilepticus. Important risk factors for acute renal failure from hyperuricemia are dehydration and/or acidemia.

Many pharmacologic agents increase uric acid excretion. Some, such as the diuretic ticrynafen, have produced acute renal failure. Radiographic contrast agents also markedly increase uric acid excretion and should be avoided, or used with caution, during hyperuricemia.

Urinary flow drops dramatically in patients with acute uric acid nephropathy. Oliguria results from renal tubular obstruction by the precipitation of uric acid in collecting tubules *(28)*. As a result of intraluminal obstruction of the distal nephron, dilatation of proximal tubules occurs. As discussed previously, uric acid is least soluble in highly

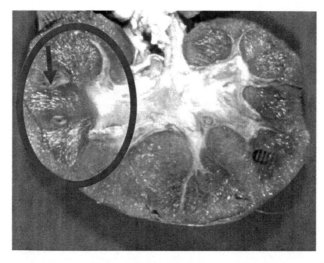

Fig. 3. This figure shows columns of uric acid crystals in the renal medulla of a child who died with a serum uric acid of 62 mg/dL.

concentrated urine of low pH and, predictably, uric acid precipitation occurs in the renal medulla and papilla in acute uric acid nephropathy (Fig. 3). Uric acid precipitation may also occur in the vasa recti supplying the distal nephron. Histological studies of kidneys during acute urate nephropathy show minimal interstitial cellular infiltration, and the pathologic changes of acute urate nephropathy are reversible.

Renal function in acute uric acid nephropathy correlates with the rate of urinary excretion of urate, rather than the serum urate level. Precipitation of uric acid in the distal renal tubules and distal renal microvasculature results in increased proximal tubule and distal tubule pressure, and a marked increase in peritubular capillary vascular resistance. In patients with hyperuricemia and leukemia, inulin clearance (C_{IN}) a measure of GFR, and para-amino hippurate (PAH) clearance, a measure of renal plasma flow, are decreased (29). The filtration fraction (C_{IN}/C_{PAH}) is also decreased. Studies of acute hyperuricemia in laboratory animal models have shown similar alterations in C_{IN} and renal blood flow. Urinary flow is almost always markedly diminished.

6. PHARMACOLOGIC AGENTS AFFECTING URIC ACID METABOLISM

A wide variety of pharmacologic agents are known to affect uric acid metabolism (30). Hyperuricemia may result from either inhibition of tubular secretion or from enhanced tubular reabsorption (Table 2). Conversely, hypouricemia may develop when tubular reabsorption is inhibited or tubular secretion is increased.

Table 2
Drugs That Decrease Uric Acid Excretion

Diuretics	Ethanol
Acetazolamide	Laxative abuse
Amiloride	Levodopa
Chlorthalidone	Methoxy flurano
Furosemide	Nicotinic acid
Thiazides	Pyrazinamide
Triamterene	Salicylates (low dose)
Ethambutol	

7. PATHOPHYSIOLOGY OF HYPOURICEMIA WITH HYPERURICOSURIA

Idiopathic hyperuricosuria may result from altered renal tubular urate transport. With renal urate wasting, serum uric acid concentrations are decreased (<2 mg/dL). Decreased tubular reabsorption of urate is the most frequent transport defect in patients with renal hyperuricosuria (31–33). Uric acid is reabsorbed in both the early and late segments of the proximal tubule. It appears that most defects in urate reabsorption occur in the early or "pre-secretory" segments. Less commonly, some children have increased tubular secretion of uric acid (32). Idiopathic renal hyperuricosuria may affect multiple family members and is frequently asymptomatic. Other etiologies of renal urate wasting include the Fanconi syndrome, cystinosis, Wilson's disease, and parenteral hyperalimentation *(34)*. A substantial number of pharmacological agents increase urinary uric acid excretion (Table 3). Obviously, any cause of increased uric acid production with hyperuricemia may result in hyperuricosuria. An approach to the patient with hypouricemia is shown in Fig. 4.

Table 3
Selected Drugs That Increase Uric Acid Excretion

Acetohexamide	Hyperosmolar contrast media
Ascorbic acid	Iodopyracet
Benzbromarone	Iopanoic acid
Calcium ipodate	Meglumine iodipamide
Chlorprothixene	Ticrynafen
Cinchophen	Orotic acid
Citrate	Outdated tetracycline
Dicumerol	Phenylbutazone
Most diuretics	Phenolsulfonphthalein
Estrogens	Probenecid
Glycerol guaiacolate	Salicylate
Glycine	Sodium diatrizoate
Halofenate	Zoxazolamine

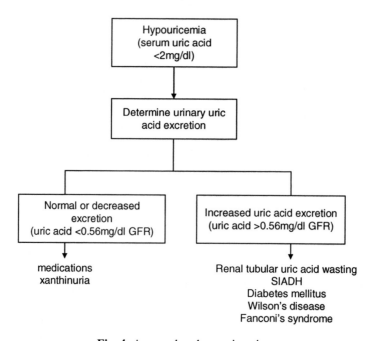

Fig. 4. Approach to hypouricemia.

8. THERAPY FOR ACUTE SEVERE HYPERURICEMIA
WITH NEPHROPATHY

Although the mortality in acute urate nephropathy was once nearly 45%, current dialysis therapies have dramatically improved survival. Mortality is now related almost exclusively to the underlying disease process. Medical therapy for patients at risk for urate nephropathy is directed toward reducing intrarenal precipitation of uric acid by maintaining a high urine flow rate with as much hydration as the level of renal function allows *(35)*.

To prevent acute uric acid nephropathy in patients undergoing induction antineoplastic therapy, intravenous fluid administration is begun at 3000 mL/m^2 body surface area per day in both children and adults, when extracellular fluid volume allows. In patients with extracellular fluid volume depletion, replacement of fluid deficits must precede high volume maintenance. An alkaline urine is maintained with intravenous sodium bicarbonate infusions. When the urine pH cannot be maintained above a pH of 7.0, acetazolamide may also be given orally (provided systemic acidosis is not present). The relative protective roles of urinary flow rate, urine osmolality, and urine pH in the prevention of acute urate nephropathy have been examined in laboratory settings *(36)*. These studies suggest that a high tubular fluid flow rate, regardless of urine pH or osmolality, offers the maximal protection against urate nephropathy. As aforementioned, use of uricosuric drugs, especially radiographic contrast agents, should be avoided in patients with hyperuricemia (Fig. 3).

During cytotoxic therapy or in patients with a sustained source of urate overproduction, the filtered urate load is reduced by administering either intravenous or oral allopurinol. Allopurinol is an inhibitor of xanthine oxidase and is effective in reducing the concentration of uric acid in the serum. Urinary oxypurine excretion is markedly increased during allopurinol therapy and renal failure secondary to xanthine precipitation has been observed rarely during allopurinol therapy *(37)*.

Dialysis or hemofiltration is effective in reducing the serum uric acid concentration and in treating the metabolic consequences of acute renal failure *(38)*. The clearance of uric acid by hemodialysis is 10 times greater than with peritoneal dialysis; therefore, hemodialysis is the dialysis treatment of choice for acute renal failure from uric acid nephropathy. Hemodialysis should be the initial treatment if oliguria or life-threatening hyperkalemia are present when renal failure is discovered. Occasionally, acute renal failure resolves after one or two dialysis treatments *(26)*. Due to the tremendous production of uric acid with initial cytotoxic therapy, frequent hemodialysis therapies may be required. When time and the initial metabolic derangements allow, continuous arteriovenous or venovenous hemofiltration or hemodiafiltration has been shown to be advantageous as renal replacement therapy for patients with acute tumor lysis syndrome. Continuous hemodiafiltration allows for the provision of intravenous nutrition and more flexibility in management. Allopurinol is removed by hemodialysis, and a dose should be given at the conclusion of dialysis treatment.

Uricolysis therapy with the intravenous administration of the enzyme, uricase (uric acid oxidase), is an exciting advance in the treatment and prevention of urate nephropathy during cytotoxic therapies *(34)*. Uric acid is degraded to allantoin in the presence of uricase. Allantoin is extremely soluble, is filtered by the glomerular membrane, and has no known nephrotoxicity. Intravenous administration of uricase in doses of 0.15–0.2 mg/kg, diluted in saline, is administered over 1–2 h during the first 5–7 days of chemotherapy. This regimen is superior to allopurinol in reducing serum uric acid concentrations and preventing oliguric acute renal failure in children with leukemia. Some patients (<5%) receiving the nonrecombinant uricase develop bronchospasm, hives, and other hypersensitivity reactions. Uricase should not be administered to patients with G6PD deficiency. Enzymatic uricolysis therapy may replace the initial use of allopurinol and dramatically reduce the need for dialysis therapies in patients with tumor lysis syndrome.

8.1. Hyperuricemia in the Pathogenesis of Hypertension and Progression of Chronic Kidney Disease

Individuals with hypertension and chronic kidney disease frequently have increased serum concentrations of uric acid. Traditional thinking has considered hyperuricemia in these settings as a secondary phenomenon and has not considered a primary pathogenetic mechanism related to uric acid *(7)*. Recent studies have hypothesized that uric acid is toxic to vascular endothelial cells and may result in the development of essential hypertension and progressive loss of renal function *(39, 40)*. This interesting hypothesis is currently the focus of rigorous study and potentially offers new therapeutic options in these conditions.

8.2. Summary

1. Serum uric acid and urinary uric acid values vary during childhood and differ from adult values.
2. Serum uric acid concentrations are altered by changes in extracellular fluid volumes.
3. Unexplained extreme hyperuricemia in an otherwise normally developing child should raise the possibility of leukemia or lymphoma, regardless of the peripheral white blood cell count.
4. Hyperuricemia is an important cause of acute renal failure in children undergoing acute tumor lysis.
5. Chronic hyperuricemia may contribute to the development of hypertension and progression of chronic kidney disease.

REFERENCES

1. Wyngaarden JB, Kelley WN. Gout. In: Stanbury JB, Wyngaarden JB, Fredrickson DS (eds.). The Metabolic Basis of Inherited Disease. New York, McGraw-Hill, 1983, p. 1043.
2. Maesaka JK, Fishbane S. Regulation of renal urate excretion: A critical review. Am J Kidney Dis 1998;32:917–933.
3. Cameron JS, Maro F, Simmonds HA. Gout, uric acid and purine metabolism in paediatric nephrology. Pediatr Nephrol 1993;7:105–118.
4. Rieselbach RE, Steele TH. Influence of the kidney upon urate homeostasis in health and disease. Am J Med 1974;56:665–672.
5. Tune BM, Burg MB, Patla KS. Characteristics of p-aminohippurate transport in proximal tubules. Am J Physiol 1969;217:1057–1063.

6. Anzai N, Kanai Y, Endou H. New insights into renal transport of urate. Curr Opin Rheumatol 2007;19:151–157.

7. Meisel AD, Diamond HS. Inhibition of probenecid uricosuria by pyrazinamide and paraaminohippurate. Am J Physiol 1976;32:F222–229.

8. Stapleton FB. Renal uric acid clearance in human neonates. J Pediatr 1983;103:290–295.

9. Stapleton FB, Linshaw MA, Hassanein K. Uric acid excretion in normal children. J Pediatr 1978;92:911–915.

10. Stapleton FB, Nash DA. A screening test for hyperuricosuria. J Pediatr 1983;102:88–91.

11. Raivio KO. Neonatal hyperuricemia. J Pediatr 1976;88:625–627.

12. Stapleton FB, Kennedy J, Nousia-Arvanitakis S, et al. Hyperuricosuria due to high dose pancreatic extract therapy in cystic fibrosis. N Engl J Med 1976;295:246–250.

13. Stapleton FB, Nyhan WL, Borden M, et al. Renal pathogenesis of familial hyperuricemia: Studies in two kindreds. Pediatr Res 1981;1447–1454.

14. Manuel MA, Steele TH. Pyrazinamide suppression of the uricosuric response to sodium chloride infusion. J Lab Clin Med 1974;83:417–422.

15. Weinman EJ, Eknoyan E, Suki WN. The influence of the extracellular fluid volume on the tubular reabsorption if uric acid. J Clin Invest 1975;55:283–290.

16. Adler R, Robinson R, Pasdral P, et al. Hyperuricemia in diarrheal dehydration. Am J Dis Child 1982;136:211–214.

17. Engle JE, Steele TH. Variation of urate excretion with urine flow in normal man. Nephron 1976;16:52–58.

18. Beck LH. Hypouricemia in the syndrome of inappropriate secretion of antidiuretic hormone. N Engl J Med 1979;301:528–530.

19. Maesaka JK, Miyawaki N, Palata T, et al. Renal salt wasting without cerebral disease: Diagnostic value of urate determinations in hyponatremia. Kidney Int 2007;71:822–826.

20. Assadi FK, et al. Hypouricemia in neonates with syndrome of inappropriate secretion of antidiuretic hormone. Pediatr Res 1985;19:424–428.

21. Burch RE, Kurlee N. The effect of lactate infusion on serum uric acid. Proc Soc Exp Biol 1968;127:17–20.

22. Greene HL, Wilson FA, Hefferan P, et al. ATP depletion, a possible role in the pathogenesis of hyperuricemia in glycogen storage disease, Type I. J Clin Invest 1978;62:321–328.

23. Padova J, Patchefsky A, Onesti G, et al. The effect of glucose loads on renal uric acid excretion in diabetic patients. Metabolism 1964;13:507–511.

24. Shichiri M, Iwamoto H, Shiifai T. Diabetic renal hypouricemia. Arch Intern Med 1987;147:225–231.

25. Jones DP, Stapleton FB, Kawinsky D, et al. Renal dysfunction and hyperuricemia at presentation and relapse of acute lymphoblastic leukemia. Med Pediatr Oncol 1990;18:283–286.

26. Stapleton FB, Strother DR, Roy III S, et al. Acute renal failure at onset of therapy for advanced stage Burkitt lymphoma and B cell acute lymphoblastic lymphoma. Pediatrics 1988;82:863–869.

27. Tsokos GC, Balow JE, Speigel RJ, et al. Renal and metabolic complications of undifferentiated and lymphoblastic lymphomas. Medicine 1981;67:218–227.

28. Spencer HW, Yarger WE, Robinson RR. Alterations of renal function during dietary-induced hyperuricemia in the rat. Kidney Int 1976;9:489–496.

29. Conger JD, Falk SA, Guggenheim SJ, et al. A micropuncture study of the early phase of acute urate nephropathy. J Clin Invest 1976;58:681–686.

35. Baldree LA, Stapleton FB. Uric acid metabolism in children. Pediatr Clin North Am 1990;2:391–418.

36. Weitz R, Sperling O. Hereditary renal hypouricemia: Isolated tubular defect of urate reabsorption. J Pediatr 1980;96:850–853.

37. Tofuku Y, Kuroda M, Takeda R. Hypouricemia due to renal urate wasting: Two types of tubular transport defect. Nephron 1982;30:39–45.

38. Nakajima H, Gomi M, Iida S, et al. Familial renal hypouricemia with intact reabsorption of uric acid. Nephron 1987;45:40–48.

34. Pui CH. Urate oxidase in the prophylaxis or treatment of hyperuricemia: The United States experience. Semin Hematol 2001;38 (Suppl 10):13–21.

30. Jeha S. Tumor lysis syndrome. Semin Hematol 2001;38 (Suppl 10):4–8.
31. Conger JD, Falk SA. Intrarenal dynamics in the pathogenesis and prevention of acute urate nephropa-
    thy. J Clin Invest 1977;59:786–796.
32. Andreoli SP, et al. Purine excretion during tumor lysis in children with acute lymphocytic leukemia
    receiving allopurinol: Relationship to acute renal failure. J Pediatr 1986;109:292.
33. Agha-Razil M, Amyot SL, Pichette V, Cardinal J, Ouimet D, Loblanc M. Continuous veno-venous
    hemodiafiltration for the treatment of spontaneous tumor lysis syndrome complicated by acute renal
    failure and severe hyperuricemia. Clin Nephrol 2000;54:59–63.
39. Feig DI, Nakagawa T, KarumachiSA et al. Hypothesis: uric acid, nephron number, and the pathogen-
    esis of essential hypertension. Kidney Int. 2004; 66:281–287.
40. Perelstein TS, Gumeniak O, Williams GH et al. Uric acid and the development of hypertension: the
    normative aging study. Hypertension. 2006; 48:1031–1036.

18 Special Situations in the NICU

Sheri L. Nemerofsky
and Deborah E. Campbell

Key Points

1. Total body water decreases significantly throughout gestation and the first year of life from 95 to 60%.
2. Postnatal weight loss in the first week of life is physiologically normal in all gestational ages.
3. Mature renal function is not achieved until approximately 2 years of life.
4. Gestational age is the major factor in the degree of insensible water loss due to transepidermal water loss, respiratory loss, and urinary losses.
5. Thermoregulation of newborns decreases morbidity and mortality.

   Key Words: Body fluids; fluid balance; water loss; electrolyte balance; acid–base metabolism

1. INTRODUCTION

The physiologic processes that occur as the newborn infant transitions from intrauterine to extrauterine life are complex and involve changes in body composition, fluid distribution, and skin, kidney, and neuroendocrine system functions. Alterations in acid–base and fluid balances are prominent during this period. In newborn infants, the skin primarily regulates fluid and electrolyte balance. In utero, the fetus is able to maintain almost all of its acid–base physiology, except for the carbon dioxide (CO_2) that diffuses across the placenta. Therefore, fetal acid–base balance may be affected by placental disturbances, such as a change in blood flow or umbilical cord compression. This may be caused by maternal factors such as hypertensive diseases of pregnancy (hypertension, preeclampsia) or placental abruption. Careful attention is required during management of neonatal fluids and acid–base balance. Both are affected by gestational age, maternal complications, mode of delivery, congenital anomalies, insensible water loss, the environment, and medications. Management of the newborn infant, particularly infants admitted to the neonatal intensive care unit will be reviewed.

From: *Nutrition and Health: Fluid and Electrolytes in Pediatrics*
Edited by: L. G. Feld, F. J. Kaskel, DOI 10.1007/978-1-60327-225-4_18,
© Humana Press, a part of Springer Science+Business Media, LLC 2010

2. BODY FLUIDS

Body composition, specifically fluid distribution, changes drastically throughout the human life span. The most significant changes occur during fetal development and throughout the first year of life (Fig. 1). Total body water (TBW) is the sum of extracellular fluid and intracellular fluid. The extracellular water (ECW) is further broken down into two parts, the interstitial fluid and plasma (not including red and white blood cells). The major cation in the ECW is sodium (Na^+) and the major anions are chloride (Cl^-) and bicarbonate (HCO_3^-). The major cations in the intracellular water (ICW) are potassium (K^+) and magnesium (Mg^{2+}) and the major anions are protein and organic phosphates.

In the first trimester, the TBW comprises about 95% of the total body weight. When gestation enters the second trimester, the TBW declines to approximately 85%. This continues to decrease until birth. Water and electrolyte exchange between the mother,

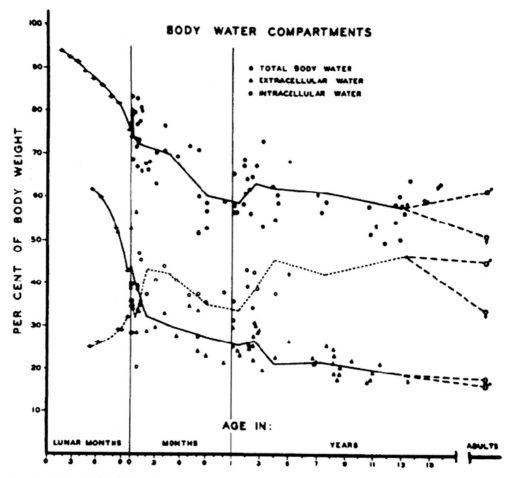

Fig. 1. TBW, ECW, ICW as percentages of body weight in infants and children, compared to corresponding values for the fetus and adults. Reproduced with permission from Friis-Hansen *(3)*.

fetus, and placenta influence fetal body composition and fluid balance. The placenta provides nutrients and electrolytes for the developing fetus. Positive electrolyte balance is required for appropriate weight gain during the third trimester.

A key factor that causes the change in ECW during pregnancy and early in gestation is the increased plasma volume. During the second trimester the blood volume of the fetus is about 160 ml/kg; this decreases to approximately 80 ml/kg at term gestation (1, 2). As gestation advances, the fetal hemoglobin rises. This contributes to a decrease in plasma volume and therefore, a decrease in ECW and an increase in ICW. There are also clinical scenarios that may cause a more substantial rise in hemoglobin concentration in a newborn infant. These include infants who are born to a diabetic mother, born after a hypoxic event near the time of delivery or affected in utero leading to intrauterine growth restriction, which may increase bone marrow red cell production leading to polycythemia.

At birth the percentage of TBW to total body weight exceeds that of an adult. The TBW of the term infant is 75% of the birth weight. Infants who are born preterm will have a higher TBW and larger extracellular compartments than babies born at term. As the ECW decreases during gestation, the ICW compartment steadily increases. By the second trimester the ICW makes up about 25% of the total body weight and by 3 months postnatal age the ICW has almost reached its peak at 40%. After this time, the intracellular volume steadily declines to about 25% at 1 year of age (3) (Fig. 1).

There are a number of factors that can affect the changes in TBW, ECW, and ICW in utero and throughout the first year of life. Fluid changes begin early in pregnancy. As maternal weight increases throughout pregnancy there is a significant increase in TBW of the mother. The TBW compartment comprises about 50% of the pregnancy weight gain (4). As the fetus develops in utero, there is a steady increase in fat and muscle with a concurrent decrease in the percentage of TBW and ECW as the gestation advances. The fetus and premature infant have a very large body surface area relative to their size. This also has a major effect on fluid balance.

Rapid changes in body water distribution also occur after birth in the full-term infant. The intracellular and extracellular compartments are inversely proportional to each other. As the ECW decreases, the ICW increases. Contraction of the extracellular compartment (interstitial tissue space) is dependent on the total body sodium content and exceeds the concurrent degree of intracellular compartment expansion that occurs after birth. This results in a total reduction of TBW. From 3 months of age onward ECW continues to decline but at a much slower rate as does the proportion of TBW. By 1 year of age, the TBW is about 60% and the ECW compartment comprises about 25% of the total body weight.

The kidneys have a major effect on fetal and neonatal fluid balance. During fetal life, the kidney function and the number of nephrons are low. The function and number of nephrons increase with advancing gestational and postnatal age (5). Mature (adult) renal function is achieved by 2 years of age. There are other factors that affect fluid and electrolyte balance in the postnatal period, including hormonal, maternal medications, and umbilical cord clamping. Changes in fetal hormone (catecholamines, vasopressin, and cortisol) levels in preparation for labor and delivery occur in conjunction with intrapartum-induced alterations in capillary permeability and the shifting of fluid from the intravascular to the interstitial space of the fetus. These physiologic processes are important for normal adaptation that occurs during the first 48 h of life. Postnatally, increased oxygenation and changes in hormone production shift fluid from the interstitium back into the intravascular space. Intrapartum events and the timing of umbilical cord clamping can also affect postnatal fluid balance. A delay in clamping the umbilical cord can increase the hematocrit of the newborn infant by 25–50% (6). There are instances where neonatal hyponatremia may develop in response to maternal treatment with indomethacin or fluid overload. Fetal hydration may also be impaired by placental insufficiency or in response to maternal diuretic therapy.

Postnatal weight loss in the healthy term infant occurs primarily in response to contraction of the extracellular compartment. Among infants who are born extremely preterm, transepidermal water loss contributes to changes in serum osmolality, and early neonatal weight loss. Immaturity in organ function of the heart, kidneys, skin and endocrine systems impair regulation of extracellular fluid and electrolyte balance. As fluid moves from the interstitial to intravascular compartments there is an increase in atrial natriuretic peptide and a decrease in other hormones that enhance the normal physiological renal sodium and water excretion characteristic of premature infants. In the immature infant there is a limited ability to respond to acute volume loads. Although the kidneys regulate the extracellular volume and osmolality, renal glomerular development (nephrogenesis) is not complete until 34–36 weeks' gestation. Renal tubular growth continues throughout the first few years of life.

The rate of sodium, bicarbonate, free water excretion, and renal concentrating capacity are determined by the degree of tubular immaturity. Maturation of renal tubular function and glomerular filtration rate are necessary to promote positive sodium balance that is critical for growth during infancy. Significant fluid and electrolyte disturbances may occur in extremely immature infants who are susceptible to fluid overload. This includes hypernatremia, hyponatremia, hyperkalemia, hypoglycemia, and hyperglycemia due to renal immaturity. Edema may develop in response to excess sodium or a volume load. Renal sodium losses leading to hyponatremia during the first week of life typically result in a negative sodium balance in preterm infants born before 33 weeks' gestation. Hypertonic dehydration may also occur in the very preterm infant in response to increased free water losses through immature skin that is not fully cornified.

Weight loss is typical in all newborn infants during the first week of life. The estimated median degree of neonatal weight loss in full-term infants is reported to be 3.5% in formula-fed infants and 6.6% in breastfed infants (7). The upper limit of normal postnatal weight loss varies in both formula feeding and breastfeeding infants, ranging from 9.5 to 12.8%, respectively. The median length of time to maximal weight loss is approximately 2–3 days. Recovery of birth weight is achieved between 6 and 9 days for most infants. A longer period to regain birth weight is more frequently required among breastfeeding infants and premature infants. The length of time to regain birth weight can also vary widely; a small percentage of infants experience limited weight gain and may take up to 3 weeks to reach their birth weight. The magnitude of postnatal weight loss is influenced not only by the normal physiologic postnatal extracellular fluid contraction, but also by the hydration status and caloric intake of the infant. Higher birth weights and exclusive formula feeding are associated with less postnatal weight loss (8). For most full-term infants during the first week of life a 10% weight loss should trigger an assessment of the hydration status and the risk for hypernatremia and/or non-hemolytic jaundice by the pediatric provider.

Colostrum is the first milk produced late in pregnancy and during the first few days after birth. Mature breast milk production typically begins 48 h after delivery. A breast-feeding infant should be fed 8–12 times a day to ensure adequate fluid and nutritional intake. Weight loss in the full-term infant who is breastfeeding usually continues until the 3rd–5th day of life *(9)*. Inadequate breastfeeding poses a potential risk for the development of hypernatremic dehydration in the neonate. However, hypernatremic dehydration is often difficult to diagnose solely on the basis of clinical examination. In the otherwise healthy neonate, skin turgor, urine output, and anterior fontanelle fullness are typically maintained even in the infant who is 10–15% dehydrated *(10, 11)*. Risk factors for excessive weight loss and dehydration in a full-term infant with a normal delivery in the newborn nursery include an inexperienced mother who is breastfeeding, inadequate frequency of breastfeeding, and poor oral-motor coordination.

3. RENAL ASPECTS OF FLUID BALANCE

The kidneys begin to function early in gestation, but nephrogenesis is not complete until 34 weeks' gestation (or 34 weeks postmenstrual age for infants born preterm). Fetal urine production increases significantly from 20 weeks gestation until birth *(12)*. At term, the newborn kidney functions at approximately 25% of the adult level and in the vast majority of newborns this degree of initial postnatal renal function is sufficient. After birth, there is a decrease in renal vascular resistance with a concurrent increase in renal blood flow and glomerular filtration. During the first 24 h, there is a three-fold increase in the glomerular filtration rate that is unrelated to the total renal blood flow or systemic blood pressure. The term neonate is able to concentrate urine to an osmolality of 600–700 mOsm/L. However, the premature newborn has limited urine concentrating ability caused by the relatively low renal medullary osmolality. In comparison, the older child or adult can achieve a urine osmolality of 1200 mOsm/L.

Other key factors influencing fluid balance include arginine vasopressin (antidiuretic hormone, ADH), prostaglandins, atrial natriuretic factor, aldosterone, and the renin–angiotensin system. Antidiuretic hormone, also known as arginine vasopressin, is produced in the posterior pituitary gland by the 11th week of gestation *(13)*. Its purpose is to conserve body water. ADH acts on the collecting tubules to reduce water loss in the urine. Infants with hypoxic-ischemic encephalopathy or a central nervous system infection experience an increase in ADH production. When the syndrome of inappropriate antidiuretic hormone (SIADH) develops urinary output decreases and there is increased permeability of the collecting ducts causing hyponatremia and an elevation in blood pressure due to arteriolar vasoconstriction. Prostaglandins are another important regulator of fetal renal blood flow that cause vasodilatation and help maintain the glomerular filtration rate. The atrial myocytes produce the atrial natriuretic factor. This hormone has potent diuretic, natriuretic, and vasodilatory effects *(14)*. The mineralocorticoid aldosterone is secreted by the adrenal cortex of the fetus *(15)*. This acts on the distal renal tubules to reabsorb sodium and excrete potassium. The renin–angiotensin system is a hormonal system that also helps regulate extracellular fluid. Renin is synthesized in the kidney and acts on angiotensin to form angiotensin II that leads to arteriolar vasoconstriction to maintain blood pressure, tubular reabsorption of sodium, and tubular excretion of potassium and aldosterone secretion.

Postnatal sodium and water balance depend on renal tubular reabsorption of sodium and water and is affected by hydrostatic and oncotic forces on the renal tubule. Fluids must be carefully balanced because preterm and full-term infants have difficulty responding to fluid deprivation and fluid overload. Postnatally, fluid and electrolyte imbalance that may occur are caused by a number of factors including renal dysfunction, renal agenesis, prematurity, congenital defects, such as abdominal wall defects and intestinal atresias, and electrolyte loss from the intestines due to vomiting or diarrhea.

All neonates are vulnerable to developing renal insufficiency; however, preterm infants are at a significantly higher risk than their full-term counterparts. It has been reported that up to 22% of preterm newborns develop acute renal failure *(16)*. Acute renal failure in the newborn often leads to water and electrolyte imbalance. The causes of renal failure may be classified by disease origin: pre-renal, renal, or post-renal. Pre-renal failure is caused by decreased perfusion of the kidney that may develop in response to hypotension, dehydration, or hypovolemia. Intrinsic renal failure is usually caused by an acute physiological event such as shock, ischemia, or renal tubular dysfunction. Post-renal failure is caused by urinary tract obstruction that usually requires surgery for definitive treatment (Fig. 2).

Pre-renal	Renal	Post-renal
Congestive Heart Failure	Acute Tubular Necrosis	*Congenital Anomalies
Dehydration	Polycystic kidney disease	Bilateral uretopelvic junction obstruction
Drugs	Renal dysplasia	Bilateral ureterovesical junction obstruction
Hemorrhage	Renal venous thrombosis	Posterior urethral valves
Necrotizing Enterocolitis	Transient acute renal	Obstructive nephrolithiasis
Sepsis	insufficiency of the newborn	Neurogenic bladder

*newborn infants < 1wk old

Fig. 2. Causes of renal failure.

Renal tubular acidosis (RTA) is common among preterm infants and is typically a transient condition in most neonates. RTA develops when the kidneys are unable to excrete acids into the urine and unable to reabsorb HCO_3^-. There are three main types of RTA: classic or distal (I), proximal (II), and hypoaldosterone (IV). Distal (I) RTA usually occurs in early in life. It is caused by diminished distal H^+ secretion and causes vomiting, polyuria, dehydration, and hypokalemia. This can be caused by a sporadic mutation, autosomal recessive or autosomal dominant disorder and is a permanent defect. Proximal (II) RTA causes a decrease in HCO_3^- reabsorption in the proximal tubule. This may be genetic, but often occurs in premature infants and is temporary. With maturation the amount of reabsorption of HCO_3^- increases. Type IV RTA results in hyperkalemia due to abnormalities in aldosterone production. Treatment for these infants usually includes mineralocorticoid supplementation.

4. INSENSIBLE WATER LOSSES

Insensible water loss is fluid loss due to transepidermal water loss (TEWL), respiratory losses, and/or urinary losses. Gestational age is the major factor in the degree of insensible water loss. The TEWL is inversely proportional to the gestational of the infant: the more immature the infant, the greater the TEWL will occur. In the extremely premature infant (<26 weeks), transepidermal water loss may be as high as 90 ml/kg/day. As the gestational age increases, transepidermal water loss will decrease. By about 28 weeks' gestation, it may be as low as 40 ml/kg/day. Transepidermal water loss plateaus around 31 weeks' gestation onward with about 10 ml/kg/day (17). This is primarily due to the large body surface area of the infant relative to the body weight and a more immature epidermal skin barrier, both of which occur in the extremely premature infant.

4.1. Transepidermal Water Loss

The purpose of the skin is to prevent fluid loss and protect the infant from infection (18). The outermost layer of the skin, the stratum corneum, helps with both of these functions. A well-developed stratum corneum that is keratinized will protect an infant against excess water loss. Keratinization begins during the second trimester and is not homogenous in its development (18). It is not well developed until about 34 weeks' gestation (19). The skin of the abdomen and back are the last to cornify. As a consequence, TEWL is very high in extremely premature infants. The relative humidity of the environment surrounding the infant, in particular the premature neonate, is an additional significant factor in the degree of TEWL. Appropriate humidification will reduce both transepidermal water and heat losses.

Postnatal age and skin maturation are important factors that affect the amount of water loss through evaporation. The stratum corneum develops much more rapidly postnatally than in utero. Within 2–3 weeks of birth of an extremely premature infant, the stratum corneum is usually thickened and less permeable (19). For instance, a 2-week-old infant born at 25 weeks' gestation will exhibit a lower rate of TEWL than a newborn infant at 27 weeks' gestation. Fluid requirement will vary daily because of the significant changes in TEWL that occur in the first week of life of a premature infant (20) (Table 1).

Sweating is an infrequent mode of transepidermal water loss in the newborn. Although sweat glands are present in the preterm infant from 28 weeks' gestation,

Table 1
Fluid Requirements for Newborn Infants (17), (21)

Gestational age	Day 0	Days 1–3	Days 3–7
<28 weeks	80–120	100–150	140–160
29–33 weeks	80–100	100–150	120–160
>34 weeks	60–80	60–100	80–120

thermal sweating does not occur prior to 30 weeks of development. Among full-term neonates sweating is also very limited in response to a thermal stimulus.

4.2. Respiratory Loss

Respiratory insensible water loss occurs in the infant, child, and adult as inspired air becomes saturated with water in the upper respiratory tract. Water loss via this route is variable and dependent on minute ventilation, ambient temperature, and humidity. The greater the humidity of inspired air, the lower the respiratory water loss during breathing *(22)*. In general, respiratory water loss accounts for about 40% of the insensible water loss in the full-term infant. Respiratory water losses will be higher in an infant who is ill and tachypneic. Lack of humidification of the inspired air increases the amount of respiratory water loss. If an infant requires respiratory support (mechanical ventilation, nasal continuous positive airway pressure, or supplemental oxygen delivered via nasal cannula or head box), heated and humidified respiratory gases should be used in order to limit or eliminate insensible losses via the respiratory tract *(23)*.

5. ENVIRONMENTAL FACTORS

It is important to maintain stable thermoregulation for infants to minimize heat loss and oxygen consumption. Heat loss is an important contributor to insensible water loss and is influenced by 4 factors: radiation, conduction, evaporation, and convection. Newborn infants may be cared for in a variety of conditions and environments. These include skin-to-skin contact, open-air bassinettes, incubators (humidified or non-humidified), and an open radiant warmer. Each one of these has their strengths and weaknesses on the basis of the maturity level, skin integrity, degree of illness, and metabolic state of the infant.

Skin-to-skin contact is defined as a naked infant lying on the bare chest of a caregiver. It has been shown to help maintain body temperature, even among preterm infants *(24)*. An open bassinette should be reserved for those infants who can maintain their own body temperature since it does not provide thermoregulation. An incubator typically provides a temperature-regulated enclosed environment with portholes to permit easy access to the infant. The air circulating through the incubator is heated and may or may not be humidified. Incubators, also referred to as isolettes, may be single or double walled. The latter will further limit the insensible water and heat loss experienced by the infant. Radiant warmers are commonly used in the delivery room. These warmers allow for easy access to the newborn and facilitate resuscitative care, stabilization, and the performance of procedures, such as intubation, and umbilical vessel catheterization. The radiant warmer should be heated prior to placing the infant on the warmer bed. Once the infant is placed on the warmer, the temperature can be set at 36.6°C and the temperature probe placed on the infant's abdomen. The infant's axillary temperature should be maintained between 36.0 and 37.0°C *(25)*. When the baby is warmed and the skin reaches the preset warmer temperature, the warmer will automatically lower its heat output. Because the temperature and humidity of the surrounding air are not controlled, convective and evaporative heat losses and insensible water losses are increased *(26)*. Radiant heat may increase insensible water loss by as much as 90% *(27)*. Compared to an incubator, heat loss in a radiant warmer can be more than twice as high *(28)*. In addition, TEWL is also significantly higher in infants cared for in this environment compared to the infant in a non-humidified incubator *(29)*. The lower ambient humidity is also responsible for the higher water loss associated with radiant warmer use *(30)*.

A higher ambient humidity decreases evaporative heat loss, thereby decreasing fluid losses. There is an inverse relationship between the humidity level in the surrounding environment and insensible water losses *(31)*. High ambient humidity may decrease insensible water loss by up to 50% *(32)*. Even extremely low birth weight infants (<1000 g) have a lower fluid requirement when using a humidified incubator for care *(33)*. For decades, there has been a concern about the use of humidification in an incubator because increased rates of infection, specifically *Pseudomonas (34)*. Since this was recognized, the practice of frequently changing the water supply and periodically changing the incubator to permit thorough cleaning has dramatically reduced infection rates. Humidification of the incubators also aids in controlling body temperature *(35)*. By decreasing evaporative water losses, humidification allows premature infants to maintain their temperature more easily.

Another method to aid in decreasing evaporative heat loss and TEWL in infants less than 28 weeks' gestation is by using polyethylene bags in the delivery room during stabilization. After delivery, the premature infant is immediately placed up to their neck into a polyethylene bag as a technique to prevent heat loss *(36)*. An alternative method to prevent heat loss is done by wrapping the infant in a non-occlusive plastic blanket.

6. SENSIBLE WATER LOSSES

Sensible losses include urine and stool water losses. Because of its small amount, stool water loss is usually negligible. Voiding occurs within 12 h of life in half of all newborns and in 92% by 24 h of life *(37)*. If an infant has not voided within 48 h, an assessment regarding fluid intake and possible renal anomalies should be undertaken. Healthy full-term infants undergo a progressive increase in urine output as enteral feeds increase. For the premature infant there are three phases of urinary output in the newborn infant. These include the pre-diuretic, diuretic, and post-diuretic phase *(38, 39)*. The pre-diuretic phase typically occurs during the first 2 days of life with urine output about 1–2 ml/kg/h and is always lower than intake. By day 3 of life, there is a significant increase in urine output as weight loss continues *(40)*. Diuresis, or the diuretic phase, is defined as a high urine output, greater than 5 ml/kg/h. This phase appears to be independent of fluid intake *(38)*. During this phase, infants are at risk for hypernatremia and hyponatremia. Hypernatremia may occur due to the high free water loss. On the other hand, hyponatremia can occur due to the high fractional excretion of sodium (FE_{Na}) in the urine caused by a decreased reabsorption of sodium in the proximal tubules of the kidney. Finally, during the post-diuretic phase, the kidneys begin to equilibrate and respond to the amount of fluid intake and urine output is usually within 1–3 ml/kg/h.

7. FLUID AND ELECTROLYTE MANAGEMENT

Attention to the components of fluid management is critical in caring for the newborn infant. All newborn infants, irrespective of their level of maturity or degree of illness, should be weighed after birth. This initial weight measurement and assessment of gestational age are important in determining the fluid requirements and risks for water and metabolic imbalances of the infant (Table 1). Most infants are weighed daily during their newborn nursery hospitalization, but this may not be necessary in the full-term infant who is well hydrated, feeding, and voiding well. Electrolyte changes and free water loss may be more extreme depending on the gestational age of the infant and severity of the illness. Therefore, laboratory tests may need to be done more frequently (Table 2).

Table 2
Electrolyte Testing Intervals (hours) for Preterm Infants

Gestational age	Day 1	Day 2	Day 3
23–25 weeks	6–8	8–12	12–24
26–29 weeks	8–12	12–24	12–24
30–34 weeks	12–18	12–24	12–24

During the initial stages of physiologic transition in preterm infants, considerable changes occur that affect the water and electrolyte balance. The goal of treatment during this period is to allow for some weight loss (10–15% during the first week of life or approximately 2–3% per day). Due to the risk of hypernatremia from significant TEWL sodium supplementation is usually withheld until adequate urine output has been established (>2.5 ml/kg/h).

Potassium is the major intracellular cation. In very premature infants, potassium supplementation is not provided during the first few days of life because of the risk of hyperkalemia. The cause of hyperkalemia is unclear, but may be due to decreased renal function, low glomerular filtration rate, increased red cell breakdown, and/or acidosis. Potassium should also be withheld until diuresis begins. Hyperkalemia may still occur in extremely premature infants even without potassium supplementation and despite adequate urine output (non-oliguric hyperkalemia). Hyperkalemia is defined as a potassium concentration > 6.5 mEq/L and may require treatment when it is greater than 7.0 mEq/L *(41)*. Possible treatment approaches include the use of furosemide, insulin/glucose infusions to stimulate the intracellular uptake of potassium, $NaHCO_3$ to shift potassium into cells, and a cation exchange resin (Kayexalate) to bind and excrete potassium through the stools (this is not used in premature infants).

Calcium supplementation is usually started on the first day of life in the high-risk infants such as premature infants and asphyxiated infants. Infants of diabetic mothers (IDM) usually do not require supplemental calcium; however, because of the risk for a blunted parathyroid response following the normal physiologic decline in ionized calcium in IDM they are at a greater risk for hypocalcemia at 24 h of life. Calcium is a routine additive in parenteral nutrition solutions when an infant is not feeding enterally, but due to the risk of sloughing of the skin that may be caused by an infiltrated intravenous line, calcium should be added to peripheral lines with caution. Magnesium is also added to parenteral nutrition fluids within the first few days of life unless the mother of the infant received supplemental magnesium prior to delivery for maternal indications, such as preeclampsia or hypertension. In these instances, it may be necessary to check the infant's serum magnesium level before supplementation is provided (Table 3).

Table 3
Electrolyte Requirements

	Day 0	Days 1–3	>Day 3
Sodium (mEq/kg/day)	0	1–3	2–5
Potassium (mEq/kg/day)	0	0–1	2–4
Calcium (mg/kg/day)	200–400	200–400	200–400
Magnesium (mg/kg/day)	0*, 0.25–0.4	0.25–0.4	0.25–0.4

*If maternal magnesium was provided prior to delivery (42), (43)

Excessive gastrointestinal losses may also cause electrolyte imbalances. Gastrointestinal losses may occur from infections, congenital malformations, or injury to the bowel that causes malabsorption. Common gastrointestinal infections caused by viruses and bacteria, such as rotavirus and *Salmonella*, frequently affect infants and toddlers and lead to extreme water loss from diarrhea. Congenital malformations such as an omphalocele and gastroschisis also cause excessive evaporative water loss and electrolyte imbalances that contribute to dehydration. Infants with damaged bowel who require bowel resections and stoma placement are predisposed to chronic intestinal fluid and electrolyte losses. These infants need close monitoring of their electrolytes and often need parenteral replacement of sodium, potassium, and chloride.

8. SPECIAL CONSIDERATIONS IN THE CARE OF THE NEWBORN REQUIRING SURGERY

There are many considerations to be undertaken with the infant who requires surgery. It is important to continue the maintenance fluid in addition to providing fluid for any additional losses during the surgical procedure. Infants are often given isotonic or hypotonic solution during surgery. Blood pressure and heart rate are monitored regularly throughout the procedure to ensure adequate perfusion and if more volume is needed, the infant's fluid support is adjusted.

After surgery, fluid often accumulates causing edema. There is often an increase in capillary permeability with leakage of protein or albumin that causes a decrease in colloid osmotic pressure. This fluid shifting is referred to as third spacing, when fluid shifts into non-functional compartments. Weight gain after surgery is common and may be as much as 30% of pre-surgical weight. Peri-operatively, fluids should be carefully monitored in order to avoid fluid overload. At times, fluid restriction may be necessary. However, it is important to watch for signs of hypovolemia, which include hypotension, tachycardia, and decreased urinary output (caused by decreased renal perfusion).

The intravascular fluid will continue to leak into the interstitial tissue space and across capillaries until the oncotic pressure improves and hydrostatic/oncotic balance is restored. Albumin or synthetic colloid infusions have been used in the past, but in randomized studies of critically ill adults it has been shown that it may contribute to an increase in mortality (44). Clinical improvement will be appreciated as the urine output increases and the infant begins to lose weight.

9. DIURETICS

Diuretics are often administered to infants in the neonatal intensive care unit. They are used in the treatment of peripheral edema, congestive heart failure, hypertension, pulmonary edema, decreased urine output, and bronchopulmonary dysplasia. Loop diuretics, such as furosemide, are often the first line of treatment. These medications bind to one of the two chlorides on the sodium/potassium/chloride co-transporter. This results in decreased reabsorption of sodium and chloride in the thick ascending loop of Henle. It also prevents reabsorption of potassium, magnesium, and calcium. If furosemide is used for a long period of time, the patient should be monitored for electrolyte imbalances such as hyponatremia, hypokalemia, hypochloremia, hypomagnesemia, and hypocalcemia. Nephrocalcinosis and ototoxicity are also known complications of loop diuretic therapy in neonates.

Thiazide diuretics, such as chlorothiazide and hydrochlorothiazide, are also frequently used in the neonatal intensive care unit. These medications block the sodium–chloride transporter at the distal convoluted tubules and collecting tubules. In addition, thiazides may actually increase reabsorption of calcium leading to hypercalcemia. Both furosemide and chlorothiazide may be given either intravenously and enterally, which make them easy to administer to infants. Some infants may require sodium, potassium, or chloride supplementation while on diuretic therapy. Serum electrolytes and renal function should be checked before initiating diuretic therapy and again after a few days of therapy to look for any abnormalities. Potassium chloride supplements are often needed when an infant is on diuretics to avoid hypokalemia and hypochloremia.

10. GLUCOSE HOMEOSTASIS

All infants require glucose after birth to avoid hypoglycemia. In healthy full-term infants this is provided by breast milk or infant formula. In premature infants, it is usually supplied intravenously. At birth the newborn infant's glucose level will be approximately 70–80% of the mother's blood sugar level. Following the birth the newborn must rely on endogenous stores of glycogen and intrinsic metabolic pathways to maintain glucose homeostasis. Most healthy, normal term infants have a sufficient amount of stored glycogen to maintain glucose homeostasis for several hours. There is a normal decline in serum glucose after birth, typically reaching a nadir between 30 and 90 min of life (45). Although transient hypoglycemia in the immediate newborn period is common, it is typically a self-limited process and spontaneously resolves within 2–3 h, even if early enteral feeding is not provided. Therefore, routine glucose monitoring is not recommended for the healthy full-term infant in the first 2 h after birth (46, 47). In the healthy term infant who is breastfeeding a marked ketogenic response occurs during periods in which low blood sugar develops as a result of prolonged intervals between breastfeeding. Ketone production provides the neonatal brain with a glucose sparing energy source that helps to protect the brain from injury. Whether an infant is breast-feeding, formula feeding or a combination of the two, glucose levels gradually rise over the first 96 h of life.

The definition of hypoglycemia in a newborn infant is controversial because of the difficulty in correlating glucose levels, clinical symptoms, and long-term outcomes. Also, glucose concentrations vary by the test method used and whether the sample tested is whole blood, plasma, or serum. Plasma and serum glucose concentrations are 10–15% higher than blood glucose concentrations. A recent population-based meta-analysis of low glucose levels in healthy newborn infants suggested low plasma glucose thresh-old levels (<5th percentile) of 28 mg/dL (1.6 mmol/L), 40 mg/dL (2.2 mmol/L), and 48 mg/dL (2.7 mmol/L) at 1–2 h (nadir), 3–47 h, and 48–72 h of life, respectively *(48)*. Approximately, 10% of newborns develop hypoglycemia if the initial feeding is delayed for more than 4 h *(49)*.

Glucose screening should be performed on high-risk infants and those with abnormal clinical signs. Among infants at risk for developing hypoglycemia in the immediate newborn period are babies who have an inadequate intake or production of glucose and babies who have an excessive use of glucose. The latter group includes infants who are hyperinsulinemic. At risk infants who should have routine glucose monitoring include babies who are born preterm, low birth weight, growth restricted, large for gestational age, and those whose mothers are diagnosed with either gestational or pre-gestational diabetes. In addition, infants with an increased metabolic rate due to perinatal stress, sepsis, hypothermia, drug withdrawal or polycythemia, or whose mothers were treated with oral hypoglycemics, beta blockers, or terbutaline are also at risk. Clinical signs of hypoglycemia include tremors, seizures, respiratory distress, cyanosis, irritability, apnea, and poor feeding *(50)*.

Blood glucose levels should be monitored for at risk infants within 1 h of birth, 2–3 h after birth, and before feeding for 24–36 h if there are any abnormal signs *(51)*. Among infants who develop hypoglycemia, it is recommended that blood sugar levels be maintained greater than 47 mg/dL (2.6 mmol/L) *(50)*. This can usually be achieved by early, frequent feedings of breast milk or formula. However, a symptomatic infant whose blood sugar level cannot be maintained above 47 mg/dL with enteral feeding should be given an intravenous infusion of 10% dextrose (200 mg/kg glucose) *(52)*. Within 24 h the blood glucose usually improves and remains >50 mg/dL *(53)*. Hypoglycemia in the new-born period may have a deleterious effect on the neurodevelopmental outcome and some recommend that plasma glucose levels should be maintained greater than 60 mg/dL *(54, 55)*.

Among infants who are ill, glucose should be provided through an intravenous glu-cose infusion. The estimated glucose requirement of a full-term infant is 4–6 mg/kg/min *(56)*. This is higher than the endogenous hepatic output for the older child or adult because of the increased reliance of the newborn brain on glucose for the early energy needs. Glycogen synthesis is initiated in the second trimester of gestation and storage does not begin until the third trimester *(56)*. Therefore, not all premature infants have a reserve and require glucose infusion soon after birth. Infants who are intrauterine growth restricted are also at risk for hypoglycemia because of their decreased glycogen stores and decreased rate of gluconeogenesis.

The glucose infusion rate requried is usually 4–6 mg/kg/min in the first day of life. The exogenous glucose infusion rate provided by an intravenous infusion is determined by the following equation: rate of IV fluid X % of dextrose x 0.167/weight of the infant (kg). As long as the infant remains euglycemic, 75–120 mg/dL, the glucose infusion rate may be increased (usually up to 11–13 mg/kg/min) in order to increase caloric intake. Premature infants have a decreased amount of glucose reabsorption by the kidneys compared to that of full-term infants and a high glucose infusion rate may lead to more glycosuria (57).

Hyperglycemia is to be avoided as well and may be caused by sepsis stress, insulin resistance, or a high glucose infusion rate. Severe hyperglycemia, ≥ 180 mg/dL, during the first 3 days of life in extremely low birth weight infants was found to be associated with an increased risk of death and sepsis (58).

11. ACID–BASE METABOLISM

The cells of the body work optimally with a normal pH. This range is very narrow and should be maintained closely in newborns, children, and adults (Table 4). As the pH drops below 7.35, acidosis worsens and conversely, as the pH rises above 7.45, the blood becomes more alkalotic. The acid–base diagram demonstrates the shifting of the pH in the blood with each diagnosis (Fig. 3).

Table 4
Normal Blood Gas Parameters

	Arterial blood
pH	7.35–7.45
pCO_2	35–45 mmHg
pO_2	75–100 mmHg
HCO_3^-	22–30 mmol/L
BE	± 3 mmol/L

The following equation explains the acid–base system in the body. A hydrogen ion (H^+) combines with a bicarbonate anion (HCO_3^-) to form carbonic acid (H_2CO_3). Ultimately, carbonic acid disassociates to become water (H_2O) and carbon dioxide (CO_2).

$$H^+ + HCO_3^- \leftrightarrow H_2CO_3 \leftrightarrow H_2O + CO_2.$$

Carbonic anhydrase is the activating enzyme for this reaction. When the $[H^+]$ increases in the body due to acidosis the equation will shift to the right and cause an increase in $[CO_2]$. Conversely, if the $[CO_2]$ increases in response to respiratory depression this will shift the equation to the left and cause an increase in $[HCO_3^-]$ to

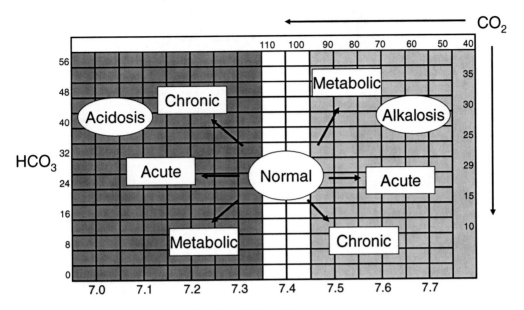

Fig. 3. Acid–base diagram.

compensate for the decrease in pH. The Henderson–Hasselbalch equation represents the relationship between the pH and bicarbonate buffering system.

$$pH = pK^+ \log([HCO_3^-]/[H_2CO_3]).$$

For easier use and understanding, there is a modified Henderson equation:

$$[H^+] = 24 \times [pCO_2/HCO_3^-].$$

When the ratio of pCO_2 and HCO_3^- changes, the $[H^+]$ changes. At times it may be difficult to look at the acid–base status of a patient at one moment in time because acute changes in clinical status may drastically affect the pH. Therefore, blood gases looking at the acid–base status of patients are often looked at over a continuum of time.

In utero, the placenta responds to changes in the acid–base milieu by removing the carbon dioxide from the blood of the fetus. A disturbance in the pH can develop when the mother experiences a medical complication or placental function is impaired. Hypovolemia, hypertension, and poor blood flow through the placenta can cause fetal acidosis. The umbilical cord has 3 vessels, two arteries, and one vein. Often times, umbilical cord blood gases are obtained from the placenta following the delivery of a high risk infant. The umbilical arterial blood is deoxygenated blood that comes from the fetus and reflects the acid–base status of the fetus. The umbilical venous blood is oxygenated coming from the mother via the placenta to the fetus to provide nutrients. The venous blood gas will always have a slightly higher pH and a lower pCO_2 than the arterial blood gas *(59, 60)* (Table 5). In response to medical–legal concerns, many hospitals and obstetricians are sending umbilical cord blood gas specimens for analysis to document evidence of the fetal status at delivery. The pH obtained on blood gas analysis is a

Table 5
Normal Cord Blood Gas Parameters (59)

	Venous	Arterial
pH	7.34(±0.06)	7.27(±0.07)
pCO_2	40(±7)	50(±10)
pO_2	25(±9)	17(±6)
Base	−3(±4)	−4(±4)

function of the pCO_2 and any accumulated metabolic acids. Since the pH is a log of the equation, the base excess may be more helpful to appreciate the severity of illness of the patient.

$$pH = pK_a + \log_{10}[A^-]/[HA].$$

A metabolic acidosis is demonstrated by the base deficit. It is recommended that infants with a base deficit greater than 12 on their umbilical cord gas be observed closely for altered neurological signs during the first 48 h of life (61). If severe metabolic acidosis (BD > −16 mmol/L) is shown on the umbilical arterial blood gas, the infant usually requires assessment and closer monitoring. This includes maternal and birth histories, examination of the infant to assess the infant's perfusion, hemodynamic stability, and for any evidence of neurologic dysfunction (tone abnormalities, altered state of consciousness, irritability, jitteriness, or seizures). The infant should have a repeat of the blood gas within the hour to assess the degree of residual acidosis. After birth, the respiratory and renal systems take over the placental functions and maintain most of the buffering for the infant. A pH < 7.0 and an Apgar score < 5 at 5 min are additional factors that necessitate careful monitoring of the newborn in a special-care nursery or neonatal intensive care unit.

11.1. Acidosis

Acidosis (pH < 7.35) may either be caused by an increase in pCO_2 (respiratory acidosis) or an increase in [H⁺] (metabolic acidosis). An infant with poor respiratory effort or poor gas exchange has an increase in pCO_2 that leads to respiratory acidosis. In a situation with primary respiratory acidosis, the pH and pCO_2 move in opposite directions. For every 10 mmHg change in pCO_2 there is a 0.08 change in pH. For example, a newborn infant has an arterial blood gas with a pH 7.39 and a pCO_2 43 mmHg. Within 6 h of births, the infant has respiratory distress and the next arterial blood gas has a pCO_2 63 mmHg. In this case the pH will be 7.23, a decrease of 0.16 (Table 6).

When there is a metabolic abnormality the [HCO_3^-] changes in the same direction as the pH. Metabolic acidosis may occur for many reasons. After the diagnosis of metabolic acidosis is made it is imperative to determine its cause for adequate treatment. Metabolic acidosis can be divided into 3 categories according to the anion gap: increased (>18),

Table 6
Acid–Base Disturbances and [HCO_3^-] Compensation

	[HCO_3^-]
Acute respiratory acidosis	↑ 1 mmol/L for each 10 > 40 mmHg
Chronic respiratory acidosis	↑ 4 mmol/L for each 10 > 40 mmHg
Acute respiratory alkalosis	↓ 2 mmol/L for each 10 < 40 mmHg
Chronic respiratory alkalosis	↓ 5 mmol/L for each 10 < 40 mmHg

normal (8–18), or low (<8). The anion gap is a value of all the unmeasured anions in the plasma and it is a valuable indicator to determine the cause of the metabolic acidosis.

$$\text{Anion gap} = [Na^+] - [Cl^-] - [HCO_3^-].$$

A normal anion gap indicates that the loss of [HCO_3^-] is being compensated by an increase in [Cl^-]. Excessive diarrhea that may occur in response to bacterial or viral infections in the neonate and infant causes a normal anion gap metabolic acidosis (8–18) due to the loss of HCO_3^-. An increased anion gap (>18) is caused by excess in inorganic, organic, and exogenous acid with no [Cl^-] compensation. A low anion gap is rare, but may occur in the setting of hypoalbuminemia, which frequently occurs in premature infants. Due to low albumin concentrations in premature infants, it is sometimes difficult to interpret the anion gap. There may be times, due to the low albumin level, when the anion gap is normal, but should be high. There is an extensive list of possible diagnoses to consider based on the calculated anion gap in an infant with metabolic acidosis (Fig. 4). It is helpful to obtain urine electrolytes when a diagnosis of metabolic acidosis is made to help determine whether there is involvement from the kidneys.

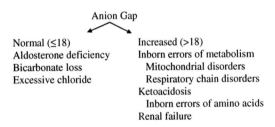

Fig. 4. Causes of anion gap acidosis

11.2. Alkalosis

Alkalosis occurs when the pH exceeds 7.45. Respiratory alkalosis in the neonate is rare, but it is sometimes seen in the critically ill patient on a mechanical ventilator. This occurs when the infant is over-ventilated with excessive CO_2 removal. When this occurs it can usually be corrected by adjusting the ventilator. Infants without intrinsic lung disease who are tachypnea can also develop respiratory alkalosis. This may occur in those infants who are responding to a metabolic acidosis or who are withdrawing from in utero narcotic exposure. Metabolic alkalosis may also be due to a loss in $[H^+]$ or an increase in $[HCO_3^-]$. Common causes of metabolic alkalosis in the non-ventilated neonate include vomiting, diuretic use, and bicarbonate administration.

Parietal cells in the stomach secrete HCl and absorb HCO_3^-. Prolonged vomiting due to obstruction or intestinal atresia can cause a loss in [HCl] leading to metabolic alkalosis. Therefore, newborns and infants with gastrointestinal atresia, gastric perforations, necrotizing enterocolitis, and pyloric stenosis need to be monitored very closely.

11.3. Compensation

Metabolic compensation occurs when there is respiratory acidosis and the kidneys respond by increasing its reabsorption of HCO_3^-. Approximately 70% of the plasma bicarbonate is absorbed in the proximal tubules of the kidneys. However, the premature kidney does not function as well as a full-term kidney and therefore, may not be able to fully compensate for the acidosis. The respiratory system will compensate for metabolic acidosis, but also is unable to completely correct for it. When there is an increase in $[H^+]$ concentration the respiratory rate of the infant will increase to lower the pCO_2 and help to normalize the pH (Table 6).

11.3.1. ACID–BASE DISTURBANCES AND $[HCO_3^-]$ COMPENSATION

To determine whether the lungs are compensating for the metabolic acidosis, the expected and measured pCO_2 must be calculated:

$$Expected\, pCO_2 = (1.5 \times [HCO_3^-]) + 8 \pm 2.$$

When the measured pCO_2 is lower than expected, there is respiratory compensation; however, when the measured and expected pCO_2 are about the same, compensation has not occurred. Blood gases are frequently monitored on patients who require respiratory support such as mechanical ventilation. Most medical caregivers draw a blood gas within an hour of each change made on the ventilator to confirm stability of the patient or more urgently if there is a change in the patient's clinical status.

12. CASE SCENARIOS

Case Scenario 1

A full-term infant is born via vaginal delivery to a 24-year-old woman. Her prenatal labs include A negative blood type. The baby has Apgar scores of 9 and 9 at 1 and 5 min, respectively, and transitions without difficulty. Her birth weight is 3.2 kg and she rooms-in with her mother. The mother understands the importance of breastfeeding and is exclusively breastfeeding the baby. The baby's blood type is B+ and the indirect Coombs' test is positive. At 24 h the infant is jaundiced with a rapidly rising bilirubin level requiring intensive phototherapy. How does phototherapy alter the fluid requirements for an infant? What are the considerations in managing fluid intake in the infant?

A full-term infant who is feeding, voiding, stooling, and well hydrated prior to commencing phototherapy does not require any supplementation. Phototherapy will not affect insensible water loss in a thermally stable infant *(62)*. Newer phototherapy devices emit a narrow band of high-intensity blue light via blue light emitting diodes (LEDs) in the range of 400–550 nm, which corresponds to the absorption of light by bilirubin. Hydration status and hyperbilirubinemia were studied and no difference in bilirubin decline was found when comparing oral hydration versus supplemental intravenous hydration *(63)*.

However, if the infant is premature and halogen phototherapy lights are used, maintenance fluids may need to be increased by 7 mL/kg/day to compensate for the increased TEWL *(64)*. A recent study showed there was no significant increase in TEWL in preterm infants with the use of LED phototherapy for hyperbilirubinemia *(65)*.

At 3 days of age the phototherapy treatment has ended and the mother is preparing to take the baby home. After reviewing the record the baby now weighs 2.9 kg. Is there a reason to be concerned? What is the total body water of this infant? What are the considerations? Are there any laboratory tests to be done?

Weight loss in most newborns during the first week of life is normal adaptive behavior. Because this infant is full term, her total body water is about 75% of her birth weight. After birth the shifting of fluid should continue and the total body water and extracellular fluid will decrease. Newborn babies' average weight loss in the first 4 days of life is about 6%, but they may lose as much as 10% of birth weight in the first week of life. Breastfed infants may lose closer to 15% of birth weight. This infant has lost 9.5% of her birth weight, which is an acceptable weight loss during this period of time. Even though she has lost 300 g she may continue to lose weight. An additional weight loss up to another 180 g may be acceptable as long as the infant remains active, alert, well hydrated, is feeding well, and voiding. This infant should be followed up closely within 1–3 days of discharge for assessment of hydration, adequacy of maternal milk production, and infant feeding skills *(66)*. On follow-up evaluation, if the infant loses more weight, develops signs of dehydration or there are observed difficulties with the mother's milk production or the infant's feeding efficiency, a serum electrolyte panel may be warranted to assess for hypernatremia and the need for nutritional supplementation.

Breastfeeding infants may lose more weight because of the small volume of the early colostrum feedings. Colostrum is usually produced during the first 3–5 postnatal days. The volume of colostrum at each feeding varies from 2 to 20 ml *(67)*. Due to small volume feeding, breastfeeding infants should be fed frequently during the immediate postnatal period at least 8–12 times per day until breastfeeding is fully established. It is also important that the infant has enough time on each breast to feed, which usually takes 10–15 min. Transitional milk follows colostrum and continues into the second week post-partum until finally mature milk is produced.

Once the frequency and adequacy of the infant's intake have been reviewed, her output should be assessed. Urine output is usually low in the first day or two of life and increases by day 3. At this point, three to five wet diapers would be acceptable and by the end of the first week the infant will likely have up to seven or eight wet diapers in a day.

Case Scenario 2

The delivery of a 26 week gestation infant is expected. What environmental factors must be considered in the infant's initial stabilization? How does this infant's prematurity influence the initial approach to fluid management? How much fluid and what electrolytes will this infant require in the first 72 h of life?

As soon as the baby is delivered the body temperature needs to be maintained and TEWL minimized. Hypothermia in a preterm infant is common and increases the risks of morbidity and mortality. Once the baby is delivered and handed to the pediatric team he should be swaddled with a plastic wrap or placed in a plastic bag up to his neck under a pre-heated radiant warmer. These measures will reduce evaporative heat and water loss and facilitate maintenance of the infant's body temperature. As noted in Table 1, the initial free water requirement for an extremely premature infant is in the range of 80–120 ml/kg/day with the appropriate environmental humidification between 70 and 80%. It would be ideal to maintain the ambient humidity at 80% to decrease the amount of insensible water losses and maintain his body temperature. This baby will also require respiratory support due to lung immaturity. Whether the infant is intubated or requires nasal CPAP (continuous positive airway pressure), the device circuit temperature should be set to deliver $37°C$ with a high relative humidity. Since this infant will receive enteral feedings initially, enteral nutrition should be established as soon as possible. A premature infant requires 4–6 mg/kg/min of glucose infusion to meet the endogenous hepatic output required for optimal function. Glucose levels should be monitored closely until stable. Sodium supplementation during the first 24–48 h of life is not required. Extreme premature infants experience large extracellular fluid losses placing the infant at risk for dehydration and hypernatremia. Also, potassium supplementation is not required until the infant establishes good urine output (>1.5 ml/kg/h). Frequent monitoring of serum electrolytes is necessary with frequent adjustments of the total fluid intake, glucose infusion rate, and electrolyte supplementation (Table 2).

Four weeks later, the infant remains on continuous positive airway pressure for respiratory support and now tolerates all of his nutritional needs enterally. What are his fluid requirements now?

Initially, one of the main reasons an extremely premature infant has a high TEWL is due to the immature skin and very thin layer of stratum corneum. However, the stratum corneum usually develops within 1–2 weeks after birth. Thereafter, these infants typically do not require extra fluids because there is no more risk of extreme water loss. Since this baby is now receiving full enteral feeds, the feeding goal is 150–160 ml/kg/day. Premature infants usually receive 24 kcal/oz formula or fortified breast milk (24 kcal/oz) while in the intensive care unit to maximize growth and nutritional needs. This volume gives the infant about 120–130 kcal/kg/day, which is usually enough for adequate daily growth (15–20 g/kg/day). Premature formula or human milk fortifier supplements added to breast milk provide the infant with additional calcium and phosphorus to help maintain adequate bone growth and prevent osteopenia of prematurity.

One week later the infant develops necrotizing enterocolitis. The blood culture is positive for Escherichia coli. His arterial blood gas shows a pH 7.15, pCO_2 40 mmHg, HCO_3–15mmol/L and base deficit of –10 mmol/L 12 mEq/L. The chemistry panel on the infant showed the following: sodium 134 mEq/L, chloride 101 mEq/L, and potassium 4.3 mEq/L. The infant is intubated for airway management and going to the operating room for an exploratory laparotomy because of peritoneal air noted on an abdominal roentgenogram. What information does the infant's blood gas provide? Is there an anion gap? If so, why? What are the fluid and electrolyte considerations in the post-operative care for this infant? What if the infant's blood gas is pH 7.15, pCO_2 55 mEq/L, HCO_3–17 mmol/L and a base deficit of –10 mmol/L

A pH <7.35 represents acidosis (Fig. 3). When the HCO_3^- has fallen below 22 mmol/L it demonstrates metabolic acidosis. The anion gap, the sodium [139] minus the sum of the chloride and potassium (101 + 4), equals 25. This infant has an anion gap metabolic acidosis (Fig. 4). This episode of sepsis caused by *E. coli* led to bowel hypoxia and ultimately necrosis that caused the metabolic acidosis. It is important to determine the cause of the acidosis to ensure the proper treatment. Antibiotics were started when the infant initially decompensated. Since there are positive blood cultures and sensitivities are obtained, the antibiotics may be changed for better coverage. In addition, the infant requires close blood pressure monitoring because of the risk of hypotension due to sepsis and hypovolemia caused by third spacing of fluid. A fluid bolus might be necessary to correct the underlying hypovolemic state and the resultant metabolic acidosis.

During surgery, the baby will be paralyzed and sedated. After surgery, there is often an increase in capillary permeability causing a decrease in colloid osmotic pressure leading to third spacing. Fluid needs to be strictly monitored to avoid fluid overload. Blood pressure must also be watched carefully to ensure hypotension does not occur due to hypovolemia and urine output must be carefully monitored to confirm good renal perfusion.

During the surgery, 15 cm of the ileum was removed and an ileostomy is created. How will this affect the fluid management of the infant? What concerns are there when part of the small intestine is removed?

When a part of the intestinal tract is removed, there is always a concern about the potential for malabsorption or short-gut syndrome. Each section of the intestine is responsible for reabsorption and secretion of certain electrolytes. The ileum is one of the primary sites of water, sodium, and potassium reabsorption. After surgery, once the infant is stable, feeding can be reinstated and slowly increased up to about 160 ml/kg/day as tolerated. The weight and ostomy output should be carefully monitored. Often times, the infants may not gain weight or may even lose weight after recovery from surgery. When the ostomy output exceeds 20–30 ml/kg/day often the fluid is replaced parenterally. The electrolytes should also be monitored closely to determine whether there are any electrolyte deficits. The intravenous fluid should be determined using the results of the chemistry panel and knowing the daily electrolyte requirements (Table 3).

Case Scenario 3

A full-term infant is born via cesarean section due to poor fetal tracing. At delivery, there is no spontaneous cry and the heart rate is less than 100. The infant is intubated and the heart rate improves. The Apgar scores are 3 and 4 at 1 and 5 min, respectively. The arterial cord blood gas shows a pH 6.9, pCO_2 50 mmHg, and a base deficit of –17 mEq/L. The infant develops seizures at 6 h of life and is hypotensive. How should the fluids be managed in an infant with neonatal encephalopathy (NE)?

There is always a concern for cerebral edema with the diagnosis of neonatal encephalopathy. Fluid administration is often restricted in these patients to 40–60 ml/kg/day (insensible water loss and urine output). Severe asphyxia may lead to multiple organ involvement, affecting the liver and kidneys while blood flow is preserved to the brain. Urine output should be monitored closely. In cases of severe NE there can be marked serum electrolyte abnormalities due to associated abnormal renal function. The kidney damage that accompanies encephalopathy often manifests as oliguria or anuria *(68)*. The key to managing these infants with renal disease caused by asphyxia is to avoid fluid overload. Once the infant begins to void, it may be helpful to check the urine electrolytes. These infants often have a polyuric phase during which time the renal tubules are not functioning properly with enhanced electrolyte loss. Urine electrolytes and serum creatinine are usually measured in these circumstances. After abnormalities are appreciated they can be replaced parenterally. Oliguria or anuria may also occur in these babies due to the inappropriate secretion of antidiuretic hormone. This will cause hyponatremia, hypokalemia, hypochloremia, and fluid overload.

Case Scenario 4

A 29 weeks' gestation infant with respiratory distress syndrome on a mechanical ventilator has an arterial blood gas that shows pH 7.49, pCO_2 32 mmHg, HCO_3^- 24 mmol/L and a base excess of mEq/L. Is this infant acidotic or alkalotic? Is it respiratory or metabolic? Is treatment necessary? If so, what should be done?

This pH in this blood gas is >7.45, which defines alkalosis (Fig. 3). The pCO_2 is below normal values indicating this is a respiratory alkalosis. The HCO_3^- is just below the normal range and means this is an acute respiratory alkalosis. Since this infant is mechanically ventilated, the ventilator settings should be adjusted to reduce the infant's minute ventilation.

REFERENCES

1. Morris JA, Hustead RF, Robinson RG, Haswell GL. Measurement of Fetoplacental Blood Volume in the Human Previable Fetus. Am J Obstet Gynecol 1974;118:927–934.
2. Mollison PL, Veall N, Gutbush M. Red Cell and Plasma Volume in Newborn Infants. Arch Dis Child 1950;25:242–253.
3. Friis-Hansen B. Body Water Compartments in Children: Changes During Growth and Related Changes in Body Composition: Kenneth D. Blackfan Memorial Lecture. Pediatrics 1961;28:169–181.
4. Lukaski HC, Siders Wa, Nielsen EJ, Hall CB. Total Body Water in Pregnancy: Assessment by Using Bioelectrical Impedance. Am J Clin Nutr 1994;59:578–585.

5. Guignard JP. The Neonatal Stressed Kidney. In: Gruskin AB, Norman ME, eds. Pediatric Nephrology. Martinus Nijhoff, 1981.

6. Ceriani Cernadas JM, Carroli G, Pellegrini L, Otaño L, Ferreria M, Ricci C, Casas O, Giordano D and Larizabal L. The Effect of Timing of Cord Clamping on Neonatal Venous Hematocrit Values and Clinical Outcome at Term: A Randomized, Controlled Trial. Pediatrics 2006 Apr;117(4):e779-e786.

7. Macdonald PD, Ross SRM, Grant L, Young D. Neonatal Weight Loss in Breast and Formula Fed Infants. Arch Dis Child Fetal Neonatal Ed 2003;88:F472–476.

8. Martens PJ, Romphf L. Factors Associated with Newborn In-Hospital Weight Loss: Comparisons by Feeding Method, Demographics and Birthing Procedures. J Hum Lact 2007;23:233–241.

9. American Academy of Pediatrics Section on Breastfeeding. Breastfeeding and the Use of Human Milk. Pediatrics 2005; 115:496–506.

10. Laing IA, Wong CM. Hypernatremia in the First Few Days: Is the Incidence Rising? Arch Dis Child Fetal Neonatal Ed 2002;87:F158–F162.

11. Oddie S, Richmond S, Coulthard M. Hypernatremic Dehydration and Breastfeeding: A Populations Study. Arch Dis Child 2001;85:318–320.

12. Rabinowitz R, Peters MT, Vyas S, Campbell S, Nicolaides KH. Measurement of Fetal Urine Production in Normal Pregnancy by Real-time Ultrasonography. Amer J Obst Gynec 1989;161:1264–1266.

13. Modi N. Hyponatraemia in the Newborn. Arch Dis Child Fetal Neonatal Ed 1998;78:F81–F84.

14. de Bold AJ. Atrial Natriuretic Factor: An Overview. Fed Proc 1986;45:2081–2085.

15. Bayard F, Ances IG, Tapper AJ, Weldon VV, Kowarski A, Migeon CJ. Transplacental Passage and Fetal Secretion of Aldosterone. J Clin Invest 1970;49:1389–1393.

16. Kavvadia V, Greenough A, Dimitriou G, Hooper R. Randomised Trial of Fluid Restriction in Ventilated Very Low Birthweight Infants. Arch Dis Child Retal Neonatal Ed 2000;83:F91–F96.

17. Hammarlund K, Sedin G. Transepidermal Water Loss in Newborn Infants III. Relation to Gestational Age. Acta Paediatr Scan 1979;68:795–801.

18. Cartlidge P. The Epidermal Barrier. Semin Neonatol 2000;4:273–280.

19. Evans N, Rutter N. Development of the Epidermis in the Newborn. Biol Neonate 1986;49:74–80.

20. Hammarlund K, Sedin G, Stromberg B. Transepidermal Water Loss in Newborn Infants: VIII. Relation to Gestational Age and Post-natal Age in Appropriate and Small for Gestational Age Infants. Acta Paediatr Scand 1983;72:721.

21. *Rutter N, Hull D. Water Loss from the Skin of Term and Preterm Babies. Arch Dis Child 1979;54:858–868.*

22. Lee RC. Relationship Between Insensible Loss of Weight and Heat Production of the Rabbit. J Nutr 1940;20:297–304.

23. Sosulski R, Polin R, Baumgart S. Respiratory Water Loss and Heat Balance in Intubated Infants Receiving Humidified Air. J Pediatr 1983;103:307–310.

24. Bauer K, Uhrig C, Sperling P, Pasel K, Wieland C, Versmold H. Body Temperatures and Oxygen Consumption During Skin-to-Skin (kangaroo) Care in Stable Preterm Infants Weighing less than 1500 Grams. J Pediatr 1997;130:240–244.

25. Thermal Protection of Low Birth Weight and Sick Newborns. In: Thermal Protection of the Newborn: A Practical Guide. World Health Organization, Geneva: 1997:26–37.

26. Bell EF. Infant Incubators and Radiant Warmers. Early Hum Dev 1983;8:351–375.

27. Wu PY, Hodgman JE. Insensible Water Loss in Preterm Infants: Changes with Postnatal Development and Non-Ionizing Radiant Energy. Pediatrics 1974;54:704–712.

28. Hammarlund K, Sedin G. Water Evaporation and Heat Exchange with the Environment in Newborn Infants. Acta Paediatr Scand Suppl 1983;305:32–35.

29. Maayan-Metzger A, Yosipovitch G, Hadad E, Sivota L. Effect of Radiant Warmer on Transepidermal Water Loss (TEWL) and Skin Hydration in Preterm Infants. J Perinat 2004;24:372–375.

30. Kjartansson S, Arsan S, Hammarlund K, Sjors G, Sedin G. Water Loss from the Skin of Term and Preterm Infants Nursed Under a Radiant Heater. Pediat Res 1995;37:233–238.

31. Hammarlund K, Sedin G. Transepidermal Water Loss in Newborn Infants III. Relation to Gestational Age. Acta Paediatr Scan 1979;68:795–801.

32. Hey EN, Katz G. Evaporative Water Loss in the New-Born Baby. J Physiol 1969;200:605–619.
33. Gaylord MS, Wright K, Lorch K, Lorch V, Walker E. Improved Fluid Management Utilizing Humidified Incubators in Extremely Low Birth Weight Infants. J Perinat 2001;21:438–443.
34. Hoffman MA, Finberg L. Pseudomonas Infections in Infants Associated with High-Humidity Environments. J Pediatr 1995;46:626–630.
35. Harpin VA, Rutter N. Humidification on Incubators. Arch of Dis Child 1985;60:219–224.
36. Vohra S, Roberts RS, Zhang B, Janes M, Schmidt B. Heat Loss Prevention (HELP) in the Delivery Room: A Randomized Controlled Trial of Polyethylene Occlusive Skin Wrapping in Very Preterm Infants. J Pediatr 2004;145:750–753.
37. Clark DA. Times of First Void and First Stool in 500 Newborns. Pediatrics 1977;60:457–459.
38. Lorenz JM, Kleinman LI, Ahmed G, Markarian K. Phases of Fluid and Electrolyte Homeostasis in the Extremely Low Birth Weight Infant. Pediatrics 1995;96:484–489.
39. Lorenz JM, Kleinman LI, Kotagal UR, Reller MD. Water Balance in Very Low-Birth-Weight Infants: Relationship to Water and Sodium Intake and Effect on Outcome. J Pediatr 1982;101:423–432.
40. Iacobelli S, Addabbo F, Bonsante F, Procino G, Tamma A, Acito L, Esposito M, Svelto M, Valenti G. Aquaporin-2 Excretion and Renal Function During the 1st Week of Life in Preterm Newborn Infants. Nephr Physiol 2006;104:121–125.
41. Shaffer SG, Kilbride HW, Hayen LK, Meade VM, Warady BA. Hyperkalemia in Very Low Birth Weight Infants. J Pediatr 1992;121:275–279.
42. Nutrition Committee, Canadian Paediatric Society. Nutrient Needs and Feeding of Premature Infants. Can Med Assoc J 1995;152:1765–1785.
43. Costarino AT, Gruskay JA, Corcoran L, Polin RA, Baumgart S. Sodium Restriction Versus Daily Maintenance Replacement in very Low Birth Weight Premature Neonates: A Randomized, Blind Therapeutic Trail. J Pediatr 1992;120;99-106.
44. Schierhout G, Roberts I. Fluid Resuscitation with Colloid or Crystalloid Solutions in Critically Ill Patients: A Systematic Review of Randomized Trials. BMJ 1998;613:961–964.
45. Srinivasan G, Pilders RS, Cattamanchi G, Voora S, Lilien LD. Plasma Glucose Values in Normal Neonates: A New Look. J Pediatr 1986;109:114–117.
46. Williams AF. Hypoglycaemia of the Newborn: A Review. Bull World Health Organ 1997;75:261–290.
47. Wright N, Marinelli KA; Academy of Breastfeeding Medicine Protocol Committee. ABM Clinical Protocol #1: Guidelines for Glucose Monitoring and Treatments of Hypoglycemia in Breastfed Neonates. Breastfeeding Medic 2006;3:178–184.
48. Alkalay AL, Sarnat HB, Flores-Sarnat L, Elashoff JD, Farber SJ, Simmons CF. Population Meta-analysis of Low Plasma Glucose Thresholds in Full-Term Normal Newborns. Am J Perinat 2006 Feb;23(2):115–119.
49. Lubchenco LO, Bard H. Incidence of Hypoglycemia in Newborn Infants Classified by Birth Weight and Gestational Age. Pediatrics 1971;47:831–838.
50. Cornblath M, Hawdon JM, Williams AF, Aynsley-Green A, Ward-Platt MP, Schwartz R, Kalhan SC. Controversies Regarding Definition of Neonatal Hypoglycemia: Suggested Operational Thresholds. Pediatrics 2000;105:1141–1145.
51. Fetus and Newborn Committee, Canadian Paediatric Society Paediatrics & Child Health 2004; 723–729.
52. Hypoglycaemia of the Newborn. Review of the Literature. World Health Organization. Geneva 1997.
53. Cornblath M. Hypoglycemia in the Neonate. Semin Perinatol 2000;24:136–149.
54. Lucas A, Morley R, Cole TJ. Adverse Neurodevelopmental Outcome of Moderate Neonatal Hypoglycaemia. BMJ. 1988;297:1304–1308.
55. Stanley CA, Baker L. The Causes of Neonatal Hypoglycemia. NEJM 1999;340:1200–1201.
56. Mitanchez D. Glucose Regulation in Preterm Newborn Infants. Horm Res 2007;68:265–271.
57. Arant BS Jr. Developmental Patterns of Renal Functional Maturational Compared in the Human Infant. J Pediatr 1978;92:705–712.
58. Kao LS, Morris BH, Lally KP, Stewart CD, Huseby V, Kennedy KA. Hyperglycemia and Morbidity and Mortality in Extremely Low Birth Weight Infants. J Perinat 2006 Dec;26(12):730–736.

59. Helwig JT, Parer JT, Kilpatrick SJ, Laros RK Jr. Umbilical Cord Blood Acid–Base State: What is Normal? Am J Obstet Gynecol 1996;174:1807–1814.
60. Yeomans ER, Hauth JC, Gilstrap LC III, Strickland DM. Umbilical Cord pH, PCO2, and Bicarbonate Following Uncomplicated Term Vaginal Deliveries. Am J Obstet Gynecol 1985;151:798–800.
61. Low JA, Lindsay BG, Derrick EJ. Threshold of Metabolic Acidosis Associated with Newborn Complications. Am J Obstet Gynecol 1997;177:1391–1394.
62. Kjartansson S, Hammarlund K, Sedin G. Insensible Water Loss from the Skin During Phototherapy in Term and Preterm Infants. Acta Paediatr 1992;81:764–768.
63. Boo N-Y, Lee H-T. Randomized Controlled Trial of Oral Versus Intravenous Fluid Supplementation on Serum Bilirubin Level During Phototherapy of Term Infants with Severe Hyperbilirubinemia. J Pediatr Child Health 2002;38:151–155.
64. Grünhagen DJ, de Boer MG, de Beaufort AJ, Walther FJ. Transepidermal Water Loss during Halogen Spotlight Phototherapy in Preterm Infants. Pediatr Res 2002;51:402–405.
65. Bertini G, Perugi S, Elia S, Pratesi S, Dani C, Rubaltelli FF. Transepidermal Water Loss and Cerebral Hemodynamic in Preterm Infants: Conventional versus LED Phototherapy. Eur J Pediatr 2008;167: 37–42.
66. American Academy of Pediatrics Subcommittee on Hyperbilirubinemia. Management of Hyperbilirubinemia in the Newborn Infant 35 or More Weeks of Gestation. Pediatrics 2004;144:297–316.
67. Simpson KR, Creehan PA. Perinatal Nursing. Lippincott Williams & Wilkins, 2007, p. 587.
68. Oh W. Renal Function and Fluid Therapy in High-Risk Infants. Biol Neonate 1988;53:230–236.

Subject Index

From: *Nutrition and Health: Fluid and Electrolytes in Pediatrics*
Edited by: L. G. Feld, F. J. Kaskel, DOI 10.1007/978-1-60327-225-4,
© Humana Press, a part of Springer Science+Business Media, LLC 2010

About the Editors

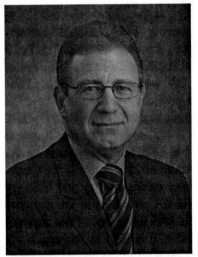

Leonard G. Feld, is the Sara H. Bissell & Howard C. Bissell Endowed Chair in Pediatrics and Chief Medical Officer at the Levine Children's Hospital at Carolinas Medical Center, and Clinical Professor of Pediatrics at UNC School of Medicine The Levine Children's Hospital is the largest children's hospital between Washington DC and Atlanta with 12 floors and 234 beds.

Prior to joining the Carolinas Healthcare System, Dr. Feld was chairman of pediatrics for the Atlantic Health System and physician-in-chief of the Goryeb Children's Hospital in New Jersey from 1997 to 2006. He was also Professor of Pediatrics at UMDNJ-New Jersey Medical School. Prior to 1997, he served as Chief of Pediatric Nephrology in the Department of Pediatrics at Children's Hospital in Buffalo, vice chairman of pediatrics and professor of pediatrics at the State University of New York at the Buffalo School of Medicine. Dr. Feld received his medical degree and Ph.D. from the State University of New York at Buffalo, School of Medicine. He continued his postgraduate training in pediatrics and pediatric nephrology at the Albert Einstein College of Medicine in New York. Dr. Feld also has a Masters in Medical Management from Carnegie Mellon University.

Dr. Feld has published 120 articles, 45 monographs/chapters, an editor or contributing editor to 9 books, and 103 abstracts. He is co-editor of the textbook – *Fast Facts in Pediatrics* and is co-editor-in-chief of *Consensus in Pediatrics*. He is also co-editor for an issue of "Pediatric Clinics of North American on Pediatric Quality" published in August 2009.

He also serves on the editorial board of Pediatrics in Review (American Academy of Pediatrics) and is a member of the Board of Directors of Horizon Blue Cross/Blue Shield of New Jersey. Dr. Feld is listed in the *Best Doctors in America*, *How to Find the Best Doctors* and *A Guide to America's Top Pediatricians*.

His areas of clinical interest include diabetic nephropathy, hypertension, and fluid/electrolyte management in pediatrics.

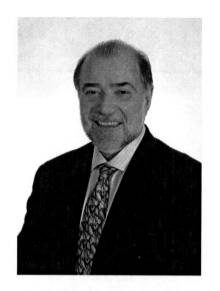

Dr. Frederick J. Kaskel is a renowned national and international physician-investigator in the field of Nephrology. He is a Pediatric Nephrologist and a past President of the American Society of Pediatric Nephrology, a Professor of Pediatrics at the Albert Einstein College of Medicine, a Vice Chairman of Pediatrics and Director of the Division of Pediatric Nephrology at the Children's Hospital at Montefiore, and Director of the National Institutes of Health supported Training Program in Pediatric Nephrology at the Albert Einstein College of Medicine, Bronx, NY, where he received his Residency training in pediatrics and nephrology. Dr. Kaskel was a co-chairman of the important FSGS in Children Task Force created by the National Institutes of Health in 2000 to discuss plans for the current FSGS clinical trials funded by the National Institute of Health. He is the Chairman of the Council of Pediatric Nephrology and Urology of the Kidney and Urology Foundation of America, a former Chairman of the Enuresis Committee of the National Kidney Foundation, and the Congress President for the 15th Congress of the International Pediatric Nephrology Association to be held in New York City in August, 2010. He is also the Medical Director of the Ruth Gottscho Children's Kidney Program at Frost Valley YMCA, which allows children on dialysis, in CKD or who have received a kidney transplant to mainstream at summer camp. He is listed in the Best Doctors in New York and America, and has received numerous recognitions included Distinguished Alumni of Monmouth College (Illinois) and the University of Cincinnati College of Medicine.

He is the Principal Investigator on the National Institutes of Health (NIH) multi-center clinical study of focal segmental glomerulosclerosis (FSGS) in children and co-PI on the Chronic Kidney Disease in Children Study (NIH).

Dr. Kaskel lives in Mamaroneck New York with his wife Phyllis and they have 4 daughters and one granddaughter. In his free time, Dr. Kaskel likes to relax by reading, sailing and hiking.

About the Series Editor

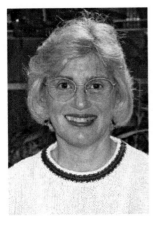

Dr. Adrianne Bendich is Clinical Director, Medical Affairs at GlaxoSmithKline (GSK) Consumer Healthcare, where she is responsible for leading the innovation and medical programs in support of many well-known brands, including TUMS and Os-Cal. Dr. Bendich had primary responsibility for GSK's support for the Women's Health Initiative (WHI) intervention study. Prior to joining GSK, Dr. Bendich was at Roche Vitamins, Inc. and was involved with the groundbreaking clinical studies showing that folic acid-containing multivitamins significantly reduced major classes of birth defects. Dr. Bendich has co-authored over 100 major clinical research studies in the area of preventive nutrition. Dr. Bendich is recognized as a leading authority on antioxidants, nutrition and immunity and pregnancy outcomes, vitamin safety and the cost-effectiveness of vitamin/mineral supplementation.

Dr. Bendich is the editor of nine books, including *Preventive Nutrition: The Comprehensive Guide For Health Professionals* coedited with Dr. Richard Deckelbaum, and is Series Editor of "Nutrition and Health" for Humana Press with 32 published volumes, including *Probiotics in Pediatric Medicine* edited by Dr. Sonia Michail and Dr. Philip Sherman; *Handbook of Nutrition and Pregnancy* edited by Dr. Carol Lammi-Keefe, Dr. Sarah Couch, and Dr. Elliot Philipson; *Nutrition and Rheumatic Disease* edited by Dr. Laura Coleman; *Nutrition and Kidney Disease* edited by Dr. Laura Byham-Grey, Dr. Jerrilynn Burrowes, and Dr. Glenn Chertow; *Nutrition and Health in Developing Countries* edited by Dr. Richard Semba and Dr. Martin Bloem; *Calcium in Human Health* edited by Dr. Robert Heaney and Dr. Connie Weaver, and *Nutrition and Bone Health* edited by Dr. Michael Holick and Dr. Bess Dawson-Hughes.

Dr. Bendich served as associate editor for "Nutrition," the International Journal, served on the editorial board of the Journal of Women's Health and Gender-Based Medicine, and was a member of the Board of Directors of the American College of Nutrition.

Dr. Bendich was the recipient of the Roche Research Award, is a *Tribute to Women and Industry* Awardee, and was a recipient of the Burroughs Wellcome Visiting Professorship in Basic Medical Sciences, 2000–2001. In 2008, Dr. Bendich was given the Council for Responsible Nutrition (CRN) Apple Award in recognition of her many contributions to the scientific understanding of dietary supplements. Dr. Bendich holds academic appointments as adjunct professor in the Department of Preventive Medicine and Community Health at UMDNJ and has an adjunct appointment at the Institute of Nutrition, Columbia University P&S, and is an Adjunct Research Professor, Rutgers University, Newark Campus. She is listed in *Who's Who in American Women*.

LaVergne, TN USA
30 December 2009
168523LV00005B/8/P

9 781603 272247